Pleural Disease

Editors

DAVID FELLER-KOPMAN
FABIEN MALDONADO

CLINICS IN
CHEST MEDICINE

www.chestmed.theclinics.com

December 2021 • Volume 42 • Number 4

ELSEVIER

1600 John F. Kennedy Boulevard • Suite 1800 • Philadelphia, Pennsylvania, 19103-2899

http://www.theclinics.com

CLINICS IN CHEST MEDICINE Volume 42, Number 4
December 2021 ISSN 0272-5231, ISBN-13: 978-0-323-81313-6

Editor: Joanna Collett
Developmental Editor: Karen Justine Solomon

Clinics in Chest Medicine (ISSN 0272-5231) is published quarterly by Elsevier Inc., 360 Park Avenue South, New York, NY 10010-1710. Months of issue are March, June, September, and December. Periodicals postage paid at New York, NY and additional mailing offices. Subscription prices are $396.00 per year (domestic individuals), $1009.00 per year (domestic institutions), $100.00 per year (domestic students/residents), $423.00 per year (Canadian individuals), $1075.00 per year (Canadian institutions), $484.00 per year (international individuals), $1075.00 per year (international institutions), $100.00 per year (Canadian Students), and $230.00 per year (International Students). International air speed delivery is included in all Clinics subscription prices. All prices are subject to change without notice. **POSTMASTER:** Send address changes to Clinics in Chest Medicine, Elsevier Health Sciences Division, Subscription Customer Service, 3251 Riverport Lane, Maryland Heights, MO 63043. **Customer Service: Telephone: 1-800-654-2452** (U.S. and Canada); **1-314-447-8871** (outside U.S. and Canada). **Fax: 1-314-447-8029.** E-mail: **journalscustomerservice-usa@elsevier.com (for print support); journalsonlinesupport-usa@elsevier.com (for online support).**

Reprints. For copies of 100 or more of articles in this publication, please contact the Commercial Reprints Department, Elsevier Inc., 360 Park Avenue South, New York, NY 10010-1710. Tel.: 212-633-3874; Fax: 212-633-3820; E-mail: reprints@elsevier. com.

Clinics in Chest Medicine is covered in *MEDLINE/PubMed (Index Medicus), Current Contents/Clinical Medicine, EMBASE/ Excerpta Medica, Science Citation Index,* and *ISI/BIOMED.*

Contributors

EDITORS

DAVID FELLER-KOPMAN, MD
Chief, Section of Pulmonary and Critical Care
Medicine, Dartmouth-Hitchcock Medical
Center, Professor of Medicine, Dartmouth
Geisel School of Medicine, Lebanon, New
Hampshire, USA

FABIEN MALDONADO, MD, FCCP
Professor of Medicine and Thoracic Surgery,
Vanderbilt University Medical Center,
Nashville, Tennessee, USA

AUTHORS

DINESH N. ADDALA, BA, BMBCH, MRCP
Oxford University Hospitals NHS Foundation
Trust, Department of Respiratory Medicine,
Churchill Hospital, Headington, Oxford, United
Kingdom

SAMEER K. AVASARALA, MD
Division of Pulmonary, Critical Care, and Sleep
Medicine, University Hospitals, Assistant
Professor of Medicine, Case Western Reserve
University School of Medicine, Cleveland,
Ohio, USA

EIHAB O. BEDAWI, MBBS, MRCP
Oxford University Hospitals NHS Foundation
Trust, Department of Respiratory Medicine,
Churchill Hospital, Headington, Oxford, United
Kingdom

KYLE T. BRAMLEY, MD
Assistant Professor of Medicine, Pulmonary,
Critical Care and Sleep Medicine, Yale
University, New Haven, Connecticut, USA

CASSANDRA M. BRAUN, MD
Division of Pulmonary and Critical Care
Medicine, Mayo Clinic College of Medicine,
Rochester, Minnesota, USA

ERIN M. DEBIASI, MD
Assistant Professor of Medicine, Division of
Pulmonary, Critical Care and Sleep Medicine,
Yale School of Medicine, New Haven,
Connecticut, USA

ANDREW DEMAIO, MD
Fellow, Interventional Pulmonology, Johns
Hopkins Hospital, Sheikh Zayed
Cardiovascular Critical Care Tower, Baltimore,
Maryland, USA

DAVID FELLER-KOPMAN, MD
Chief, Section of Pulmonary and Critical Care
Medicine, Dartmouth-Hitchcock Medical
Center, Professor of Medicine, Dartmouth
Geisel School of Medicine, Lebanon, New
Hampshire, USA

**Y.C. GARY LEE, MBChB, PhD, FRACP,
FCCP, FRCP**
Respiratory Medicine, Sir Charles Gairdner
Hospital, Pleural Medicine Unit, Institute for
Respiratory Health, School of Medical and
Health Sciences, Edith Cowan University,
School of Medicine, The University of Western
Australia, Perth, Western Australia

MARK GODFREY, MD
Clinical Fellow, Division of Pulmonary, Critical
Care and Sleep Medicine, Yale School of
Medicine, New Haven, Connecticut, USA

ROB HALLIFAX, PhD, MRCP
Department of Respiratory Medicine,
University of Oxford, Churchill Hospital,
Oxford, United Kingdom

NAI-CHIEN HUAN, MBBS, MRCP
Department of Pulmonology, Serdang
Hospital, Kajang, Malaysia

CHRISTOPHER M. KAPP, MD
Department of Medicine, Division of
Pulmonary, Critical Care, Sleep and Allergy
Medicine, University of Illinois at Chicago,
Chicago, Illinois, USA

**COENRAAD F.N. KOEGELENBERG,
MBChB, MMed (Int), FCP (SA), FRCP (UK),
Cert Pulm (SA), PhD**
Professor, Division of Pulmonology,
Department of Medicine, Faculty of Medicine
and Health Sciences, Stellenbosch University
and Tygerberg Academic Hospital, Cape
Town, South Africa

HANS J. LEE, MD
Section of Interventional Pulmonology, Division
of Pulmonary and Critical Care Medicine,
Johns Hopkins University, Baltimore,
Maryland, USA

ROBERT J. LENTZ, MD
Assistant Professor, Division of Allergy,
Pulmonary and Critical Care Medicine,
Departments of Internal Medicine, and
Thoracic Surgery, Vanderbilt University
Medical Center, Assistant Professor,
Vanderbilt University School of Medicine,
Nashville, Tennessee, USA

†RICHARD W. LIGHT, MD, FCCP
Division of Allergy, Pulmonary and Critical
Care, Vanderbilt University, Nashville,
Tennessee, USA

AMBER LOUW, MBBS
Pleural Medicine Unit, Institute for Respiratory
Health, School of Medical and Health
Sciences, Edith Cowan University, National
Centre for Asbestos Related Diseases, The
University of Western Australia, Perth, Western
Australia

FABIEN MALDONADO, MD, FCCP
Professor of Medicine and Thoracic Surgery,
Vanderbilt University Medical Center,
Nashville, Tennessee, USA

NICK MASKELL, MD
Professor of Respiratory Medicine, Bristol
Academic Respiratory Unit, North Bristol NHS

Trust, England; University of Bristol, Bristol,
England

HELEN MCDILL, MBBS, BSc
Respiratory SpR, Bristol Academic Respiratory
Unit, North Bristol NHS Trust, England

SHAIKH M. NOOR HUSNAIN, MD
Division of Pulmonary and Critical Care
Medicine, Henry Ford Hospital, Detroit,
Michigan, USA

DAVID E. OST, MD, MPH
Professor, Department of Pulmonary Medicine,
The University of Texas MD Anderson Cancer
Center, Houston, Texas, USA

JOSÉ M. PORCEL, MD, FCCP, FACP, FERS
Pleural Medicine Unit, Department of Internal
Medicine, Arnau de Vilanova University
Hospital, IRBLleida, University of Lleida, Lleida,
Spain

JONATHAN PUCHALSKI, MD, MEd
Associate Professor of Medicine, Division of
Pulmonary, Critical Care and Sleep Medicine,
Yale School of Medicine, New Haven,
Connecticut, USA

NAJIB M. RAHMAN, MD, DPhil
Professor, Oxford University Hospitals NHS
Foundation Trust, Oxford NIHR Biomedical
Research Centre, John Radcliffe Hospital,
Headington, United Kingdom

LANCE ROLLER, MS
Research Coordinator, Division of Allergy,
Pulmonary, and Critical Care Medicine,
Vanderbilt University Medical Center,
Nashville, Tennessee, USA

JAY H. RYU, MD
Division of Pulmonary and Critical Care
Medicine, Mayo Clinic College of Medicine,
Rochester, Minnesota, USA

AUDRA J. SCHWALK, MD, MBA
Assistant Professor, Division of Pulmonary and
Critical Care, The University of Texas
Southwestern Medical Center, Dallas, Texas,
USA

ROY SEMAAN, MD
Assistant Professor of Medicine, Director,
Interventional Pulmonology, University of

Pittsburgh Medical Center, Montefiore Hospital, Pittsburgh, Pennsylvania, USA

JANE A. SHAW, MBChB, MMed (Int), MPhil (Pulm), FCP (SA), Cert Pulm (SA)
DST-NRF Centre of Excellence for Biomedical Tuberculosis Research, South African Medical Research Council Centre for Tuberculosis Research, Division of Molecular Biology and Human Genetics, Faculty of Medicine and Health Sciences, Stellenbosch University, Cape Town, South Africa

SAMIRA SHOJAEE, MD, MPH
Department of Pulmonary and Critical Care Medicine, Section of Interventional Pulmonology, Virginia Commonwealth University Health System, Richmond, Virginia, USA

CALVIN SIDHU, MBBS, FRACP
Department of Respiratory Medicine, Sir Charles Gairdner Hospital, Pleural Medicine Unit, Institute for Respiratory Health, School of

Medical and Health Sciences, Edith Cowan University, Perth, Western Australia

JEFFREY THIBOUTOT, MD
Assistant Professor of Medicine, Pulmonary and Critical Care Medicine, Johns Hopkins University, Baltimore, Maryland, USA

RAJESH THOMAS, MBBS, PhD, FRACP
Clinical Associate Professor, Department of Respiratory Medicine, Sir Charles Gairdner Hospital, School of Medicine, The University of Western Australia, Perth, Australia

MARIA TSAKOK, BM, BCh, BA (Hons), FRCR
Department of Radiology, Oxford University Hospitals NHS Foundation Trust, Churchill Hospital, Oxford, United Kingdom

LONNY B. YARMUS, DO, MBA
Associate Professor, Division of Pulmonary and Critical Care Medicine, Johns Hopkins University School of Medicine, Baltimore, Maryland, USA

Contents

Section 1: Pleural Basics

The unique anatomy and physiology of the pleural space provides tight regulation of liquid within the space under normal physiologic conditions. When this balance is disrupted and pleural effusions develop, there can be significant impacts on the respiratory system. Drainage of effusions can lead to meaningful improvement in symptoms, primarily owing to improvement in the length–tension relationship of the respiratory muscles. Ultrasound examination to evaluate the movement and function of the diaphragm, as well as pleural manometry, have provided a greater understanding of the impact of pleural effusion and thoracentesis.

Pleural disease affects more than 300 people per 100,000 population each year and leads to more than 150 admissions per 100,000 population/y (costing >$10 billion in the United States alone). Radiological investigation is key in establishing a diagnosis for patients presenting with pleural effusion, thickening, masses, and pneumothorax. Radiological findings also often determine the initial management options and monitoring for ongoing management. Chest radiography remains the initial modality of choice for the investigation of pleural disease. Further imaging includes thoracic ultrasonography, computed tomography, MRI, and PET, which have important roles in further investigation, but appropriate modality selection is critical.

Pleural diseases are frequently encountered across multiple inpatient and outpatient settings, making pleural drainage and sampling one of the most common medical procedures. With the widespread adoption of bedside ultrasound examination, ultrasound machines are now readily available in many clinical settings, providing both diagnostic and procedural guidance. The modern management of pleural disease is dominated by ultrasound assessment with strong evidence supporting its use to guide pleural interventions. Here, we review the current landscape of ultrasound use to guide pleural drainage, pneumothorax management, and pleural biopsy.

Section 2: Non-Malignant Pleural Disease

Pleural tuberculosis (TB) is common and often follows a benign course but may result in serious long-term morbidity. Diagnosis is challenging because of the paucibacillary nature of the condition. Advances in Mycobacterium culture media and PCR-based techniques have increased the yield from mycobacteriologic tests. Surrogate biomarkers perform well in diagnostic accuracy studies but must be interpreted in the context of the pretest probability in the individual patient. Confirming the diagnosis often requires biopsy, which may be acquired through thoracoscopy or image-guided closed pleural biopsy. Treatment is standard anti-TB therapy, with optional drainage and intrapleural fibrinolytics or surgery in complicated cases.

Classically, both chylothorax and pseudochylothorax present as a pleural effusion with a characteristic milky white appearance to the pleural fluid. Although both are rare causes of pleural effusion, they have distinct etiologies and clinical implications, and as a result require different management strategies. Pleural fluid analysis of cholesterol and triglyceride levels is key to differentiating the 2 entities from one another and then guide the clinician to determine the best next steps in evaluation and management.

Thoracentesis is a common bedside procedure, which has a low risk of complications when performed with thoracic ultrasound and by experienced operators. In critically ill or mechanically ventilated patients, or in patients with bleeding risks due to medications or other coagulopathies, the complication rate remains low. Drainage of pleural effusion in the intensive care unit has diagnostic and therapeutic utility, and perceived bleeding risks should be one part of an individualized and comprehensive risk-benefit analysis.

Section 3: Pleural Malignancy

Malignant pleural effusions have a significant burden on patients and the health care system. Diagnosis is typically via thoracentesis, although other times more invasive procedures are required. Management centers around relief of dyspnea and patient quality of life and can be done via serial thoracentesis, indwelling pleural catheter, or pleurodesis. This article focuses on the diagnosis and management of malignant pleural effusion.

The global incidence of malignant pleural mesothelioma continues to rise. Most patients present first to pulmonologists who need to be aware of the diagnosis, and new developments in the molecular diagnosis of the disease, especially targeting BAP-1 and CDKN2A. This review also outlines recent advances in treatment of mesothelioma (such as immunotherapy) and related presentations, especially malignant pleural effusions. We review current practice and knowledge gaps in the management (including supportive care) of patients with mesothelioma.

Section 4: Pneumothorax

Pneumothorax is a common problem worldwide. Pneumothorax develops secondary to diverse aetiologies; in many cases, there may be no recognizable lung abnormality. The pathogenetic mechanism(s) causing spontaneous pneumothorax may be related to an interplay between lung-related abnormalities and environmental factors such as smoking. Tobacco smoking is a major risk factor for primary spontaneous pneumothorax; chronic obstructive pulmonary disease is most frequently associated with secondary spontaneous pneumothorax. This review article provides an overview of the historical perspective, epidemiology, classification, and aetiology of pneumothorax. It also aims to highlight current knowledge and understanding of underlying risks and pathophysiological mechanisms in pneumothorax development.

Pneumothorax is a common medical condition encountered in a wide variety of clinical presentations, ranging from asymptomatic to life threatening. When symptomatic, it is important to remove air from the pleural space and provide re-expansion of the lung. Additionally, patients who experience a spontaneous pneumothorax are at high risk for recurrence, so treatment goals also include recurrence prevention. Several recent studies have evaluated less invasive management strategies for pneumothorax, including conservative or outpatient management. Future studies may help to identify who is greatest at risk for recurrence and direct earlier definitive management strategies, including thoracoscopic surgery, to those patients.

Section 5: Minimally Invasive Definitive Pleural Intervention

Recurrent, symptomatic pleural effusions are common and can contribute to significant morbidity in affected patients. Various management options are available and indwelling pleural catheter placement is becoming more commonplace and is the preferred option in certain clinical scenarios. The body of literature pertaining to indwelling pleural catheter use has grown substantially over the last decade and the purpose of this review is to summarize the best available evidence.

Sameer K. Avasarala, Robert J. Lentz, and Fabien Maldonado

> Medical thoracoscopy is an effective and safe modality to visualize and sample contents of the pleural cavity. It is an outpatient procedure that can be performed while the patient is spontaneously breathing, with the use of local anesthesia and intravenous medications for sedation and analgesia. Medical thoracoscopy has indications in the management of a variety of pleural diseases. It is most commonly performed as a diagnostic procedure but has therapeutic applications as well. Although it has its advantages, management strategies of certain pleural diseases should take place within a multidisciplinary environment including general pulmonologists, interventional pulmonologists, and thoracic surgeons.

Section 6: The Future of Pleural Disease

Lance Roller, Lonny B. Yarmus, and Robert J. Lentz

> This article details the pros, cons, challenges/pitfalls, and elements required for the successful conduct of multicenter randomized trials, with specific focus on trials related to pleural diseases. Several networks dedicated to the multicenter study of important pleural conditions have developed, yielding practice-changing studies in pleural disease. This review describes the importance of multicenter trials, major elements required for the conduct of such trials, and lessons learned from the ongoing development of the Interventional Pulmonary Outcomes Group, a consortium of interventional pulmonologists dedicated to advancing diagnostic and management strategies in pleural, pulmonary parenchymal, and airway disease by generating high-quality multicenter evidence.

CLINICS IN CHEST MEDICINE

SERIES OF RELATED INTEREST

Cardiology Clinics
Available at: https://www.cardiology.theclinics.com/

THE CLINICS ARE AVAILABLE ONLINE!
Access your subscription at:
www.theclinics.com

Preface

State-of-the-Art in Pleural Disease: A Tribute to Dr Richard Light

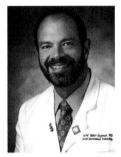 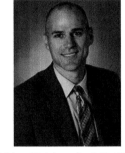

David Feller-Kopman, MD   Fabien Maldonado, MD, FCCP

Editors

Diseases of the pleura affect almost two million patients each year in the United States alone, often with debilitating symptoms. Over the last several years, there has been a renewed interest in pleural disease, with multiple large multicenter randomized trials having been published in our top journals. We have achieved a better understanding of pleural pathophysiology, the importance of dedicated pleural imaging, and the advantages of ultrasound-guided pleural interventions, among many others. Through collaborations between pulmonologists, radiologists, and thoracic surgeons, multidisciplinary pleural disease services have become indispensable and continue to improve the care of patients around the world. We have learned that patients with nonmalignant pleural effusions can have worse outcomes than those with malignant pleural effusions, primarily due to the severity of their underlying disease process, and

that palliative interventions in both of these populations should focus on patient-centered outcomes. Key principles of this approach consist of selecting minimally invasive interventions that will improve symptoms and minimize interactions with the health care system while simultaneously maximizing the quality of life of our patients and those who help provide their care.

So much of our understanding of pleural disease is a direct result of Dr Richard Light's legacy. Since his seminal paper defining transudative and exudative effusions in 1972,[1] Dr Light has published more than 380 articles and has edited the definitive texts on pleural disease. He has lectured in almost 80 countries and throughout his travels has always been generous with his time, insights, and humor. Perhaps even more importantly, he has personally impacted the lives of patients and medical professionals around the world. This is

Clin Chest Med 42 (2021) xiii–xiv
https://doi.org/10.1016/j.ccm.2021.08.013
0272-5231/21/© 2021 Published by Elsevier Inc.

specifically true for all of the authors in this issue of *Clinics in Chest Medicine* whose careers and academic interests have been profoundly influenced by Dr Light's research, mentorship, and friendship.

It is with a mixture of sadness over Dr Light's recent death as well as joy in our memories of the times we have shared that we dedicate this issue to Dr Light. He was, and will always be, an inspiration to those interested in pleural disease, and we are forever grateful.

David Feller-Kopman, MD
Section of Pulmonary and Critical Care Medicine
Dartmouth-Hitchcock Medical Center
Geisel School of Medicine
One Medical Center Drive
Lebanon, NH 03756, USA

Fabien Maldonado, MD, FCCP
Vanderbilt University Medical Center
T-1218 Medical Center North, 1161 21st Avenue
South
Nashville, TN 37232, USA

E-mail addresses:
David.J.Feller-Kopman@Hitchcock.org (D. Feller-Kopman)
Fabien.Maldonado@vumc.org (F. Maldonado)

REFERENCE

1. Light RW, Macgregor MI, Luchsinger PC, et al. Pleural effusions: the diagnostic separation of transudates and exudates. Ann InternMed 1972;77(4):507–13.

Section 1: Pleural Basics

Anatomy and Applied Physiology of the Pleural Space

Erin M. DeBiasi, MD[a],*, David Feller-Kopman, MD[b]

KEYWORDS

- Pleural anatomy • Pleural effusion • Thoracentesis • Pleural manometry

KEY POINTS

- Accumulation of liquid in the pleural space depends on the the balance of forces determining production and resorption.
- Lymphatics on the parietal pleura play a crucial role in the resorption of pleural liquid.
- Pleural effusions cause dyspnea primarily by affecting the length-tension relationship of the diaphragm.
- Measurement of pleural pressure can be used to predict lung expansion with drainage of pleural fluid.

INTRODUCTION

The human pleural space is a fluid-filled cavity located between the mediastinum, diaphragmatic dome, chest wall, and lung surface. The thin layer of liquid within this space is of vital importance to the respiratory system. It provides mechanical coupling of the chest wall and lung during the respiratory cycle, as well as lubrication between the 2 structures during respiration. Additionally, the negative intrapleural pressure relative to atmospheric pressure results in a positive transpulmonary pressure preventing atelectasis at end-exhalation and allowing the lung to inflate during inspiration. The amount of liquid present in the pleural space under normal circumstances is highly regulated owing to unique features of the pleural surfaces. Disruption of the pleural membranes, or within the pleural space, either by excess fluid or by air can result in significant physiologic consequences.

PLEURAL ANATOMY

There are 2 layers of the pleura. The visceral layer overlies the lung surface (including the fissures) and the parietal layer overlies the chest wall, mediastinal structures, and diaphragmatic dome. The surface area in humans is about 4000 cm^2 in a 70 kg man. The pleura is composed of mesothelial cells and underlying connective tissue containing blood vessels and lymphatics. Mesothelial cells of the pleura are flat, squamous-like cells that are 1 to 4 μm thick.[1] They contain microtubules, microfilaments, vesicles, vacuoles, a few Golgi apparatus, and rough endoplasmic reticulum. The luminal surface has a well-developed microvillus border.

Pleural mesothelial cells have several active metabolic and structural functions. Phospholipids, both saturated and unsaturated, as well as hyaluronan, a large molecular weight glycosaminoglycan, are synthesized by pleural mesothelial cells and secreted into the pleural space. These substances act to decrease friction and provide lubrication of the pleural surfaces.[2,3] Additionally, mesothelial cells can secrete a variety of chemokines, cytokines, prostaglandins, prostacyclins, and growth factors that can play a role in postinflammatory tissue remodeling.[4] Mesothelial cells

[a] Division of Pulmonary, Critical Care and Sleep Medicine, Yale University School of Medicine, New Haven, CT 06510, USA; [b] Division of Pulmonary and Critical Care Medicine, Dartmouth-Hitchcock Medical Center, Lebanon, NH, USA
* Corresponding author.
E-mail address: Erin.debiasi@yale.edu

Clin Chest Med 42 (2021) 567–576
https://doi.org/10.1016/j.ccm.2021.08.005
0272-5231/21/© 2021 Elsevier Inc. All rights reserved.

are active sources of components of the extracellular matrix of the interstitial space.[5] The parietal pleura is supplied by the systemic blood capillaries, whereas the visceral pleura is supplied by the bronchial circulation.

The lymphatic system of the pleura, in particular the parietal pleura, is quite unique. Stomata, cylindrical-like openings with a diameter of 0.5 to 20.0 µm, are formed by discontinuities of the parietal mesothelium and submesothelial interstitial space and are the origins of the parietal pleural lymphatic system.[6,7] They are most prevalent on the diaphragm, although they are found throughout the parietal pleura.[6] Peripheral branches of the pulmonary lymphatic system extend to the in the submesothelial layer of the visceral pleura (**Fig. 1**). There are not stomata in the visceral mesothelium.[8]

PLEURAL PHYSIOLOGY

At functional residual capacity (FRC) the pleural pressure is approximately –6 cm H_2O. The negative intrapleural pressure is created by the elastic recoil force of the lung opposed to the tendency of the chest wall to expand. There is a vertical gradient related to gravity of about 0.2 cm H_2O/cm of lung height.[9] During inspiration, a decrease in pleural pressure is generated via contraction of the diaphragm and external intercostal muscles, with subsequent enlargement in the thoracic cage volume. This process translates into a negative intrapulmonary pressure and inspiratory

airflow. Conversely, during expiration, the elastic recoil forces of the lung inward and chest wall outward with relaxation of the diaphragm and inspiratory muscles result in a slightly higher pleural (although still negative) pressure (–3 to –5 cm H_2O at FRC). This negative intrapleural pressure maintains the lungs at their inflated state. When this negative intrapleural pressure is eliminated, for example, in the setting of pneumothorax or a large pleural effusion, the lungs may collapse owing to their own elastic recoil.

PLEURAL FLUID

The typical volume of pleural liquid in healthy humans is 0.26 mL/kg^{-1}.[10] Fluid is constantly filtered and then drained from the pleural space. The egress of pleural fluid occurs through several mechanisms.[1,11,12] Passive fluid flow down a pressure gradient through the visceral pleura occurs, but is felt to account for only a small proportion of fluid egress owing to the relatively tight adherens junctions between the visceral mesothelial cells.[1] Similarly, active solute coupled fluid absorption also likely accounts for a small proportion of fluid egress.[11] Transcytosis through small vesicles called caveolae is a pressure-independent process and also may occur. The primary mechanism of pleural drainage is through the extensive pleural lymphatic system. The flow of fluid from the pleural space into the parietal pleural stomata occurs when the pressure within the pleural lymphatics decreases to less than the pleural liquid

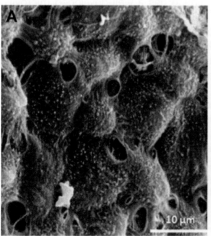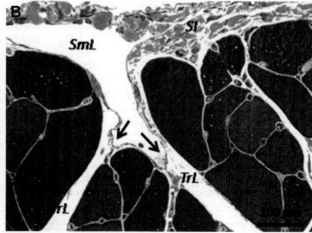

Fig. 1. (*A*) Scanning electron microscopy image of the diaphragm with lymphatic stomata at junctions between mesothelial cells which are covered in microvilli. (*B*) Cross-section of the diaphragmatic pleura with large submesothelial lymphatic (SmL) that collects pleural fluid from stomata and submesothelial interstitium (SI) and drains through transverse lymphatics (TrL) of skeletal muscle cells (SkM). One way valves of lymphatics indicated by *arrows*. (*From* Negrini D and Moriondo A. Pleural function and lymphatics. Acta Physiol 2013;207(2)247; with permission.)

pressure. Subatmospheric pressure within the pleural lymphatics occurs at times during the cardiorespiratory cycle.[12] Spontaneous breathing produces pressure within the pleural lymphatics of values between -0.5 cm H_2O at end expiration and -24 cm H_2O at end inspiration.[12] This cyclical oscillation of pressure is responsible for propulsion of fluid through the pleural lymphatic system.

Effusions develop when pleural fluid filtration occurs in excess of absorption. Excess fluid filtration through the parietal mesothelium can occur in the setting of systemic hypertension or decreased plasma protein concentration, although with normal hydraulic conductivity of the parietal pleura, this process is not common. Increased fluid filtration from the pulmonary capillaries and through the visceral mesothelium can occur in the setting of pulmonary edema.[13,14] Initially, in the setting of mild edema, pulmonary interstitial fluid is removed via the pulmonary lymphatics. However, with increasing edema, this drainage can become saturated and fluid accumulates in the interstitial space, resulting in increasing pressure driving fluid into the pleural space. Primary lymphatic disorders, thoracic duct injury, and other etiologies leading leakage of leak lymph fluid can result in chylothorax.

PHYSIOLOGIC IMPACT OF PLEURAL EFFUSION
Effect on Gas Exchange

Hypoxemia can be observed in patients with pleural effusions. Low arterial oxygenation is most likely owing to the presence of mild intrapulmonary shunt resulting in ventilation/perfusion mismatch.[15,16] Using a multiple inert gas elimination technique, Agusti and colleagues demonstrated in a series of 9 patients that the degree of arterial hypoxemia was related to the amount of intrapulmonary shunt.[15] Thoracentesis improved shunt fraction resulting in slightly improved partial pressure of oxygen (Pao_2). Similarly, in a porcine model, the volume of pleural effusion was directly related to the increase in intrapulmonary shunt and a decrease in Pao_2.[16] After thoracentesis, both shunting and the Pao_2 improved. Pneumothorax can sometimes lead to hypoxemia. The etiology is also most likely related to worsened shunting.[17] Early studies demonstrated that shunt fraction did not increase until pneumothorax volume was greater than 25% of the thoracic cage volume. The degree of shunting is related to the size of the pneumothorax.

Clinically, observation of the impact of thoracentesis on oxygenation has been mixed.[15,18–25] These conflicting reports may in part be due to the when oxygenation is measured after thoracentesis, with a less significant and/or no improvement observed when oxygenation is measured more proximally to the procedure.[15,19,24,25] This finding may be due to delayed improvement in shunt fraction immediately after thoracentesis.

In contrast, when oxygenation is measured at a later time point, more significant changes may be observed.[21,22,26,27] In nonmechanically ventilated patients, Perpina demonstrated a significant increase in Pao_2 after 24 hours.[22] In 20 mechanically ventilated patients after thoracentesis, Razazi and associates[21] demonstrated an improved Pao_2:-fraction of inspired oxygen (Fio_2) at 3 hours and 24 hours after thoracentesis. Similarly, Sakurai and colleagues[26] demonstrated a significant increase in the Pao_2:Fio_2 at 24 hours after thoracentesis in 22 patients. This effect was sustained for up to 1 week only in patients with a lower baseline Pao_2:Fio_2 (<174).

Chen and colleagues[28] postulated that the lack of observed change in oxygenation immediately after thoracentesis may be due to confounding factors such as intrinsic lung disease. In a cohort of 26 mechanically ventilated patients with congestive heart failure-associated pleural effusions, the Pao_2 and Pao_2:Fio_2 improved in all patients. Patients with normal pleural elastance had a greater improvement in oxygenation. Other investigators have postulated that the volume of effusion removed may account for the variable effect on oxygenation.[21,23,25,29] However, clinically, the relationship between the volume of fluid removed and oxygenation is also variable. This difference may be due to heterogenicity in the cohorts. In mechanically ventilated patients, Roch and colleagues[23] found that the Pao_2:Fio_2 improved only when more than 500 mL of fluid was drained. However, in a cohort of 122 nonmechanically ventilated patients, patients with smaller amounts removed (mean, 716 mL) had more significant increase in Pao_2 compared with those drained for a greater amount.[25] Razazi and coworkers[21] found that, after large volume thoracentesis, improved oxygenation was significantly correlated with an increase in end-expiratory lung volume rather than volume of fluid withdrawn.

Effect on Pulmonary Function, Lung Volumes, and Lung Mechanics

Excess pleural fluid is accommodated in the chest primarily by an increased thoracic cage volume owing to a greater anteroposterior and lateral rib cage diameter and, most important, the downward displacement of the diaphragm.[30,31] Animal models have quantified that approximately two-thirds of the volume of effusion is accommodated by an increase in chest wall volume, with only a one-third decrease in the FRC[30] (**Fig. 2**). Not unsurprisingly, after thoracentesis there are only modest changes noted in lung volumes. In a study of 9 patients, Brown and associates[18] demonstrated a small improvement in FRC and total lung capacity 3 hours after thoracentesis. This finding did not correlate with any symptom improvement or gas exchange. Several studies demonstrated small improvement in vital capacity after thoracentesis.[32,33]

After thoracentesis, patients can experience a significant improvement in dyspnea despite only small improvement in lung volumes. Palliation of dyspnea occurs primarily through the optimization of respiratory mechanics rather than a change in lung volume. Animal models suggest this process is due to improvement in the length–tension relationship of the respiratory muscles. In Estenne and colleagues'[33] early studies, drainage of effusion produced a significant improvement in the inspiratory muscles' ability to generate negative pressure for a given lung volume. There was not a consistent improvement of lung volumes. Measurements of respiratory muscle strength including maximal inspiratory pressure and maximal expiratory pressure as well as forced expiratory volume in 1 second and forced vital capacity may all improve after thoracentesis.[34–36]

Increased access to quality bedside ultrasound examination has increased our understanding of

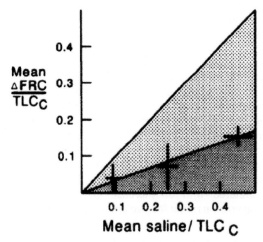

Fig. 2. Change in FRC with saline infusion into pleural space of the dog. Mean decrease in FRC (*dark gray*) as a fraction of total lung capacity (TLC) (*y*-axis) versus volume of saline as a fraction of TLC (*x*-axis). Light gray represents increase in chest wall. (*From* Krell WS, Rodarte JR. Effects of acute pleural effusion on respiratory system mechanics in dogs. Journal of applied physiology (Bethesda, Md: 1985). 1985;59(5):1458-1463.)

diaphragm function in relation to the presence of pleural effusion.[36–42] A large pleural effusion may lead to flattening, eversion, or paradoxic movement of the hemidiaphragm. In patients with paradoxic movement of the diaphragm, Wang and coworkers[42] noted a significant improvement in post-thoracentesis metrics including dyspnea, oxygenation, forced expiratory volume in 1 second, and forced vital capacity. These effects were less significant in patients without paradoxic movement. In mechanically ventilated patients, the impact of thoracentesis was similar; Umbrello and associates[38] demonstrated improved contractile force of the diaphragm and improved tidal volumes. In a large multifaceted study evaluating the physiologic effects of thoracentesis on 145 symptomatic patients with pleural effusion, Muruganandan and colleagues[36] found a significant association of diaphragm shape and movement with post-thoracentesis outcomes. Before thoracentesis, one-half of the patients had either flattened or everted diaphragms noted on ultrasound examination. A normal, dome-shaped diaphragm was noted after thoracentesis in 94%. Ultrasound examination demonstrated abnormal (48%) or decreased (21%) movement of the diaphragm before thoracentesis in most patients. Thoracentesis improved this dysfunction in 97% of patients. Relief of dyspnea after thoracentesis was strongly associated with abnormal or paradoxic diaphragm movement before thoracentesis (odds ratio, 4.37). Similarly, Skaarup and colleagues[40] demonstrated that thoracentesis led to both an improvement in qualitative and quantitative measurements of diaphragm movement. Using an area method with ultrasound examination to calculate diaphragm movement, they demonstrated that the affected hemidiaphragm movement increased to the level similar to the contralateral side without effusion after thoracentesis. This finding was associated with significant improvement of dyspnea as measured by the Borg scale.

Aguilera Garcia and colleagues[41] recently described the relationship with pleural elastance and diaphragm movement during thoracentesis. Using M-mode ultrasound examination, they measured both diaphragm excursion and the velocity of diaphragm contraction before and after thoracentesis. Pleural manometry was used to measure pleural pressure serially. There were significant improvements in both the velocity of diaphragm contraction and diaphragm excursion in patients with expandable lung. This improvement was positively correlated with an increase in the respirophasic changes in pleural pressure. Improvement in diaphragm function was felt to be due to improvement in the length–tension relationship of the diaphragm after thoracentesis and lung expansion. In those with nonexpandable lung, there were no significant changes in either. This finding was possibly due to removal of a smaller volume of effusion versus the restriction of the inspiratory movement of the diaphragm owing to nonexpandable lung.

Other Symptoms

Dyspnea is the most common patient-reported symptom of pleural effusion and can significantly improve after thoracentesis.[35,36,43–46] The modified BORG (mBORG) score is the most commonly used scale to quantify dyspnea, although other scores including the dyspnea-12 and visual analog scale (VAS) are also used. Boshuizen and associates[46] demonstrated that daily dyspnea assessments performed by patients after thoracentesis using the mBORG score can help to predict the need for reintervention. Similar to the delay noted in improvement in oxygenation, patients noted maximal relief of dyspnea 1.9 days after thoracentesis.

Muruganandan and colleagues[36] recently published one of the largest, most comprehensive studies to date of patient reported outcomes after thoracentesis. The Pleural Effusion And Symptom Evaluation (PLEASE) study found that thoracentesis improved dyspnea as measured by the mBORG, dyspnea-12 and VAS in the majority of the 145 participants studied (**Fig. 3**). Using the VAS alone, 73% of patients had a significant improvement in dyspnea after thoracentesis. The most significant predictor of improvement was degree of baseline dyspnea. In another large cohort of 163 patients, Argento and colleagues[47]

described a sustained improvement in the mBORG 30 days after thoracentesis in the majority of patients. Several other smaller studies have demonstrated significant improvement in the mBORG score after thoracentesis.[35,45]

Effusion-related dyspnea is often more severe with exertion.[35,36,46] This factor can lead to a decrease in physical activity and worsening performance status.[48] Boshuizen and colleagues[46] reported that dyspnea was decreased more markedly after thoracentesis during exercise. In the PLEASE study described elsewhere in this article, thoracentesis improved dyspnea both at rest and after a 6-minute walk test, but the mean change in the mBORG was more significant after the 6-minute walk test.[36] Additionally, patients were able to walk a mean of 29.7 m further 24 to 36 hours after thoracentesis. Cartaxo and co-workers[35] found a similar improvement in a cohort of 25 patients after thoracentesis. Six-minute walk distances improved by a mean of 63 m at 48 hours after thoracentesis and were correlated with improved forced vital capacity and forced expiratory volume in 1 second. The maximal mBORG improvement was noted post-thoracentesis with exertion.

Poor sleep quality is often subjectively described by patients with pleural effusions.[45] Marcondes and colleagues[45] performed full night polysomnography on patients before and after thoracentesis. Polysomnography after thoracentesis was notable for improved sleep efficiency, total sleep time, and percentage of rapid eye movement sleep. This study did not demonstrate any significant change in nocturnal desaturation events after thoracentesis.

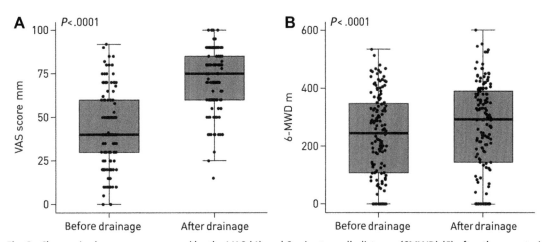

Fig. 3. Change in dyspnea as measured by the VAS (*A*) and 6-minute walk distance (6MWD) (*B*) after thoracentesis in 145 patients. (*Reproduced* with permission of the © ERS 2021: *From* Muruganandan S, Azzopardi M, Thomas R, et al. The Pleural Effusion And Symptom Evaluation (PLEASE) study of breathlessness in patients with a symptomatic pleural effusion. The European respiratory journal. 2020;55(5) 1900980; 10.1183/13993003.00980-2019. Published 14 May 2020.)

PLEURAL PRESSURE

Liquid in the pleural space generally leads to an increase in the pleural pressure. Owing to the hydrostatic pressure of the fluid column, this pressure is not equally distributed within the pleural space; rather, there is a vertical gradient of 1 cm H_2O/cm height, with more basilar areas having a higher pleural pressure than more apical regions.[15,49] Various methods can be used to measure pleural pressure and have led to a greater understanding of pleural elastance, or the change in pleural pressure at a given change in pleural volume.[50–56]

Using a simple U-tube manometer, Light and coworkers[54] were the first to describe 3 characteristic pleural elastance curves: normal, trapped, and entrapped (**Fig. 4**). When pleural elastance is normal, before thoracentesis, pleural pressure is typically positive. As fluid is drained, the pressure–volume curve is monophasic and the slope is slightly downward. The final pleural pressure is −3 to −5 cm H_2O and the pleural elastance is less than14.5 cm H_2O/L. Trapped lung results from long-standing pleural inflammation, which causes a fibrinous visceral pleural peel. It can be seen after cardiac surgery, hemothorax, empyema, or tuberculosis.[57] The pleural pressure may be initially negative, even in the presence of an effusion. During thoracentesis, the pressure–volume curve is steep with excessively high pleural elastance, typically more than 25 cm H_2O/L.[55,57,58] These patients tend to have minimal symptoms of dyspnea, although they often develop chest discomfort during thoracentesis.[57] An entrapped lung is typically associated with visceral pleural thickening owing to an active inflammatory process, increased lung elastic recoil, or endobronchial obstruction preventing the lung from expanding with fluid drainage. During thoracentesis, the pressure–volume curve is biphasic with an initial normal pleural elastance and slight downward trajectory followed by a marked steep decline. Patients with an entrapped lung, in contrast with those with a trapped lung, are usually symptomatically short of breath.

Pleural Pressure Monitoring and Procedural Complications

Complications of pleural fluid drainage include pneumothorax, reexpansion pulmonary edema (RPE), and chest discomfort. It has been hypothesized that these complications may be due to excessively negative intrapleural pressure during thoracentesis and that measurement of pleural pressure may mitigate these complications.[50,51,54,59]

Pneumothorax after thoracentesis may be due to direct iatrogenic pleural injury, but with the routine use of ultrasound examination, this complication is rare.[60] More commonly, it is due to a nonexpandable lung and/or transient alveolar–pleural fistulae, possibly created by excessively negative intrapleural pressure.[61] Several studies have demonstrated that pleural manometry fails to identify those that are at risk of postprocedural pneumothorax.[58,61] In a study of 193 patients undergoing thoracentesis with pleural manometry, 8 were found to have postprocedural pneumothorax owing to nonexpandable lung.[61] One-half of the patients had abnormal pleural elastance measurements, but none had an excessively negative pleural pressure (<−20 cm H_2O) during

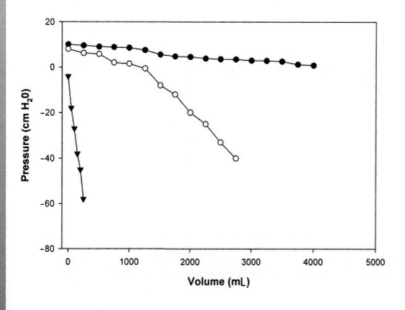

Fig. 4. Three characteristic pleural pressure/volume curves during thoracentesis in normal (*solid circles*), entrapped (*open circles*) and trapped (*triangles*) lung. (*From* Doelken P, Huggins JT, Pastis NJ, Sahn SA. Pleural manometry: technique and clinical implications. Chest. 2004;126(6):1764-1769.)

thoracentesis. Another study of 57 patients identified 9 with post-thoracentesis pneumothorax.[58] In those with pneumothorax, the most negative pleural pressure during thoracentesis was -10.8 cm H_2O in patients with an expandable lung and -17.3 cm H_2O in those with a nonexpandable lung.

RPE is noted infrequently after thoracentesis; however, when significant, it can result in high mortality.[50,62,63] RPE likely is caused by an ischemia–reperfusion injury. In a study conducted by Feller-Kopman and associates[50] of 185 patients undergoing large volume thoracentesis, there was 1 patient with clinically significant RPE and 4 with radiographic RPE. The development of RPE was not associated with pleural pressure at the start or end of the procedure, or with pleural elastance. A conservative procedure termination point of a pleural pressure of less than -20 cm H_2O may partially be the reason that no correlation was noted; prior animal models suggest that RPE is associated with more excessively negative pleural pressures.[50,64]

Chest pain during thoracentesis can be quite distressing for patients. It has been postulated that excessive chest discomfort may be correlated with the development of negative intrapleural pressure.[51,59,65] A value of -20 cm H_2O has frequently been identified as a possible cut off point for the termination of thoracentesis when using manometry. In a retrospective study of 214 patients undergoing thoracentesis with and without manometry, no significant difference was seen in the incidence of chest discomfort despite termination of the procedure if pleural pressure fell below -20 cm H_2O.[59] Lentz and colleagues[65] performed a single-blind, randomized controlled trial with 124 patients undergoing thoracentesis with or without manometry. A VAS was used to measure chest discomfort before, during, and at specified intervals after the procedure. The procedure was terminated if patients developed persistent chest discomfort, intractable cough, or if fluid was fully aspirated. If manometry was used, the procedure was also terminated if pleural pressure decreased to less than -20 cm H_2O or if there was a change in more than 10 cm H_2O between 2 readings to a value of less than -10 cm H_2O. No difference in development of chest pain at 5 and 15 minutes after thoracentesis was noted when manometry was used. Notably, in a separate study the authors validated the values reported by a VAS of chest discomfort, and found that a change in 16 mm on the VAS was a clinically significant value.[66]

In a study from Feller-Kopman and colleagues[51] of 169 patients undergoing manometry-guided thoracentesis, 11% reported chest discomfort. A significantly lower closing pleural pressure and change in pleural pressure was noted in patients with chest discomfort compared with asymptomatic patients. Chest discomfort was not associated with the volume of fluid removed, opening pleural pressure, or pleural elastance. Only a minority of patients with chest discomfort had a pleural pressure values of less than -20 cm H_2O and several asymptomatic patients developed pleural pressures of less than -20 cm H_2O.

Pleural Drainage Techniques

Although none of these studies directly demonstrated the correlation between pleural pressure and procedural outcomes, many are mindful of the generation of excessively negative pleural pressure during thoracentesis. An effusion is commonly manually aspirated during thoracentesis; other options include suction (wall or vacuum bottle) and gravity drainage. Three recent studies have evaluated the most optimum drainage technique.[67–69]

One hypothesis generated by these studies is that excessively negative pleural pressures may be inadvertently missed during thoracentesis using intermittent pleural pressure monitoring. Lentz and colleagues,[67] therefore, sought to determine whether simple gravity drainage may result in better patient-related outcomes. In their GRAVITAS study, 140 patients undergoing thoracentesis were randomized to undergo gravity drainage versus manual suction. Patient-reported chest pain at 5 minutes was the primary outcome and was no different between the arms. There were also no complications or difference noted in dyspnea. Gravity drainage took considerably longer.

Senitko and associates[68] randomized a cohort of 100 patients to manual aspiration versus vacuum drainage. No complications were noted in the manual aspiration group. There were 5 complications, including 3 pneumothoraces and 1 each of hemothorax and RPE in the vacuum group. Patients in the vacuum group also had a higher rate of chest pain. The authors concluded that the sustained pressures of -450 cm H_2O during vacuum drainage compared with peak manual aspiration pressures of -150 cm H_2O to -300 cm H_2O may lead to a higher rate of complications and procedure-related pain.

Although these studies indicate that manual aspiration may be the most ideal method to drain pleural effusions, Sagar and colleagues[69] recently shared their 14-year experience using vacuum drainage. A total of 10,344 thoracentesis were analyzed retrospectively. Thoracentesis was either performed with vacuum bottles or wall suction on the maximum setting. The procedure was terminated when the effusion was drained completely or limited by the development of chest pain or persistent cough. The pneumothorax rate was comparable with the literature (3.98% overall, 0.28% requiring intervention). Similarly, the incidence of RPE was low (0.08%). Overall, the authors concluded that despite sustained negative pressure of −700 to −800 cm H_2O generated with suction, when the procedure was terminated based on patient symptoms, it was safe to drain effusion using suction.

Practical Applications of Pleural Manometry and Future Directions

Although the measurement of pleural pressure during thoracentesis has not been shown to prevent complications of the procedure, knowledge of pleural elastance may be beneficial in determining the optimal long term management in patients with effusion, especially if malignant. Most recent guidelines for management of malignant pleural effusion support the use of talc pleurodesis when the lung is expandable.[70] This factor is often determined by evaluating post-thoracentesis chest imaging. Martin and colleagues[71] used pleural manometry upfront to try to identify patients that would have successful pleurodesis after talc slurry in their pre-EDIT (elastance-directed indwelling pleural catheter or talc slurry pleurodesis) trial. In this feasibility trial, 31 patients were randomized to standard of care talc slurry pleurodesis versus the EDIT protocol, in which an indwelling catheter was placed immediately if pleural elastance during initial large volume thoracentesis was sustained over 14.5 cm H_2O/L. The study demonstrated that pleural elastance was measured successfully in 87% of patients, and values of greater than 14.5 cm H_2O/L were 100% sensitive for a nonexpendable lung. A phase III trial of the EDIT protocol is forthcoming and may greatly impact the management of malignant pleural effusion.

SUMMARY

Pleural effusion develops when there are alterations in the typically tightly regulated fluid balance in the pleural space. The significant physiologic impairments caused by pleural effusion can be improved with thoracentesis. Disruption of the shape and function of the diaphragm is the primary cause of symptomatology associated with pleural effusion. Understanding of the change intrapleural pressure with thoracentesis can help guide the best practices of drainage and future management of recurrences.

CLINICS CARE POINTS

- The understanding of pleural anatomy and physiology directly impact the care of our patients.
- Dyspnea often improves following thoracentesis, irrespective of lung re-expansion and relates to the mechanics of diaphragmatic function.
- Re-expansion pulmonary edema is rare, and likely unrelated to volume of fluid removed.
- Studies are underway to determine if pleural manometry can be used to guide the management of patients with malignant pleural effusion.

CONFLICTS OF INTEREST

None.

REFERENCES

1. Wang NS. The regional difference of pleural mesothelial cells in rabbits. Am Rev Respir Dis 1974; 110(5):623–33.
2. Wang PM, Lai-Fook SJ. Pleural tissue hyaluronan produced by postmortem ventilation in rabbits. Lung 2000;178(1):1–12.
3. Mills PC, Chen Y, Hills YC, et al. Comparison of surfactant lipids between pleural and pulmonary lining fluids. Pulm Pharmacol Ther 2006;19(4):292–6.
4. Mutsaers SE. Mesothelial cells: their structure, function and role in serosal repair. Respirology 2002; 7(3):171–91.
5. Rennard SI, Jaurand MC, Bignon J, et al. Role of pleural mesothelial cells in the production of the submesothelial connective tissue matrix of lung. Am Rev Respir Dis 1984;130(2):267–74.
6. Negrini D, Mukenge S, Del Fabbro M, et al. Distribution of diaphragmatic lymphatic stomata. J Appl Physiol (1985) 1991;70(4):1544–9.
7. Grimaldi A, Moriondo A, Sciacca L, et al. Functional arrangement of rat diaphragmatic initial lymphatic network. Am J Physiol Heart Circ Physiol 2006; 291(2):H876–85.
8. Albertine KH, Wiener-Kronish JP, Roos PJ, et al. Structure, blood supply, and lymphatic vessels of the sheep's visceral pleura. Am J Anat 1982; 165(3):277–94.
9. Agostoni E. Mechanics of the pleural space. Physiol Rev 1972;52(1):57–128.
10. Noppen M, De Waele M, Li R, et al. Volume and cellular content of normal pleural fluid in humans

examined by pleural lavage. Am J Respir Crit Care Med 2000;162(3 Pt 1):1023–6.

11. Agostoni E, Zocchi L. Pleural liquid and its exchanges. Respir Physiol Neurobiol 2007;159(3):311–23.

12. Moriondo A, Mukenge S, Negrini D. Transmural pressure in rat initial subpleural lymphatics during spontaneous or mechanical ventilation. Am J Physiol Heart Circ Physiol 2005;289(1):H263–9.

13. Negrini D, Passi A, de Luca G, et al. Pulmonary interstitial pressure and proteoglycans during development of pulmonary edema. Am J Physiol 1996; 270(6 Pt 2):H2000–7.

14. Negrini D. Pulmonary microvascular pressure profile during development of hydrostatic edema. Microcirculation 1995;2(2):173–80.

15. Agustí AG, Cardús J, Roca J, et al. Ventilation-perfusion mismatch in patients with pleural effusion: effects of thoracentesis. Am J Respir Crit Care Med 1997;156(4 Pt 1):1205–9.

16. Nishida O, Arellano R, Cheng DC, et al. Gas exchange and hemodynamics in experimental pleural effusion. Crit Care Med 1999;27(3):583–7.

17. Norris RM, Jones JG, Bishop JM. Respiratory gas exchange in patients with spontaneous pneumothorax. Thorax 1968;23(4):427–33.

18. Brown NE, Zamel N, Aberman A. Changes in pulmonary mechanics and gas exchange following thoracocentesis. Chest 1978;74(5):540–2.

19. Doelken P, Abreu R, Sahn SA, et al. Effect of thoracentesis on respiratory mechanics and gas exchange in the patient receiving mechanical ventilation. Chest 2006;130(5):1354–61.

20. Goligher EC, Leis JA, Fowler RA, et al. Utility and safety of draining pleural effusions in mechanically ventilated patients: a systematic review and meta-analysis. Crit Care 2011;15(1):R46.

21. Razazi K, Thille AW, Carteaux G, et al. Effects of pleural effusion drainage on oxygenation, respiratory mechanics, and hemodynamics in mechanically ventilated patients. Ann Am Thorac Soc 2014;11(7):1018–24.

22. Perpina M, Benlloch E, Marco V, et al. Effect of thoracentesis on pulmonary gas exchange. Thorax 1983;38(10):747–50.

23. Roch A, Bojan M, Michelet P, et al. Usefulness of ultrasonography in predicting pleural effusions >500 mL in patients receiving mechanical ventilation. Chest 2005;127(1):224–32.

24. Karetzky MS, Kothari GA, Fourre JA, et al. Effect of thoracentesis on arterial oxygen tension. Respiration 1978;36(2):96–103.

25. Michaelides SA, Bablekos GD, Analitis A, et al. Initial size of unilateral pleural effusion determines impact of thoracocentesis on oxygenation. Postgrad Med J 2017;93(1105):691–5.

26. Sakurai M, Morinaga K, Shimoyama K, et al. Effects of pleural drainage on oxygenation in critically ill patients. Acute Med Surg 2020;7(1):e489.

27. Taylor TM, Radchenko C, Sanchez TM, et al. The impact of thoracentesis on postprocedure pulse oximetry. J Bronchology Interv Pulmonol 2021;28(3): 192–200.

28. Chen WL, Chung CL, Hsiao SH, et al. Pleural space elastance and changes in oxygenation after therapeutic thoracentesis in ventilated patients with heart failure and transudative pleural effusions. Respirology 2010;15(6):1001–8.

29. Vetrugno L, Bignami E, Orso D, et al. Utility of pleural effusion drainage in the ICU: an updated systematic review and META-analysis. J Crit Care 2019;52:22–32.

30. Krell WS, Rodarte JR. Effects of acute pleural effusion on respiratory system mechanics in dogs. J Appl Physiol (1985) 1985;59(5):1458–63.

31. Sousa AS, Moll RJ, Pontes CF, et al. Mechanical and morphometrical changes in progressive bilateral pneumothorax and pleural effusion in normal rats. Eur Respir J 1995;8(1):99–104.

32. Light RW, Stansbury DW, Brown SE. The relationship between pleural pressures and changes in pulmonary function after therapeutic thoracentesis. Am Rev Respir Dis 1986;133(4):658–61.

33. Estenne M, Yernault JC, De Troyer A. Mechanism of relief of dyspnea after thoracocentesis in patients with large pleural effusions. Am J Med 1983;74(5):813–9.

34. Michaelides SA, Bablekos GD, Analitis A, et al. Temporal evolution of thoracocentesis-induced changes in spirometry and respiratory muscle pressures. Postgrad Med J 2017;93(1102):460–4.

35. Cartaxo AM, Vargas FS, Salge JM, et al. Improvements in the 6-min walk test and spirometry following thoracentesis for symptomatic pleural effusions. Chest 2011;139(6):1424–9.

36. Muruganandan S, Azzopardi M, Thomas R, et al. The Pleural Effusion and Symptom Evaluation (PLEASE) study of breathlessness in patients with a symptomatic pleural effusion. Eur Respir J 2020; 55(5):1900980.

37. Wang JS, Tseng CH. Changes in pulmonary mechanics and gas exchange after thoracentesis on patients with inversion of a hemidiaphragm secondary to large pleural effusion. Chest 1995;107(6): 1610–4.

38. Umbrello M, Mistraletti G, Galimberti A, et al. Drainage of pleural effusion improves diaphragmatic function in mechanically ventilated patients. Crit Care Resusc 2017;19(1):64–70.

39. Garske LA, Kunarajah K, Zimmerman PV, et al. In patients with unilateral pleural effusion, restricted lung inflation is the principal predictor of increased dyspnoea. PloS one 2018;13(10):e0202621.

40. Skaarup SH, Lonni S, Quadri F, et al. Ultrasound evaluation of hemidiaphragm function following thoracentesis: a study on mechanisms of dyspnea related to pleural effusion. J Bronchology Interv Pulmonol 2020;27(3):172–8.

41. Aguilera Garcia Y, Palkar A, Koenig SJ, et al. Assessment of diaphragm function and pleural pressures during thoracentesis. Chest 2020;157(1):205–11.

42. Wang LM, Cherng JM, Wang JS. Improved lung function after thoracocentesis in patients with paradoxical movement of a hemidiaphragm secondary to a large pleural effusion. Respirology 2007;12(5):719–23.

43. Davies HE, Mishra EK, Kahan BC, et al. Effect of an indwelling pleural catheter vs chest tube and talc pleurodesis for relieving dyspnea in patients with malignant pleural effusion: the TIME2 randomized controlled trial. JAMA 2012;307(22):2383–9.

44. Lorenzo MJ, Modesto M, Perez J, et al. Quality-of-Life assessment in malignant pleural effusion treated with indwelling pleural catheter: a prospective study. Palliat Med 2014;28(4):326–34.

45. Marcondes BF, Vargas F, Paschoal FH, et al. Sleep in patients with large pleural effusion: impact of thoracentesis. Sleep Breath 2012;16(2):483–9.

46. Boshuizen RC, Vincent AD, van den Heuvel MM. Comparison of modified Borg scale and visual analog scale dyspnea scores in predicting re-intervention after drainage of malignant pleural effusion. Support Care Cancer 2013;21(11):3109–16.

47. Argento AC, Murphy TE, Pisani MA, et al. Patient-centered outcomes following thoracentesis. PLEURA 2015;2. 2373997515600404.

48. Jeffery E, Lee YG, McVeigh J, et al. Feasibility of objectively measured physical activity and sedentary behavior in patients with malignant pleural effusion. Support Care Cancer 2017;25(10):3133–41.

49. Light RW. Pleural diseases. Philadelphia: Lippincott Williams & Wilkins; 2007.

50. Feller-Kopman D, Berkowitz D, Boiselle P, et al. Large-volume thoracentesis and the risk of reexpansion pulmonary edema. Ann Thorac Surg 2007;84(5):1656–61.

51. Feller-Kopman D, Walkey A, Berkowitz D, et al. The relationship of pleural pressure to symptom development during therapeutic thoracentesis. Chest 2006;129(6):1556–60.

52. Krenke R, Guc M, Grabczak EM, et al. Development of an electronic manometer for intrapleural pressure monitoring. Respiration 2011;82(4):377–85.

53. Salamonsen M, Ware R, Fielding D. A new method for performing continuous manometry during pleural effusion drainage. Respiration 2014;88(1):61–6.

54. Light RW, Jenkinson SG, Minh VD, et al. Observations on pleural fluid pressures as fluid is withdrawn during thoracentesis. Am Rev Respir Dis 1980;121(5):799–804.

55. Doelken P, Huggins JT, Pastis NJ, et al. Pleural manometry: technique and clinical implications. Chest 2004;126(6):1764–9.

56. Lee HJ, Yarmus L, Kidd D, et al. Comparison of pleural pressure measuring instruments. Chest 2014;146(4):1007–12.

57. Huggins JT, Sahn SA, Heidecker J, et al. Characteristics of trapped lung: pleural fluid analysis, manometry, and air-contrast chest CT. Chest 2007;131(1):206–13.

58. Villena V, López-Encuentra A, Pozo F, et al. Measurement of pleural pressure during therapeutic thoracentesis. Am J Respir Crit Care Med 2000;162(4 Pt 1):1534–8.

59. Pannu J, DePew ZS, Mullon JJ, et al. Impact of pleural manometry on the development of chest discomfort during thoracentesis: a symptom-based study. J Bronchology Interv Pulmonol 2014;21(4):306–13.

60. Gordon CE, Feller-Kopman D, Balk EM, et al. Pneumothorax following thoracentesis: a systematic review and meta-analysis. Arch Intern Med 2010;170(4):332–9.

61. Heidecker J, Huggins JT, Sahn SA, et al. Pathophysiology of pneumothorax following ultrasound-guided thoracentesis. Chest 2006;130(4):1173–84.

62. Ault MJ, Rosen BT, Scher J, et al. Thoracentesis outcomes: a 12-year experience. Thorax 2015;70(2):127–32.

63. Mahfood S, Hix WR, Aaron BL, et al. Reexpansion pulmonary edema. Ann Thorac Surg 1988;45(3):340–5.

64. Pavlin J, Cheney FW Jr. Unilateral pulmonary edema in rabbits after reexpansion of collapsed lung. J Appl Physiol Respir Environ Exerc Physiol 1979;46(1):31–5.

65. Lentz RJ, Lerner AD, Pannu JK, et al. Routine monitoring with pleural manometry during therapeutic large-volume thoracentesis to prevent pleural-pressure-related complications: a multicentre, single-blind randomised controlled trial. Lancet Respir Med 2019;7(5):447–55.

66. Dahlberg GJ, Maldonado F, Chen H, et al. Minimal clinically important difference for chest discomfort in patients undergoing pleural interventions. BMJ Open Respir Res 2020;7(1):e000667.

67. Lentz RJ, Shojaee S, Grosu HB, et al. The impact of gravity vs suction-driven therapeutic thoracentesis on pressure-related complications: the GRAVITAS multicenter randomized controlled trial. Chest 2020;157(3):702–11.

68. Senitko M, Ray AS, Murphy TE, et al. Safety and tolerability of vacuum versus manual drainage during thoracentesis: a randomized trial. J Bronchology Interv Pulmonol 2019;26(3):166–71.

69. Sagar AES, Landaeta MF, Adrianza AM, et al. Complications following symptom-limited thoracentesis using suction. Eur Respir J 2020;56(5):1902356.

70. Feller-Kopman DJ, Reddy CB, DeCamp MM, et al. Management of malignant pleural effusions. An official ATS/STS/STR clinical practice guideline. Am J Respir Crit Care Med 2018;198(7):839–49.

71. Martin GA, Tsim S, Kidd AC, et al. Pre-EDIT: a randomized feasibility trial of elastance-directed intrapleural catheter or talc pleurodesis in malignant pleural effusion. Chest 2019;156(6):1204–13.

Updates in Pleural Imaging

Maria Tsakok, BM, BCh, BA (Hons), FRCR[a], Rob Hallifax, PhD, MRCP[b],*

KEYWORDS

- Radiology • Pleura • Effusion • Ultrasonography • CT

KEY POINTS

- Initial modality of choice remains CXR.
- Ultrasound is increasingly being used for point-of-care diagnostics.
- Ultrasound is vital to guide pleural procedures.
- CT provides additional diagnostic assessment of pleural disease.
- MRI and PET/CT are becoming increasingly useful.

Pleural disease affects more than 300 people per 100,000 population each year and leads to more than 150 admissions per 100,000 population/y (costing >$10 billion in the United States alone). Radiological investigation is key in establishing a diagnosis for patients presenting with pleural effusion, thickening, masses, and pneumothorax. Radiological findings also often determine the initial management options and monitoring for ongoing management. Chest radiography remains the initial modality of choice for the investigation of pleural disease. Further imaging includes thoracic ultrasonography, computed tomography, MRI, and PET, which have important roles in further investigation, but appropriate modality selection is critical.

INTRODUCTION

Pleural disease is common, affecting more than 300 people per 100,000 population each year[1] and leading to more than 150 admissions per 100,000 population/y (costing >$10 billion in the United States alone).[2] Radiological investigation is key in establishing a diagnosis for patients presenting with pleural effusion, thickening, masses, and pneumothorax. Radiological findings also often determine the initial management options and monitoring for ongoing management.

Chest radiography (CXR) remains the initial modality of choice for the investigation of pleural disease. Further imaging includes thoracic ultrasonography (US), computed tomography (CT), MRI, and PET, which have important roles in further investigation, but appropriate modality selection is critical.

This article summarizes existing techniques and provides an up-to-date review of the evidence by disease area, highlighting the benefits and applications of each imaging modality.

IMAGING TECHNIQUES
Chest Radiography

An erect posterior-anterior CXR is the most important and widely used method to show and to follow the progress of pleural disease. It should be the initial choice of investigation wherever possible. Previously, lateral CXRs were used to show small effusions, but this has largely been superseded by the widespread use of US and CT imaging. Supine CXRs are less useful than erect CXRs in the detection of air or fluid.

Ultrasonography

US is frequently used to assess pleural disease first detected on CXR. The portability and ease of use of US allows its use on patients both as outpatients in clinic or inpatients (including critically unwell patients in intensive care in whom an erect CXR may not be possible). For reasons of safety

a Department of Radiology, Oxford University Hospitals NHS Foundation Trust, Churchill Hospital, Old Road, Oxford OX3 7LE, UK; b Department of Respiratory Medicine, University of Oxford, Churchill Hospital, Old Road, Oxford OX3 7LE, UK
* Corresponding author.
E-mail address: Robert.hallifax@ndm.ox.ac.uk
Twitter: @drhallifax (R.H.)

Clin Chest Med 42 (2021) 577–590
https://doi.org/10.1016/j.ccm.2021.07.001

and efficacy, US is now mandatory when performing pleural procedures investigating pleural fluid.[3,4] US is excellent for the investigation of pleural effusions because it can provide high-fidelity images of fluid composition and pleural thickening or masses.

Computed Tomography

CT investigation of pleural disease should involve the generation of multislice thin sections (0.5–2.0 mm) to enable multiplanar reconstruction. Pleural soft tissues are best imaged using pleural-phase intravenous contrast, administered with a delay of 60 to 90 seconds. This method allows maximum pleural soft tissue enhancement.[5] Images should be reviewed using mediastinal window setting (40/400) on a soft tissue algorithm along with review of the fissures using lung window settings (−500/1500).

PET/Computed Tomography

The combination of PET/CT and CT scanning allows visualization of metabolically active tissue by detecting increased uptake of a radiolabeled glucose isotope (eg, 18-fluorodeoxyglucose [FDG]). Malignant cells are usually more metabolically active than nonmalignant cells and therefore concentrate FDG more avidly than normal tissue. However, the clinical usage of PET/CT remains limited by cost, availability, and length of examination time. Patients must fast for 4 to 6 hours before imaging and avoid strenuous activity for 24 hours, with radioisotope administration 1 hour before the scan, which takes between 30 and 60 minutes. Nevertheless, it has an important role in evaluation of pleural disease in the detection of extrathoracic metastases and now forms part of the British Thoracic Society (BTS) guidelines.[6,7]

MRI

MRI has an increasing role in evaluating pleural disease because of improvements in sequences and technique. A body coil is used initially to obtain field-of-view scout images. Specialized coils can then be used if further specific images are required. Respiratory and cardiac gating are used to minimize movement artifact.[8] Typical sequences used to image the chest are T1-weighted spin echo, proton-density and T2-weighted spin echo or fast spin echo with fat saturation, and short tau inversion recovery (STIR). T1-weighted images show excellent contrast between abnormalities in the pleural space and extrapleural fat.[9] T2-weighted images highlight pleural fluid and provide good contrast between pleural malignancy and

skeletal muscle.[9] Because of its superior soft tissue contrast resolution compared with CT, MRI is now first line for the evaluation for chest wall invasion should this influence management in the evaluation of malignant pleural disease.[6,7] Dynamic contrast-enhanced (DCE) MRI and diffusion-weighted imaging (DWI) can be used to assess malignant pleural vascularity and may predict response to chemotherapy in patients with mesothelioma.[10–12]

NORMAL APPEARANCE
Chest Radiography

In health, the parietal and visceral pleura are thin membranes and so are not visualized on CXR, except where the visceral pleura invaginates into the lung to form the fissures (eg, oblique and horizontal fissures) because they are tangential to the x-ray beam.

Ultrasonography

The normal pleura is seen as a bright echogenic line, known as the pleural stripe, comprising the parietal and visceral pleura (**Fig. 1**). This line occurs because most of the acoustic energy of the US beam is reflected at the interface between the air in the lung up to the visceral pleural. Distal to the pleural stripe, artifacts known as B lines (or comet tails) appear as vertical echogenic bands extending deep into the image. B lines are produced by any small highly reflective object in the scanning plane and may be caused by inhomogeneities (eg, small foreign bodies, foci of calcification, and discrete air collections) at the pleural surface.[13] During normal respiration, the pleural stripe appears to shimmer as inhomogeneities

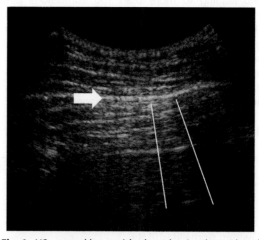

Fig. 1. US: normal lung with pleural stripe (*arrow*) and comet-tail artifacts (*white lines*).

move at the pleural interface. This effect is known as lung sliding. B lines and lung sliding signs are absent in the presence of pneumothorax.

Computed Tomography

In health, the thin visceral pleura and parietal pleura are not easily visualized on standard CT imaging. However, on high-resolution CT (HRCT), the thin layer of extrapleural fat that separates the pleura from the fascia adjacent to the parietal pleura is visible as a 1-mm to 2-mm intercostal stripe[14] (**Fig. 2**). In the absence of disease, there should be no soft tissue internal to the rib or paravertebral region. On multislice CT or HRCT, fissures appear as smooth, well-defined linear opacities, less than 1 mm in thickness.[14]

MRI

MRI can only identify pleural membranes if there is thickening or fluid present.

PLEURAL FLUID
Chest Radiography

Pleural fluid on erect CXR appears as a blunting of the costophrenic angle and a flattening of the diaphragm. CXR can appear normal with up to 500 mL.[15] As the volume of fluid increases, there is progressive homogeneous opacification of the lower chest with obliteration of the costophrenic angle and the hemidiaphragm, and characteristic meniscus sign is seen on CXR (**Fig. 3**).

Fluid can loculate between visceral and parietal layers (against the chest wall) or between visceral layers in fissures. Loculated effusions may occur in the context of empyema or hemothorax and do not move freely in the pleural space because of adhesions between the pleural layers. Therefore, the fluid does not always appear in dependent areas with sharp medial margins, but may appear in hazy lateral margins making an obtuse angle with the chest wall.[16] Occasionally, locations occurring in interlobular fissures can resemble masses (pseudotumors). Lateral CXR, US, and CT may be required to distinguish between loculated fluid and a solid mass.

In supine patients, the classic signs of pleural effusion (basal opacification and the meniscus sign) may be lost as the fluid extends posteriorly. In this case, effusions may appear as veil-like opacities over the whole or lower part of the hemithorax with preserved lung vascular markings in the overlying lung.

Ultrasonography

US is the most performed radiological investigation to evaluate effusions and should be universally used in respiratory and radiological practice. It can easily confirm the presence of an effusion and assess its character, and is mandated before any pleural intervention.[3,4] Transudative pleural fluid is hypoechoic, appearing dark on US. Echogenic effusions are always exudates, but anechoic effusions can be either transudates or exudates.[17] Exudative effusions (with high protein content) often form septations, which are fibrin strands initially appearing as thin strands that can be seen to move with movement of the fluid caused by respiration or cardiac pulsation (**Fig. 4**A). Septations are associated with infected or malignant effusion. Septations usually progress over time

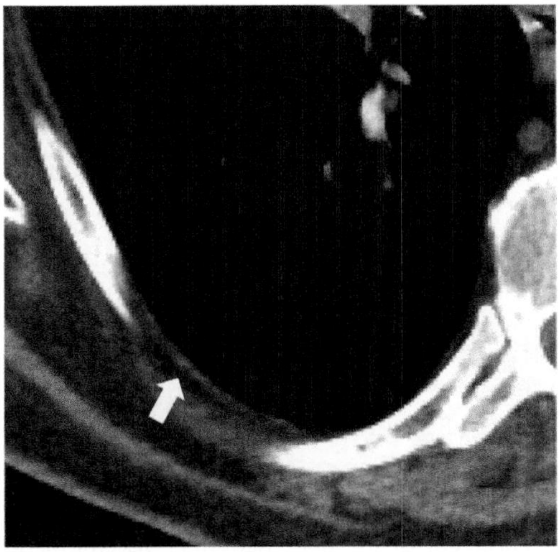

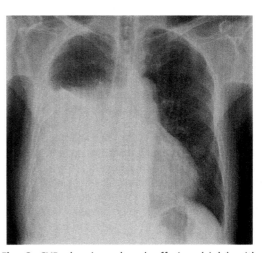

Fig. 2. Normal CT with pleural intercostal stripe (*arrow*).

Fig. 3. CXR showing pleural effusion (*right*) with meniscus sign.

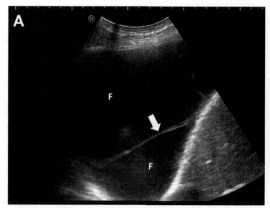
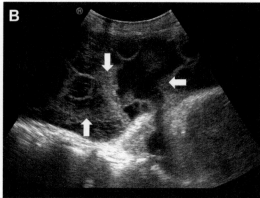

Fig. 4. (A) US showing pleural effusion (F) with early septations (*arrow*). (B) US showing organizing pleural effusion with heavy mature septations (*arrows*).

as additional fibrin is deposited. Eventually they may be thick and profuse enough to give a honeycomblike appearance of separate, noncommunicating pockets of fluid (**Fig. 4**B). Patients with septated pleural effusions have a higher morbidity and mortality compared with those without septations.[18]

Computed Tomography

CT is very sensitive in detecting pleural fluid and can distinguish between free and loculated effusions. In the investigation of the cause of an exudative pleural effusion, CT should be undertaken. CT can distinguish between parenchymal lung disease and pleural disease. Pleural phase contrast-enhanced CT scans can enable distinction between small effusions and pleural thickening that may appear similar on an unenhanced scan. CT should also be considered in those patients with suspected infected pleural fluid (empyema) who are too unwell or unsuitable for US (eg, in intensive care), or those who show significant volume loss on the CXR or lobar collapse potentially suggestive of underlying malignancy.

Empyema (as with an exudative cause of effusion) shows parietal and visceral pleural enhancement on contrast-enhanced CT scan, resulting in the split-pleura sign (**Fig. 5**). Although pleural thickening and enhancement are seen in 86% to 100% of patients with empyema, they are also seen in 60% of parapneumonic effusions.[19] In empyema, attenuation of the extrapleural fat adjacent to the fluid is also likely to be present.[19] CT can be helpful in patients not responding to conventional treatment of empyema with antibiotics and chest tube drainage by identifying nondraining locules of collection. Septations are best seen on US,

but multiple pockets of gas (with or without associated air fluid levels) on CT scanning are suggestive of septated fluid. Loculated pleural collections are often lenticular in shape with smooth margins and relatively homogeneous attenuation.[20] Enlargement of mediastinal node (<2 cm) is a common finding, but nodal involvement and increased CT-detected pleural thickening have not been shown to be predictive of outcome of empyema treatment (eg, need for surgery).[21]

It is important to differentiate between empyema and pulmonary abscesses that abut the pleura, because the former require chest tube placement for drainage, whereas inadvertent drainage of the latter may result in bronchopleural fistula formation. However, this can be difficult. On CT, abscesses often appear as spherical, thick-

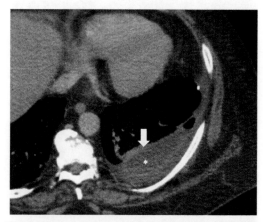

Fig. 5. CT showing empyema and split-pleura sign: enhancement of the thickened inner visceral pleura (*arrow*) and outer parietal pleura separated by pleural fluid.

walled lesions with abrupt vessel cutoff and the presence of bronchi at the interface between abscess and normal lung. In addition, pulmonary abscesses often make an acute angle with the chest wall, whereas empyema usually creates an obtuse angle.[22]

On a CT scan, hemothorax may show areas of hyperdensity or layering. The level of attenuation depends on the duration of the hemothorax because fresh blood has an attenuation of greater than 35 Hounsfield units (HU), and clotting blood of 70 HU. CT may useful in determining the cause of the hemothorax: for example, trauma (rib or sternal factures), or ruptured thoracic aneurysm.

PET/Computed Tomography

PET/CT can differentiate a transudate from an exudative effusion because the transudate is metabolically less active and so has low FDG update. However, PET/CT is rarely useful in the context of pleural infection because the effusion is highlighted as metabolically active and thus is indistinguishable from potential underlying malignancy.

MRI

Although CT imaging with pleural phase contrast remains the optimum modality for assessing malignant pleural effusions, there may be benefit for specifically designed pleural thoracic MRI protocols in certain clinical scenarios evaluating pleural effusion. Prior limitations of flow artifacts within the fluid created respiratory and cardiac movement that can now be mitigated by respiratory and electrocardiogram-gated sequences. If iodinated contrast is contraindicated or identification of chest wall invasion or septations within pleural fluid is required, MRI (with or without gadolinium contrast) may add value. Pleural fluid usually has a low signal on T1-weighted sequences and high signal on T2-weighted sequences. Therefore, T2-weighted sequences may show pleural nodularity, in the absence of contrast, because both fluid and extrapleural fat are high signal in comparison with the low-signal pleura, with high-resolution MRI now adding greater spatial and contrast resolution. T2 inversion recovery sequences with fat suppression or low b-value DWI can help further highlight nodular pleural foci, increasing sensitivity for detection. Portal-venous phase contrast administration may also show pleural enhancement and nodularity, in a similar manner to CT pleural imaging, with nodular or masslike enhancement raising suspicion for tumor. MRI may be superior to CT in differentiating transudates from exudates, with transudates usually T2 hyperintense, without pleural enhancement and no septations, whereas exudates have a lower T2 signal intensity and show greater heterogeneity, enhancement, and septae. Exudates have been shown to have lower apparent diffusion coefficient (ADC) values in some studies.[23,24] Because of the high level of triglycerides, chylous effusion can cause high signal intensity on T1-weighted images similar to subcutaneous fat. MRI is also specific for hemothorax, with bright signal intensity on T1-weighted images, surrounded by a dark rim caused by hemosiderin.

BENIGN PLEURAL THICKENING
Chest Radiography

CXR can show whether thickening is localized or diffuse, smooth or nodular, and the presence of pleural plaque. If viewed en profile, the thickening appears more or less parallel to the chest wall and forms a sharp interface with the lung. En face, thickening looks like an ill-defined veil-like opacification. Therefore, on standard posteroanterior CXR, thickening can be a subtle increase in radiographic density laterally on CXR, and often includes blunting of the costophrenic angle[25] (**Fig. 6**). Diffuse pleural thickening is seen as smooth, continuous opacification of fluid/soft tissue density extending over at least 25% of the chest wall.

Pleural plaques are areas of focal pleural thickening that usually undergo hyaline transformation and calcify. When calcified, pleural plaques are seen as white lines on tangential views parallel to the chest wall, or diaphragm, and when seen en face they produce the holly-leaf sign of irregular linear or stippled uneven calcifications.

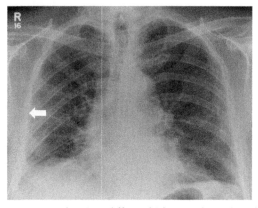

Fig. 6. CXR showing diffuse thickening (*arrow*) and blunting of costophrenic angle (*right*).

Ultrasonography

Pleural thickening can be identified on US once greater than 1 cm in depth.[26] Identification of pleural thickening can be difficult in the absence of pleural fluid because of lack of contrast between thickening, extrapleural fat, and the pleural stripe (the lung-pleura interface). Color Doppler functionality on US can sometimes usefully distinguish between thickening and small loculated effusions, because effusions may show fluid movement (eg, with cardiac pulsation).

Computed Tomography

CT is the modality of choice for the detection and characterization of pleural thickening, which is most easily assessed adjacent to ribs, where there should not normally be any soft tissue opacity. Pleural plaques commonly occur in the posterolateral aspect in the lower thorax, parietal region, and on the diaphragm. The characteristic appearance of plaques on CT are discrete, elevated lesions with steep rounded or rolled edges.[27] However, pleural plaques often increase in size and may be numerous. With time, they may involve other aspects of the parietal pleura and may become extensive, making differentiation from diffuse pleural thickening more difficult. Pleural plaques may also be associated with more subtle changes

in the lung parenchyma, appearing as interstitial lines on CT, hence being known as hairy plaques (**Fig. 7**A). Diffuse visceral pleural thickening, which may occur in the context of pleural plaques, is defined as a continuous sheet of pleural thickening greater than 5 cm wide, greater than 8 cm in craniocaudal extent, and greater than 3 mm thick,[27] and the edge is tapered[28] and is usually associated with rounded atelectasis.[29] Rounded atelectasis is the contraction and distortion of the lung adjacent to chronic pleural thickening and appears on CT as a rounded mass, with distortion of the lung seen as swirling and deviation of vessels and bronchi converging on the mass (**Fig. 7**B). It can occur with pleural thickening of any cause but is most commonly associated with asbestos-related pleural disease.

The final radiological appearances of most causes of benign pleural thickening are similar. However, certain features on CT scan may give clues as to the initial cause: extensive calcification, volume loss, thickened extrapleural fat layer, and associated parenchymal abnormality suggest prior empyema (including tuberculosis); pleural calcification with rib deformity and normal lung parenchyma could indicate previous traumatic hemothorax. The appearance after talc pleurodesis typically shows a characteristic talc sandwich of soft tissue parietal pleural thickening, high-

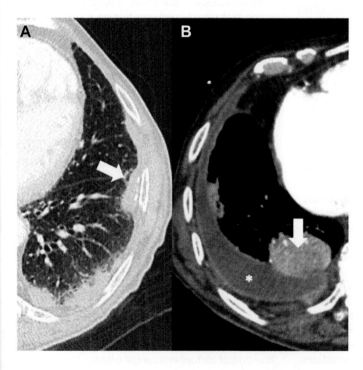

Fig. 7. (*A*) CT image showing pleural plaques with associated atelectasis and interstitial lines (hairy plaques) (*arrow*). (*B*) Rounded atelectasis (*arrow*) and pleural effusion (asterisk).

attenuation talc, and increased soft tissue visceral pleural thickening.[30]

MRI

High-resolution MRI is a good technique for assessing pleural plaques and is comparable with CT, although CT is superior in detecting calcification. On T1-weighted and T2-weighted sequences, plaques are of low signal.

MALIGNANT PLEURAL DISEASE
Chest Radiography

Metastatic disease accounts for most malignant pleural thickening. Primary pleural malignancy (mesothelioma) and metastatic disease are usually indistinguishable on imaging. However, the presence of pleural plaques provides evidence of prior asbestos exposure. Malignant pleural thickening changes seen on CXR are irregular, nodular opacities around the periphery of the lung. Pleural malignancy can be associated with pleural effusions in 60%, usually unilateral, but 5% may be bilateral.[31] Mesothelioma can be associated with volume loss in the affected hemithorax, but this is not specific for malignancy.

Ultrasonography

In the presence of a pleural effusion, pleural nodularity (parietal, visceral, or diaphragmatic) is a highly sensitive marker of pleural malignancy.[17] Contrast-enhanced thoracic US (CETUS) uses highly echogenic agents that are injected intravenously, thereby creating a blood signal that provides information on the vascularity of tissue/tumors. Therefore, CETUS may be able to distinguish benign from malignant pleural disease,[32] but its use is currently confined to a few specialist centers.

Computed Tomography

The classic features of malignant disease on CT scanning are nodular pleural thickening, mediastinal pleural thickening, parietal pleural thickening (>1 cm), and circumferential pleural thickening(- **Fig. 8**).[33] These 4 features are said to have high specificities (87%–100%, 68%–97%, 64%–98%, and 63%–100%) but low sensitivities (18%–53%, 14%–74%, 7%–47% and 7%–54%, respectively).[33–39] The presence of circumferential pleural thickening in the presence of pleural fluid is less specific for malignancy.[36] The positive predictive value of a malignant CT report is 80% but the negative predictive value (to exclude malignancy) is only 65%.[40] Therefore, clinicians should not necessarily rely on a CT scan without the classic features in patients with a high clinical suspicion

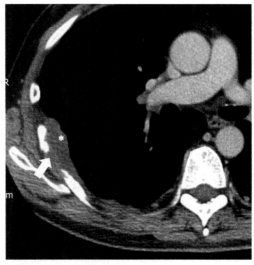

Fig. 8. CT image showing features of malignant disease: nodular thickening (asterisk) with rib invasion (*arrow*).

of malignancy. Other features, such as chest wall invasion and rib destruction, are good indicators of malignancy.

In patients being investigated for potential pleural malignancy with pleural effusion, there is no need to drain the pleural fluid before CXR or CT scan.[41]

Newer CT techniques to differentiate benign from malignant include dynamic contrast-enhanced CT (DCE-CT) and dual energy (or spectral) CT (DECT).

DCE-CT imaging describes the acquisition of a baseline image without contrast enhancement followed by a series of images acquired over time after an intravenous bolus of conventional contrast administration, and has advantage in differentiating benign from malignant disease because of the increased and often disorganized malignant tumor vascularity.[42] A recent study has shown potential utility of DCE-CT in assessing pharmacodynamic end points in the treatment of malignant pleural mesothelioma.[43] However, this technique is limited by high radiation dose.

DECT uses 2 separate x-ray photon energy spectra, allowing greater interrogation of materials that have different attenuation properties at different energies. Lower kiloelectron volt imaging enhances vessel contrast, image quality, and the detection of hypervascularized tissue, with iodine overlay imaging showing value in improved detection of occult metastases in various tumor types.[44] DECT has been shown to achieve better sensitivity and specificity than standard CT for differentiating malignant from benign disease in solitary pulmonary nodules[45] and pleural carcinomatosis.[46]

Nevertheless, a prospective large cohort validation study is required before inclusion in clinical practice.

PET/Computed Tomography

PET/CT is commonly used as a noninvasive method of determining metastatic spread in patients with cancer. In addition, PET/CT has been proposed as an imaging technique to allow differentiation between benign and malignant pleural disease (**Fig. 9**), but there is variation in the reported sensitivity (88%–100%) and specificity (35%–100%).[47–50] Clinicians should therefore be aware of the potential false-negative and false-positive findings. False-positives include infection (eg, pleural tuberculosis) or previous talc pleurodesis. PET/CT should be avoided in patients who have previously received talc pleurodesis because PET is highly avid regardless of underlying disease (see **Fig. 8**B). False-negatives could include low-grade epithelioid mesothelioma (with low metabolic activity) and small tumor size. The added value of PET/CT in pleural malignancy T-tumor staging is limited for local staging because of its poor spatial resolution; however, it has considerable value in determining nodal status and the detection of unsuspected extrathoracic metastases, which may alter treatment planning.[7]

PET/CT may be of use in determining prognosis and assessing response to chemotherapy.[51–53] Tumors with low SUV (standardized update value) on PET/CT are more likely to be epithelioid and to have a better prognosis. Data suggest that a reduction in metabolic activity after chemotherapy (as measured by SUV, metabolic tumor volume, or total glycolytic volume) correlates with increased time to progression and longer survival.[53] However, this application has not translated into routine clinical use.

Apical pleural thickening (or pleural cap) is often idiopathic and its frequency increases with age. It may be associated with previous tuberculosis, in which case CT shows an increase in apical pleural fat. However, it is important to distinguish benign pleural capping from Pancoast tumor. Malignant thickening is PET avid, with the CT component usually showing greater thickening and asymmetry and possibly associated with bony destruction.

MRI

Although CT is the imaging method of choice for investigating potential pleural malignancy, MRI may be of some additional value in differentiating benign from malignant disease[8,54–56] and determining T stage (in terms of chest wall invasion), and may have a role in treatment evaluation. Contrast-enhanced fat-saturated T1-weighted sequences may be useful in assessing focal thickening and interlobular fissures. DWI shows promise in differentiating benign from malignant disease, with malignant tissue being more structured and compact than benign. The characteristic difference in signal results in a hyperintense speckled appearance called pointillism. One study suggested that pointillism has a sensitivity of 93% and specificity of 79% in diagnosing malignant pleural disease (mainly mesothelioma),[11] with potential further benefit in guiding tumor sampling with biopsy. Diffusion-weighted MRI may identify sarcomatoid subtype of mesothelioma (lower ADC values than the epithelioid subtype), although biopsy is still required because of the considerable overlap of the biphasic subtype.

T stage in terms of chest wall invasion is superiorly evaluated on MRI compared with CT, and, where this will affect management, MRI should be performed.[7] Meanwhile, dynamic contrast-enhanced weighted images (repeated acquisition of an anatomic area through different stages of gadolinium administration) can provide extra information about tumor perfusion, vascularity, and vascular permeability, which can be correlated with tumor response to chemotherapy and therefore prognosis. Combined techniques of PET/MRI are feasible and show potential in accurately T staging mesothelioma.[57]

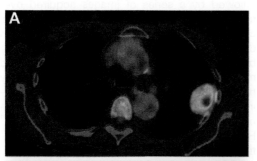
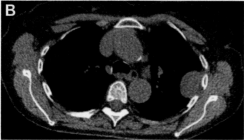

Fig. 9. CT image (*A*) and PET/CT image (*B*) confirming malignant disease (*bright red*).

RARE PLEURAL TUMORS
Fibromas

Chest radiography

Localized fibrous tumors are small rounded or oval homogeneous masses on CXR. They have a sharply delineated contour and are most commonly seen in the lower half of the chest.

Computed tomography

On unenhanced CT scan, fibromas are homogeneous, with calcification seen when large. Fibromas can vary in size, and larger tumors can displace the lung parenchyma, causing atelectasis in adjacent lung, with a smooth tapering margin and a characteristic obtuse angle at the junction of the mass and the pleura.[58] On contrast scan, up to 40% of fibromas are heterogeneous (**Fig. 10**).[59] Those with malignant change may show central necrosis on contrast-enhanced CT scan. Fibromas should be identified radiologically because seeding of pleural metastases can occur after percutaneous biopsy. Embolization of collateral circulation may be required before surgical resection.

PET/computed tomography

PET/CT may be valuable in identifying sarcomatous change within a pleural fibroma, by showing significantly increased FDG avidity.

MRI

On MRI, pleural fibromas appear as fibrous tissue masses with low to intermediate signal on T1-weighted and T2-weighted scans. Heterogeneous areas, including necrosis or hemorrhage, are seen as high signal intensity on STIR or T2-weighted images (**Fig. 10**).

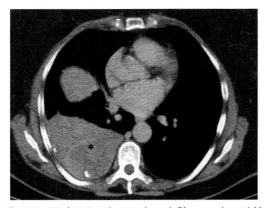

Fig. 10. CT showing large pleural fibroma (asterisk) with heterogeneous pattern postcontrast.

Lipomas and Liposarcomas

Lipomas are rare asymptomatic benign pleural tumors, usually discovered incidentally. On CT scan, lipomas appear as uniform pleural masses of fat density (<50 HU) (**Fig. 11**).[60] MRI also identifies a well-defined homogeneous mass that is hyperintense on T1-weighted and moderate intensity on T2-weighted images.

Liposarcomas

Liposarcomas are rare malignant tumors arising from fatty tissue. Unlike lipomas, patients often report chest pain and/or soft tissue swelling (if the mass extends through the chest wall). In contrast with lipomas, CT scan shows a heterogeneous mass with components of fat, fibrous septae, and nodular soft tissue,[60] and MRI shows low signal on T1-weighted and high intensity on T2-weighted images (myxoid degeneration). PET/CT can detect suspected sarcomatous change in lipomas.

PNEUMOTHORAX
Chest Radiography

Pneumothorax is usually diagnosed on erect CXR alone by visualization of the visceral pleural line (not normally seen) with an absence of parenchymal lung markings (and increased radiolucency) beyond this line (**Fig. 12**). CXR films should be taken on inspiration. There is little additional benefit in performing additional expiratory films for small pneumothorax detection.[61] CT is a more sensitive modality in these cases. Identification may be difficult in patients with bullous lung disease (who already have decreased vascular markings) and when linear shadows are generated by clothing, tubing, or skin-fold artifacts.

In supine films, identification of the deep-sulcus sign may aid pneumothorax detection: air seen anteromedially and subpulmonarily creates a lucent focus adjacent to the diaphragm.[62] In patients with suspected tension pneumothorax, decompression should be performed on clinical grounds and clinicians should not wait for this to be confirmed on imaging.

Ultrasonography

The sonographic finding of pneumothorax is a lack of the normal characteristic lung sliding.[13] M mode can be used to look for lung sliding, because it detects movement over time in a single plain. In normal patients, lung movement generates the seashore sign because lung sliding distal to the pleural line creates a granular pattern (the sand) and the static portion proximal to the pleural line creates lines (the sea) (**Fig. 13**A). If a

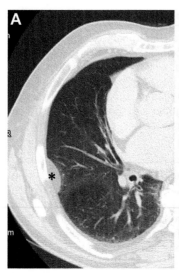
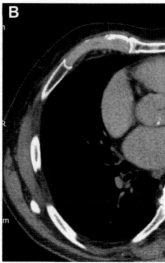

Fig. 11. CT with contrast showing pleural lipoma (asterisk). (*A*) Using lung windows; (*B*) using mediastinal windows (note low density of lipoma).

pneumothorax is present, the lack of lung sliding removes the granular pattern and the whole image becomes a series of parallel lines known as the stratosphere sign (**Fig. 13**B).[63] The lung-point sign delineating the border between normal sliding lung and pneumothorax can be used to identify and potentially determine the size of pneumothoraces. However, it has high specificity but low sensitivity because it relies on at least part of the lung being in contact with the chest wall and is therefore not seen in large pneumothoraces.[64] Horizontal reverberation artifacts (or A lines) appear as equally spaced hyperechoic repetitive lines caused by reflection from the pleura in the presence of pneumothorax and not in normal patients.

US has been reported as more sensitive than CXR in detecting pneumothorax after percutaneous lung biopsy,[13,65] after transbronchial biopsy during bronchoscopy,[66] and detecting occult traumatic pneumothoraces in emergency departments.[67] In addition, US could be useful in monitoring resolution of pneumothorax during treatment and identifying residual pneumothorax at follow-up.[68] However, by relying on an absence of signs, there is a risk of false-positives, particularly in patients with hyperinflation, air trapping, or bullous disease (such as in chronic obstructive pulmonary disease), or in those with previous pleurodesis who may have a lack of lung sliding.[69]

Computed Tomography

CT is more sensitive than CXR for small pneumothoraces, particularly when the patient is supine. From 25% to 40% of pneumothoraces after lung biopsy not detectable on CXR are present on CT.[70] In the context of trauma, CT may also provide important information such as lung contusion, infiltrates, or pericardial effusions. In patients with extensive subcutaneous emphysema, consolidation, or adult respiratory distress syndrome in intensive care, identification of pneumothorax on CXR can be difficult. In these patients, CT can assist in pneumothorax detection and determining site for chest drain insertion, and also in patients with tethered lung or if there is concern regarding the degree of pneumothorax in the context of severe bullous lung disease.

Fig. 12. CXR showing pneumothorax (*left*). Arrow shows visible visceral pleural edge.

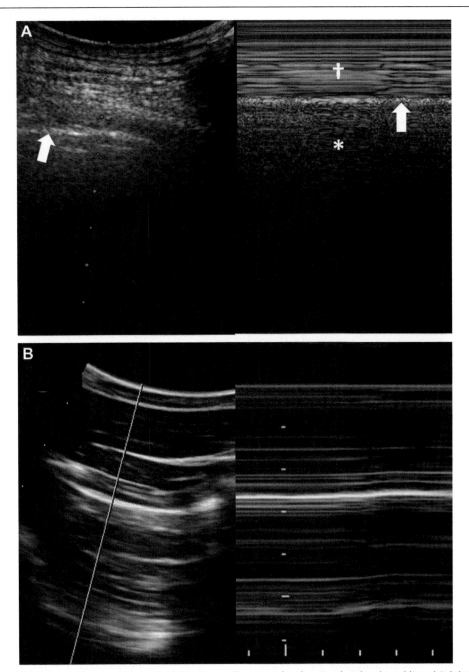

Fig. 13. (*A*) US images of normal lung: (*left*) 3.5-Hz curvilinear probe showing bright pleural line; (*right*) M-mode seashore sign: lung sliding distal to the pleural line creating granular pattern (the sand [*asterisk*]) and the static portion proximal to the pleural line creating lines (the sea [*dagger*]). (*B*) US images in pneumothorax: (*left*) 3.5-Hz curvilinear probe showing bright pleural line and also exaggerated horizontal (A-line) artifacts (*arrows*); (*right*) M-mode showing the stratosphere sign: loss of granular pattern associated with lung movement. Whole image is a series of parallel lines.

SUMMARY

CXR remains the initial investigation of choice in patients with suspected pleural disease. US is most useful in providing detailed assessment of pleural fluid and pleural nodularity, as well as being essential in guiding pleural procedures. US is increasingly used for point-of-care identification of pneumothorax, but this is highly operator dependent. CT scan is the modality of choice for further assessment of pleural disease. Newer techniques of dynamic contrast-enhanced CT and dual energy or spectral CT show potential for future use. MRI has specific utility for soft tissue abnormalities and may have a role for younger patients requiring follow-up serial imaging. MRI and PET/CT are increasingly being developed as tools to assess prognosis and response to therapy in malignant pleural disease.

CLINICS CARE POINTS

- Chest x-ray remains crucial for diagnosis and monitoring of pleural disease

- Portal venous phase contrast-enhanced CT on soft tissue algorithm allows more detailed assessment of pleural disease, its causes and complications

- PET/CT and MRI now play a crucial role in the detection of extrathoracic metastases and chest wall invasion respectively in staging and prognosis of pleural malignancy

- US is invaluable in the detection of small volume of pleural fluid (>20ml) and is particularly useful in a clinic or bedside setting

- Advances in pleural imaging the clinical utility of which is yet to be defined include:

  ○ Contrast-enhanced thoracic ultrasound – Intravenous high echogenicity contrast agents that assesses vascularity of tissue and may help distinguish benign from malignant disease but use of which remains limited to specialist centres and is highly operator-dependent

  ○ Dynamic contrast-enhanced CT - Allows more detailed vascular characterisation of tumours and may prove beneficial for determining pharmacodynamic end points in the treatment of pleural malignancy

  ○ Dual energy/spectral CT – Early potential for differentiating malignant from benign disease by enhancing vessel contrast, image quality and detection of hypervascularized tissue by use of iodine overlay maps

  ○ PET/CT – Early evidence of utility in determining prognosis and assessing response to chemotherapy by post-treatment changes in SUV, metabolic tumour volume or total glycolytic volume

  ○ Diffusion weighted imaging in MRI – Early evidence that a speckled appearance called pointillism may help diagnose pleural malignancy, guide tumour sampling and differentiate subtypes of mesothelioma

DISCLOSURE

RH is funded by an National Institute of Health Research (NIHR) Academic Clinical Lectureship.

REFERENCES

1. Du Rand I, Maskell N. Introduction and methods: British Thoracic Society pleural disease guideline. Thorax 2010;65(Suppl 2):ii1–3.
2. Mummadi SR, Stoller JK, Lopez R, et al. Epidemiology of adult pleural disease in the United States. Chest 2021. [Epub ahead of print].
3. Havelock T, Teoh R, Laws D, et al, BTS Pleural Disease Guideline Group. Pleural procedures and thoracic ultrasound: British thoracic Society pleural disease guideline 2010. Thorax 2010;65(Suppl 2):ii61–76.
4. The Royal College of Radiologists. Ultrasound training and recommendations for medical and surgical specialties. 2nd edition. London: The Royal College of Radiologists; 2012.
5. Gorg C, Bert T, Gorg K. Contrast-enhanced sonography for differential diagnosis of pleurisy and focal pleural lesions of unknown cause. Chest 2005; 128(6):3894–9.
6. Woolhouse I, Bishop L, Darlison L, et al. British Thoracic Society guideline for the investigation and management of malignant pleural mesothelioma. Thorax 2018;73(Suppl 1):i1–30.
7. Sinha S, Swift AJ, Kamil MA, et al. The role of imaging in malignant pleural mesothelioma: an update after the 2018 BTS guidelines. Clin Radiol 2020;75(6):423–32.
8. Helm EJ, Matin TN, Gleeson FV. Imaging of the pleura. J Magn Reson Imaging 2010;32(6):1275–86.
9. McLoud TC, Flower CD. Imaging the pleura: sonography, CT, and MR imaging. AJR Am J Roentgenol 1991;156(6):1145–53.
10. Giesel FL, Bischoff H, von Tengg-Kobligk H, et al. Dynamic contrast-enhanced MRI of malignant pleural mesothelioma: a feasibility study of noninvasive assessment, therapeutic follow-up, and possible predictor of improved outcome. Chest 2006;129(6):1570–6.
11. Coolen J, De Keyzer F, Nafteux P, et al. Malignant pleural mesothelioma: visual assessment by using pleural pointillism at diffusion-weighted MR imaging. Radiology 2015;274(2):576–84.

12. Vivoda Tomsic M, Bisdas S, Kovac V, et al. Dynamic contrast-enhanced MRI of malignant pleural mesothelioma: a comparative study of pharmacokinetic models and correlation with mRECIST criteria. Cancer Imaging 2019;19(1):10.

13. Goodman TR, Traill ZC, Phillips AJ, et al. Ultrasound detection of pneumothorax. Clin Radiol 1999;54(11): 736–9.

14. Im J-G, Webb WR, Rosen A, et al. Costal pleura: appearances at high-resolution CT. Radiology 1989; 171(1):125–31.

15. Blackmore CC, Black WC, Dallas RV, et al. Pleural fluid volume estimation: a chest radiograph prediction rule. Acad Radiol 1996;3(2):103–9.

16. Armstrong P, Wilson AG, Dee P, et al. Imaging diseases of the chest. 3rd edition. London: Mosby; 2000.

17. Qureshi NR, Rahman NM, Gleeson FV. Thoracic ultrasound in the diagnosis of malignant pleural effusion. Thorax 2009;64(2):139–43.

18. Chen CH, Chen W, Chen HJ, et al. Transthoracic ultrasonography in predicting the outcome of small-bore catheter drainage in empyemas or complicated parapneumonic effusions. Ultrasound Med Biol 2009; 35(9):1468–74.

19. Waite RJ, Carbonneau RJ, Balikian JP, et al. Parietal pleural changes in empyema: appearances at CT. Radiology 1990;175(1):145–50.

20. Henschke CI, Davis SD, Romano PM, et al. Pleural effusions: pathogenesis, radiologic evaluation, and therapy. J Thorac Imaging 1989;4(1):49–60.

21. Kearney SE, Davies CW, Davies RJ, et al. Computed tomography and ultrasound in parapneumonic effusions and empyema. Clin Radiol 2000;55(7):542–7.

22. Stark DD, Federle MP, Goodman PC, et al. Differentiating lung abscess and empyema: radiography and computed tomography. AJR Am J Roentgenol 1983;141(1):163–7.

23. Inan N, Arslan A, Akansel G, et al. Diffusion-weighted MRI in the characterization of pleural effusions. Diagn Interv Radiol 2009;15(1):13–8.

24. Baysal T, Bulut T, Gokirmak M, et al. Diffusion-weighted MR imaging of pleural fluid: differentiation of transudative vs exudative pleural effusions. Eur Radiol 2004;14(5):890–6.

25. McLoud TC, Woods BO, Carrington CB, et al. Diffuse pleural thickening in an asbestos-exposed population: prevalence and causes. AJR Am J Roentgenol 1985;144(1):9–18.

26. Wernecke K. Sonographic features of pleural disease. AJR Am J Roentgenol 1997;168(4):1061–6.

27. Lynch DA, Gamsu G, Aberle DR. Conventional and high resolution computed tomography in the diagnosis of asbestos-related diseases. Radiographics 1989;9(3):523–51.

28. Copley SJ, Wells AU, Rubens MB, et al. Functional consequences of pleural disease evaluated with chest radiography and CT. Radiology 2001;220(1):237–43.

29. Gevenois PA, de Maertelaer V, Madani A, et al. Asbestosis, pleural plaques and diffuse pleural thickening: three distinct benign responses to asbestos exposure. Eur Respir J 1998;11(5):1021–7.

30. Murray JG, Patz EF, Erasmus JJ, et al. CT appearance of the pleural space after talc pleurodesis. AJR Am J Roentgenol 1997;169(1):89–91.

31. Astoul P. Pleural mesothelioma. Curr Opin Pulm Med 1999;5(4):259–68.

32. Jacobsen N, Pietersen PI, Nolsoe C, et al. Clinical applications of contrast-enhanced thoracic ultrasound (CETUS) compared to standard reference tests: a systematic review. Ultraschall Med 2020. [Epub ahead of print].

33. Leung AN, Miller RR. CT in differential diagnosis of diffuse pleural disease. AJR Am J Roentgenol 1990;154(3):487–92.

34. Hierholzer J, Luo L, Bittner RC, et al. MRI and CT in the differential diagnosis of pleural disease. Chest 2000;118(3):604–9.

35. Arenas-Jiménez J, Alonso-Charterina S, Sánchez-Payá J, et al. Evaluation of CT findings for diagnosis of pleural effusions. Eur Radiol 2000;10(4):681–90.

36. Traill ZC, Davies RJ, Gleeson FV. Thoracic computed tomography in patients with suspected malignant pleural effusions. Clin Radiol 2001;56(3):193–6.

37. Metintas MUI, Elbek O, Erginel S, et al. Computed tomography features in malignant pleural mesothelioma and other commonly seen pleural diseases. Eur J Radiol 2002;41(1):1–9.

38. Yilmaz U, Polat G, Sahin N, et al. CT in differential diagnosis of benign and malignant pleural disease. Monaldi Arch Chest Dis 2005;63(1):17–22.

39. Kim JS, Shim SS, Kim Y, et al. Chest CT findings of pleural tuberculosis: differential diagnosis of pleural tuberculosis and malignant pleural dissemination. Acta Radiol 2014;55(9):1063–8.

40. Hallifax RJ, Haris M, Corcoran JP, et al. Role of CT in assessing pleural malignancy prior to thoracoscopy. Thorax 2015;70(2):192–3.

41. Corcoran JP, Acton L, Ahmed A, et al. Diagnostic value of radiological imaging pre- and post-drainage of pleural effusions. Respirology 2016;21(2):392–5.

42. Zhang M, Kono M. Solitary pulmonary nodules: evaluation of blood flow patterns with dynamic CT. Radiology 1997;205(2):471–8.

43. Gudmundsson E, Labby Z, Straus CM, et al. Dynamic contrast-enhanced CT for the assessment of tumour response in malignant pleural mesothelioma: a pilot study. Eur Radiol 2019;29(2):682–8.

44. Uhrig M, Simons D, Ganten MK, et al. Histogram analysis of iodine maps from dual energy computed tomography for monitoring targeted therapy of melanoma patients. Future Oncol 2015;11(4):591–606.

45. Zhang Y, Cheng J, Hua X, et al. Can spectral CT imaging improve the differentiation between malignant

and benign solitary pulmonary nodules? PLoS One 2016;11(2):e0147537.

46. Lennartz S, Le Blanc M, Zopfs D, et al. Dual-energy CT-derived iodine maps: use in assessing pleural carcinomatosis. Radiology 2019;290(3):796–804.

47. Duysinx B, Corhay JL, Larock MP, et al. Contribution of positron emission tomography in pleural disease. Rev Mal Respir 2010;27:e47–53.

48. Treglia G, Sadeghi R, Annunziata S, et al. Diagnostic accuracy of 18F-FDG-PET and PET/CT in the differential diagnosis between malignant and benign pleural lesions: a systematic review and meta-analysis. Acad Radiol 2014;21(1):11–20.

49. Treglia G, Sadeghi R, Annunziata S, et al. Diagnostic performance of fluorine-18-fluorodeoxyglucose positron emission tomography in the assessment of pleural abnormalities in cancer patients: a systematic review and a meta-analysis. Lung Cancer 2014;83(1):1–7.

50. Porcel JM, Hernandez P, Martinez-Alonso M, et al. Accuracy of fluorodeoxyglucose-PET imaging for differentiating benign from malignant pleural effusions: a meta-analysis. Chest 2015;147(2):502–12.

51. Gerbaudo VH, Britz-Cunningham S, Sugarbaker DJ, et al. Metabolic significance of the pattern, intensity and kinetics of 18F-FDG uptake in malignant pleural mesothelioma. Thorax 2003;58(12):1077–82.

52. Zucali PA, Lopci E, Ceresoli GL, et al. Prognostic and predictive role of [(18) F]fluorodeoxyglucose positron emission tomography (FDG-PET) in patients with unresectable malignant pleural mesothelioma (MPM) treated with up-front pemetrexed-based chemotherapy. Cancer Med 2017;6(10):2287–96.

53. Lopci E, Zucali PA, Ceresoli GL, et al. Quantitative analyses at baseline and interim PET evaluation for response assessment and outcome definition in patients with malignant pleural mesothelioma. Eur J Nucl Med Mol Imaging 2015;42(5):667–75.

54. Falaschi F, Battolla L, Zampa V, et al. [Comparison of computerized tomography and magnetic resonance in the assessment of benign and malignant pleural diseases]. Radiol Med 1996;92(6):713–8.

55. Armato SG 3rd, Francis RJ, Katz SI, et al. Imaging in pleural mesothelioma: a review of the 14th international conference of the international mesothelioma interest group. Lung Cancer 2019;130:108–14.

56. Raptis CA, McWilliams SR, Ratkowski KL, et al. Mediastinal and pleural MR imaging: practical approach for daily practice. Radiographics 2018; 38(1):37–55.

57. Murphy DJ, Mak SM, Mallia A, et al. Loco-regional staging of malignant pleural mesothelioma by integrated (18)F-FDG PET/MRI. Eur J Radiol 2019;115:46–52.

58. Dedrick CG, McLoud TC, Shepard JA, et al. Computed tomography of localized pleural mesothelioma. AJR Am J Roentgenol 1985;144(2):275–80.

59. Mendelson DS, Meary E, Buy JN, et al. Localized fibrous pleural mesothelioma: CT findings. Clin Imaging 1991;15(2):105–8.

60. Munk PL, Lee MJ, Janzen DL, et al. Lipoma and liposarcoma: evaluation using CT and MR imaging. AJR Am J Roentgenol 1997;169(2):589–94.

61. Schramel FM, Golding RP, Haakman CD, et al. Expiratory chest radiographs do not improve visibility of small apical pneumothoraces by enhanced contrast. Eur Respir J 1996;9(3):406–9.

62. Gordon R. The deep sulcus sign. Radiology 1980; 136(1):25–7.

63. Barillari A, Kiuru S. Detection of spontaneous pneumothorax with chest ultrasound in the emergency department. Intern Emerg Med 2010;5(3):253–5.

64. Lichtenstein D, Meziere G, Biderman P, et al. The "lung point": an ultrasound sign specific to pneumothorax. Intensive Care Med 2000;26(10):1434–40.

65. Sartori S, Tombesi P, Trevisani L, et al. Accuracy of transthoracic sonography in detection of pneumothorax after sonographically guided lung biopsy: prospective comparison with chest radiography. AJR Am J Roentgenol 2007;188(1):37–41.

66. Reissig A, Kroegel C. Accuracy of transthoracic sonography in excluding post-interventional pneumothorax and hydropneumothorax. Comparison to chest radiography. Eur J Radiol 2005;53(3):463–70.

67. Soldati G, Testa A, Sher S, et al. Occult traumatic pneumothorax: diagnostic accuracy of lung ultrasonography in the emergency department. Chest 2008;133(1):204–11.

68. Galbois A, Ait-Oufella H, Baudel JL, et al. Pleural ultrasound compared with chest radiographic detection of pneumothorax resolution after drainage. Chest 2010;138(3):648–55.

69. Slater A, Goodwin M, Anderson KE, et al. COPD can mimic the appearance of pneumothorax on thoracic ultrasound. Chest 2006;129(3):545–50.

70. Bungay HK, Berger J, Traill ZC, et al. Pneumothorax post CT-guided lung biopsy: a comparison between detection on chest radiographs and CT. Br J Radiol 1999;72(864):1160–3.

Ultrasound-Guided Pleural Investigations
Fluid, Air, and Biopsy

Jeffrey Thiboutot, MD[a],*, Kyle T. Bramley, MD[b]

KEYWORDS

- Pleural effusion • Pneumothorax • Thoracentesis • Ultrasound • Chest tube

KEY POINTS

- The majority of new pleural effusions require pleural drainage to help establish a diagnostic and provide symptomatic relief.
- There is strong evidence supporting ultrasound use for pleural drainage to decrease complication rates.
- Thoracic ultrasound examination is a sensitive and specific tool for the bedside diagnosis of pneumothorax.

INTRODUCTION

Pleural diseases are frequently encountered across multiple inpatient and outpatient settings, making pleural drainage and sampling one of the most common medical procedures. With the widespread adoption of bedside ultrasound examination, ultrasound machines are now readily available in many clinical settings, providing both diagnostic and procedural guidance. The modern management of pleural disease is dominated by ultrasound assessment with strong evidence supporting its use to guide pleural interventions. Here, we review the current landscape of ultrasound use to guide pleural drainage, pneumothorax management, and pleural biopsy.

INDICATIONS FOR PLEURAL FLUID DRAINAGE

Medical dogma teaches: "the sun should never rise nor fall on a pleural effusion." Although this is an overly simplistic view, the basic principle that a new pleural effusion needs prompt and thorough evaluation still holds. To determine the etiology of a pleural effusion, many physicians are quick to jump to pleural drainage. However, a thorough history and physical examination are often overlooked and may yield more valuable information than pleural fluid analysis. If, after a noninvasive assessment, there remains equipoise as to the etiology (which is often the case), or the patient is symptomatic, prompt drainage of the pleural space is indicated. Drainage can be both diagnostic and therapeutic. Indications for pleural drainage follow 1 of 2 pathways: the first is to establish a diagnosis, and the second is for therapeutic benefit (**Box 1**). Often both reasons are required.

Diagnostic Indications

The diagnostic indications for a newly discovered pleural effusion are rather broad. If an effusion can be simply explained by clinical presentation (ie, bilateral free-flowing effusion in a patient with decompensated heart failure), drainage can be deferred and the patient can be treated medically. However, any new effusion that cannot be explained otherwise should undergo sampling. For diagnostic purposes, sampling can be performed under ultrasound guidance via simple needle aspiration or thoracentesis.

[a] Pulmonary and Critical Care Medicine, Johns Hopkins University, Baltimore, MD, USA; [b] Pulmonary, Critical Care & Sleep Medicine, Yale University, 15 York Street, LCI 100, New Haven, CT 06510, USA
* Corresponding author. Johns Hopkins Hospital, Sheikh Zayed Tower 7-125, Baltimore, MD 21287.
E-mail address: jthibou1@jhmi.edu

Clin Chest Med 42 (2021) 591–597
https://doi.org/10.1016/j.ccm.2021.07.002
0272-5231/21/© 2021 Elsevier Inc. All rights reserved.

Box 1
Indications for pleural drainage
Undiagnosed
Fever
Dyspnea
Leukocytosis
Pleurisy
Immunocompromised host
Unilateral
Suspected malignancy

Therapeutics

When a patient presents symptomatic owing to a pleural effusion, most commonly owing to dyspnea, therapeutic drainage is indicated. These are often due to large or complex effusions. Therapeutic drainage is performed via ultrasound-guided thoracentesis or chest drain insertion.

ULTRASOUND-GUIDED PLEURAL FLUID DRAINAGE

Pleural drainage can be achieved via simple needle aspiration, thoracentesis, or chest drain insertion. Pleural ultrasound guidance permits the identification of anatomic structures, selection of site for insertion, real-time guidance, as well as prediction of pleural pathology (malignancy or complicated effusions). These added benefits of procedural ultrasound guidance have led to lower complication and failure rates.[1–4] For these reasons, performing pleural drainage procedures under ultrasound guidance has become the standard of care.[5,6]

Training

The British Thoracic Society guidelines and the American College of Graduate Medical Education recommend a combination of didactic lectures and simulated experience using ultrasound guidance for thoracentesis and the insertion of chest drains. Part of this process requires training from an experienced practitioner. Studies have shown that junior physicians are only able to correctly identify a safe site for insertion in 44% to 55% of cases,[7,8] level of experience and supervised insertion aided in safe site identification. A rigorous training system with structured proficiency and competency standards, including the use of ultrasound guidance, can decrease pneumothorax rates from 8% to 1%.[9] Training in pleural drainage and ultrasound examination should be taught across various training levels, including both medical undergraduate and graduate levels. The implementation of pleural drainage training programs has been shown to improve procedural competency[10] and decrease pain and anxiety for patients.[11] For these reasons, the American College of Chest Physicians, the American College of Surgeons, the American College of Emergency Physicians, and the UK Royal College of Radiologists have all published teaching curricula for pleural ultrasound competency.[12,13]

Anatomic Site Selection

Improper site selection can lead to significant harm with visceral injury to lung, heart, diaphragm, liver, and spleen. Classically a chest radiograph was needed to confirm the indication and side of procedure, although ultrasound imaging has largely replaced this requirement. Puncture site selection is likely the most critical step of performing pleural access, whether via simple aspiration, thoracentesis, or pleural drain placement. The preferred site of puncture is the triangle of safety. That said, ultrasound findings of the largest hypoechoic pocket will ultimately guide the ideal location.

The most common complication of pleural drainage of fluid is pneumothorax. Other complications include hemorrhage, infection, chest pain, diaphragmatic injury and re-expansion pulmonary edema. The use of pleural ultrasound during the drainage procedure has been shown to reduce these complication rates. There is wide variation in the reported pneumothorax rates following pleural effusion drainage, ranging from 0.9% to 15.0%.[14–17] The most common predictor of a complication is the lack of operator experience and the lack of ultrasound guidance. Diacon and colleagues[18] found that ultrasound guidance was able to locate a safe pocket for drainage when deemed unable to be performed by standard physical examination alone in 54% of cases. Ultrasound guidance prevented accidental organ puncture in 10% of cases and increased the rate of accurate site selection by 26%. In fact, the sensitivity and specificity of identifying a proper site for puncture with clinical examination alone was 77% and 60%, respectively, compared with ultrasound guidance as the gold standard. Retrospective studies have shown that the use of ultrasound examination can decrease pneumothorax rates from 10% to 5%.[3] For large effusions, the data for ultrasound use is more equivocal. Kohan and colleagues[19] showed a significant increase in the adequate performance of thoracentesis with ultrasound guidance for small effusions, but no differences were noted in large effusions. A 2010 meta-analysis including 24 studies evaluating pneumothorax rates after pleural drainage found a pooled pneumothorax rate of 6.0%.[4] Again this study finds the use of ultrasound examination significantly decreased pneumothorax rates (odds ratio, 0.3; 95% confidence interval, 0.2–0.7), and lower complication rates occur with experienced operators (3.9% vs 8.5%; $P = .04$). The use of ultrasound guidance for appropriate site selection is not limited to thoracentesis alone; there is growing literature supporting its safe and efficacious use when placing pleural drains as well (both large and small bore chest tubes).[20–22]

Volume of Fluid Removal

A feared complication of large volume fluid removal is re-expansion pulmonary edema. Although there is no definite maximum volume of fluid that can be removed safely, the frequency of re-expansion edema increases as greater volumes of fluid are drained. Attention should be paid to the signs and symptoms of re-expansion pulmonary edema, such as pain and intractable cough. Retrospective reviews have shown a mortality rate of up to 20% in patients who develop re-expansion pulmonary edema after pleural drainage.[23] The British Thoracic Society guidelines suggest drainage should be limited to 1.5 L.[5] However, in a patient with a large effusion who is asymptomatic during drainage, there are numerous studies showing that greater volumes can safely be removed.[24–26] The debated 1.5 L cutoff is based on data showing an increase in rates of pneumothorax after large volume drainage. Josephson and colleagues[27] showed in a prospective study of 735 thoracenteses, compared with a drainage of 0.8 to 1.2 L, draining 1.8 to 2.2 L was associated with an odds ratio of 3.8 (95% confidence interval, 1.3–25.0) for the development of a pneumothorax. Other smaller studies have reported an increased incidence of pneumothorax with increased volume of drainage; however, taken together the level of evidence supporting stopping drainage at a fixed volume in an asymptomatic patient is low.[17,24,28,29]

It is in fact thought that the development of complications owing to over drainage of the pleural space is not due to volume alone, but rather driven by rapid, nonuniform decreases in the pleural pressure. This point had led to investigations of pleural manometry to guide drainage. During drainage, greater decreases in pleural pressures have been associated with nonexpandable lung (with risk of pneumothorax ex vacuo). That said, the presence of more negative pleural pressures

was not able to accurately predict the development of pneumothorax ex vacuo.[30] Although pneumothorax ex vacuo is a radiographic finding of little importance to the patient and/or providers, pain is a significant complication that often accompanies a nonexpandable lung. This premise has been tested in a multicenter randomized controlled study by Lentz and colleagues,[31] comparing a manometry-guided drainage approach versus a symptom-guided drainage approach. These findings show that using manometry to guide volume of drainage did result in lower rates of pneumothorax ex vacuo; however, no significant differences in the primary outcome of pain were observed. These findings are in line with prior nonrandomized studies evaluating the usefulness of pleural manometry to guide drainage.[32,33] Pleural manometry has also been used to predict nonexpandable lung after indwelling pleural catheter placement. A study by Halford and colleagues[34] showed that patients with a nonexpandable lung had significantly lower closing pleural pressures (-15.0 vs 0.0; $P = .01$); however, the ability for the pleural pressure to predict the development of nonexpandable lung was low. Together, the data on the use of manometry during pleural drainage is equivocal and it is not recommended for routine use.

ULTRASOUND EXAMINATION TO DIAGNOSE PNEUMOTHORAX

Pneumothorax is defined as the presence of air in the chest cavity. This situation can occur spontaneously, as a consequence of underlying pulmonary disease, or result from iatrogenic or traumatic etiologies. A pneumothorax can present as a life-threatening emergency and rapid diagnosis is essential. Thoracic ultrasound examination is useful for the bedside diagnosis of pneumothorax and is readily available for rapid assessment.

There are several ultrasound findings that are both sensitive and specific to evaluate for pneumothorax. Under normal conditions, the parietal and visceral pleura are apposed, with movement of the visceral pleura throughout the respiratory cycle. This movement can be visualized easily via ultrasound examination and is referred to as "lung sliding." When a pneumothorax is present, the parietal and visceral pleura are no longer apposed, with air between the surfaces. This air scatters the ultrasound waves and lung sliding is no longer seen. This finding, coupled with A-lines (equidistant, horizontal, parallel lines that are a reverberation artifact of the parietal pleura), is diagnostic of a pneumothorax.[35]

There are also ultrasound findings that indicate the absence of pneumothorax. In a completely atelectatic lung, this pleural movement with respiration may not be visible and the clinician may instead see conducted pulsations from the heart along the pleural surface. This finding is known as a "lung pulse" and its presence confirms the absence of a pneumothorax. If the lung parenchyma contains alveolar or interstitial fluid, we may see this reflected off the pleura in the form of B lines—vertical lines arising from the pleura. The presence of B lines confirms apposition of the parietal and visceral pleural surfaces and rules out a pneumothorax.

The pathognomonic finding of a pneumothorax is the "lung point" sign, which is the visualization of the transition zone from normally apposed pleura and pneumothorax. This process is seen as a lack of lung sliding with A lines (reflecting a pneumothorax), with an area of normal lung sliding moving through the visualization window during the respiratory cycle. The lung point is not always identifiable and may be absent with large pneumothoraces. The presence of a lung point has a specificity and positive predictive value of 100%.[36]

ULTRASOUND-GUIDED CHEST TUBE PLACEMENT FOR PNEUMOTHORAX

Thoracic ultrasound examination is used widely to guide interventions in the setting of pleural effusions. There are data to support the role of ultrasound guidance to increase the safety and improve the accuracy of the placement of catheters in pleural effusion. Despite the widespread acceptance of thoracic ultrasound guidance in the diagnosis of pneumothorax, there are seemingly few descriptions of its use to guide treatment interventions. The use of the ultrasound examination in the treatment of pneumothorax has many potential advantages.

Thoracostomy tubes are generally placed in the triangle of safety, or the anatomic area bordered by the pectoralis major, latissimus dorsi, and a horizontal line at the fifth intercostal space. This location minimizes the risk of bleeding by avoiding the larger intercostal vessels that may not traverse at the inferior border of the rib posteriorly. It also helps to prevent subdiaphragmatic tube placement by suggesting a safe lower boundary. Although the anatomic boundary of the fifth intercostal space will identify the location for thoracic placement of the chest tube in most patients, this is not true for all patients. A recent study used ultrasound examination to identify the level of the diaphragm in 50 patients presenting to the emergency room. The diaphragm was seen to cross, or be located above the fifth intercostal space 20% of the time on the right side and 18% on the left, suggesting added benefit of ultrasound examination to select a location for thoracostomy placement.[37]

Thoracic ultrasound examinations can be used to screen for vulnerable intercostal arteries at bedside before procedures. A recent study of 50 patients undergoing contrast-enhanced computed tomography scans evaluated the ability to identify potentially exposed intercostal vessels with thoracic ultrasound examination. The sensitivity was 86% to 88% depending on the ultrasound system used. The negative predictive value (the probability the artery is truly behind the rib when it is not identified on ultrasound examination), was low at 0.26. Based on these data, it is reasonable to screen for vulnerable vessels in patients who are at high risk for bleeding, although a negative scan does not ensure optimal arterial location.[38,39]

In patients with smaller pneumothoraces, ultrasound examination may be used to help identify the pneumothorax pocket and aid in choosing the optimal site for tube placement. If there is ultrasound evidence of lung apposition, such as where lung sliding or B lines are seen, the risk of injury to the lung may be greater when entering the space, particularly with Seldinger-type chest tubes. Using the ultrasound examination to identify areas where there is not apposition may decrease these injuries. If a lung point is seen, a location outside of this transition zone can be chosen to potentially avoid injury to the lung.

This approach was well-described in a case report of ultrasound examination being used to identify a loculated basilar pneumothorax. Ultrasound examination was used to outline the loculated pocket by identifying a lung point superiorly and the diaphragm inferiorly, with a typical pneumothorax pattern seen in the pocket.[40] These approaches have not been studied rigorously, but are helpful clinically to guide chest tube placement.

The usefulness of ultrasound examination can be limited in certain situations. Subcutaneous emphysema can cause artifact and prevent adequate ultrasound visualization of the pleura, thus limiting the ability to obtain adequate images in these patients to guide chest tube placement.[35]

After chest tube placement, ultrasound examination seems to be effective at confirming intrathoracic placement of thoracostomy tubes. The ultrasound examination is used to scan the soft tissues of the chest wall from the tube insertion site and can follow the course of the tube. The tube will be seen to traverse into the pleural cavity with intrathoracic placement, although it can be followed for its length in the subcutaneous space if it is extrathoracic. The use of ultrasound examination to confirm placement has been shown to be feasible and accurate in limited cadaveric[41,42] and human studies.[43]

ULTRASOUND-GUIDED BIOPSIES

Thoracic ultrasound examinations can also be used to guide pleural biopsies in cases where thoracentesis alone does not yield a diagnosis or when thoracoscopy is not feasible. At one time, closed pleural biopsies were a widely used method for pleural sampling when simple thoracentesis did not yield a diagnosis. Although it has been replaced by medical pleuroscopy in many institutions, it remains a useful technique for patients who cannot undergo pleuroscopy, either because of their clinical status or institutional availability. A full discussion of medical pleuroscopy is described elsewhere in a later article.

Ultrasound-guided biopsies can be performed in a number of ways. In the case of more diffuse disease, biopsies can be obtained with reversed-bevel closed needles (closed pleural biopsies), with models named after their creators Abrams and Cope. The reported sensitivities vary widely depending on the population studied, with a large retrospective study suggesting a diagnostic yield of 51.5% for malignancy and 69.0% for tuberculous pleuritis.[44] A recent meta-analysis of 10 studies evaluating closed pleural biopsies in the diagnosis of exudative pleural effusions suggested a pooled sensitivity of 77%.[45] The role of ultrasound examination to guide these biopsies is not well-defined, with only small studies suggesting a benefit. Theoretically, we would expect pleural metastases to be more frequent inferiorly in the thorax and ultrasound examination may be able to help identify a more suitable, lower location for sampling.[46] One small study comparing a single proceduralist's diagnostic yield before and after the addition of ultrasound guidance showed a nonstatistically significant increase in diagnostic yield.[46]

If there is a discrete pleural mass or area of pleural thickening, a cutting needle biopsy can be used to obtain a core sample. A recent meta-analysis found that ultrasound-guided needle biopsies in patients with a variety of diagnoses resulted in a pooled sensitivity of 83% and specificity of 100%.[47]

Ultrasound-guided needle biopsies seem to be safe and beneficial in patients in whom thoracoscopy is not feasible. One retrospective review describes 13 patients who had failed thoracoscopy secondary to adhesions, and another 37 patients who were deemed too frail to undergo the procedure. Ultrasound-guided cutting needle biopsies were performed successfully in 47 of these patients (94%), including 11 of the 13 patients (85%) whom had a failed pleuroscopy.[48]

Tuberculous Pleuritis

The use of ultrasound-guided biopsies has been evaluated in diagnosing tuberculous pleuritis. A prospective, randomized, controlled trial compared a cutting needle biopsy with a thoracoscopic biopsy for tuberculous pleuritis. They showed a sensitivity of 82% for needle biopsy and 90% for thoracoscopy, a difference that was not statistically significant.[49] In this study, there were 6 patients who could not undergo thoracoscopic biopsy given significant adhesions. Four patients subsequently underwent successful cutting needle biopsies and were diagnosed with tuberculous pleuritis.[49] A randomized controlled trial directly compared ultrasound-guided Abrams biopsy with cutting needle biopsy in the diagnosis of tuberculous pleurisy. Each patient underwent ultrasound-guided Abrams biopsies and were more likely to contain pleural tissue (91% vs 78%) and had a higher sensitivity (82% vs 65%).[50]

Bacterial Pleural Infection

A potential new use for pleural biopsies was recently evaluated in the AUDIO study. The diagnostic yield of microbiologic cultures of pleural fluid in patients with pleural infection is low. It was hypothesized that the addition of pleural biopsies to standard cultures would improve the overall yield. In a pilot study of 20 patients with known pleural infection, ultrasound-guided pleural biopsies were obtained at the time of tube thoracostomy placement. The overall diagnostic yield of the biopsy cultures was 45%. The addition of biopsies to blood and pleural fluid cultures increased the overall yield by 25%.[51]

SUMMARY

Undifferentiated and symptomatic pleural effusions require drainage, either via simple needle aspiration, thoracentesis, or pleural drain placement. Thoracic ultrasound examination is a useful tool for the diagnostic evaluation of pleural disease, with strong evidence supporting its use during procedural pleural drainage. Ultrasound examination should be used to guide site selection for fluid drainage, evacuation of pneumothoraces, and pleural biopsy to reduce incidence of pneumothorax and nearby visceral organ injury.

CLINICS CARE POINTS

- Use of ultrasound for pleural procedures decreases complication rates.
- Ultrasound guidance should be used for site selection for pleural access and biopsy.

DISCLOSURE

J. Thiboutot and K.T. Bramley have nothing to disclose.

REFERENCES

1. Grogan DR, Irwin RS, Channick R, et al. Complications associated with thoracentesis. A prospective, randomized study comparing three different methods. Arch Intern Med 1990;150:873–7.
2. Raptopoulos V, Davis LM, Lee G, et al. Factors affecting the development of pneumothorax associated with thoracentesis. AJR Am J Roentgenol 1991; 156:917–20.
3. Barnes TW, Morgenthaler TI, Olson EJ, et al. Sonographically guided thoracentesis and rate of pneumothorax. J Clin Ultrasound 2005;33:442–6.
4. Gordon CE, Feller-Kopman D, Balk EM, et al. Pneumothorax following thoracentesis: a systematic review and meta-analysis. Arch Intern Med 2010; 170:332–9.
5. Havelock T, Teoh R, Laws D, et al. Pleural procedures and thoracic ultrasound: British thoracic Society pleural disease guideline 2010. Thorax 2010; 65(Suppl 2):ii61–76.
6. Dancel R, Schnobrich D, Puri N, et al. Recommendations on the use of ultrasound guidance for adult thoracentesis: a position statement of the Society of Hospital Medicine. J Hosp Med 2018;13:126–35.
7. Griffiths JR, Roberts N. Do junior doctors know where to insert chest drains safely? Postgrad Med J 2005;81:456–8.
8. Elsayed H, Roberts R, Emadi M, et al. Chest drain insertion is not a harmless procedure–are we doing it safely? Interactive Cardiovasc Thorac Surg 2010; 11:745–8.
9. Duncan DR, Morgenthaler TI, Ryu JH, et al. Reducing iatrogenic risk in thoracentesis: establishing best practice via experiential training in a zero-risk environment. Chest 2009;135:1315–20.
10. Wayne DB, Barsuk JH, O'Leary KJ, et al. Mastery learning of thoracentesis skills by internal medicine residents using simulation technology and deliberate practice. J Hosp Med 2008;3:48–54.
11. Luketich JD, Kiss M, Hershey J, et al. Chest tube insertion: a prospective evaluation of pain management. The Clin J pain 1998;14:152–4.
12. Mayo PH, Beaulieu Y, Doelken P, et al. American College of Chest Physicians/La Société de Réanimation de Langue Française statement on competence in critical care ultrasonography. Chest 2009;135: 1050–60.
13. American College of Emergency Physicians. Use of ultrasound imaging by emergency physicians. Ann Emerg Med 2001;38:469–70.
14. Harnsberger HR, Lee TG, Mukuno DH. Rapid, inexpensive real-time directed thoracentesis. Radiology 1983;146:545–6.
15. Collins TR, Sahn SA. Thoracocentesis. Clinical value, complications, technical problems, and patient experience. Chest 1987;91:817–22.
16. Grodzin CJ, Balk RA. Indwelling small pleural catheter needle thoracentesis in the management of large pleural effusions. Chest 1997;111:981–8.
17. Colt HG, Brewer N, Barbur E. Evaluation of patient-related and procedure-related factors contributing to pneumothorax following thoracentesis. Chest 1999;116:134–8.
18. Diacon AH, Brutsche MH, Solèr M. Accuracy of pleural puncture sites*: a prospective comparison of clinical examination with ultrasound. Chest 2003; 123:436–41.
19. Kohan JM, Poe RH, Israel RH, et al. Value of chest ultrasonography versus decubitus roentgenography for thoracentesis. Am Rev Respir Dis 1986;133:1124–6.
20. Moulton JS, Benkert RE, Weisiger KH, et al. Treatment of complicated pleural fluid collections with image-guided drainage and intracavitary urokinase. Chest 1995;108:1252–9.
21. vanSonnenberg E, Nakamoto SK, Mueller PR, et al. CT- and ultrasound-guided catheter drainage of empyemas after chest-tube failure. Radiology 1984; 151:349–53.
22. Cantin L, Chartrand-Lefebvre C, Lepanto L, et al. Chest tube drainage under radiological guidance for pleural effusion and pneumothorax in a tertiary care university teaching hospital: review of 51 cases. Can Respir J 2005;12:29–33.
23. Mahfood S, Hix WR, Aaron BL, et al. Reexpansion pulmonary edema. Ann Thorac Surg 1988;45:340–5.
24. Pihlajamaa K, Bode MK, Puumalainen T, et al. Pneumothorax and the value of chest radiography after ultrasound-guided thoracocentesis. Acta Radiol 2004;45:828–32.
25. Feller-Kopman D, Berkowitz D, Boiselle P, et al. Large-volume thoracentesis and the risk of reexpansion pulmonary edema. Ann Thorac Surg 2007;84: 1656–61.
26. Mynarek G, Brabrand K, Jakobsen JA, et al. Complications following ultrasound-guided thoracocentesis. Acta Radiol 2004;45:519–22.

27. Josephson T, Nordenskjold CA, Larsson J, et al. Amount drained at ultrasound-guided thoracentesis and risk of pneumothorax. Acta Radiol 2009;50: 42–7.

28. Heidecker J, Huggins JT, Sahn SA, et al. Pathophysiology of pneumothorax following ultrasound-guided thoracentesis. Chest 2006;130:1173–84.

29. Shechtman L, Shrem M, Kleinbaum Y, et al. Incidence and risk factors of pneumothorax following pre-procedural ultrasound-guided thoracentesis. J Thorac Dis 2020;12:942–8.

30. Chopra A, Judson MA, Doelken P, et al. The relationship of pleural manometry with postthoracentesis chest radiographic findings in malignant pleural effusion. Chest 2020;157:421–6.

31. Lentz RJ, Lerner AD, Pannu JK, et al. Routine monitoring with pleural manometry during therapeutic large-volume thoracentesis to prevent pleural-pressure-related complications: a multicentre, single-blind randomised controlled trial. Lancet Respir Med 2019;7:447–55.

32. Pannu J, DePew ZS, Mullon JJ, et al. Impact of pleural manometry on the development of chest discomfort during thoracentesis: a symptom-based study. J Bronchol Interv Pulmonol 2014;21:306–13.

33. Feller-Kopman D, Walkey A, Berkowitz D, et al. The relationship of pleural pressure to symptom development during therapeutic thoracentesis. Chest 2006;129:1556–60.

34. Halford PJ, Bhatnagar R, White P, et al. Manometry performed at indwelling pleural catheter insertion to predict unexpandable lung. J Thorac Dis 2020; 12:1374–84.

35. Volpicelli G. Sonographic diagnosis of pneumothorax. Intensive Care Med 2011;37:224–32.

36. Lichtenstein D, Meziere G, Biderman P, et al. The "lung point": an ultrasound sign specific to pneumothorax. Intensive Care Med 2000;26:1434–40.

37. Gray EJ, Cranford JA, Betcher JA, et al. Sonogram of safety: ultrasound outperforms the fifth intercostal space landmark for tube thoracostomy site selection. J Clin Ultrasound 2020;48:303–6.

38. Salamonsen M, Dobeli K, McGrath D, et al. Physician-performed ultrasound can accurately screen for a vulnerable intercostal artery prior to chest drainage procedures. Respirology 2013;18:942–7.

39. Corcoran JP, Psallidas I, Ross CL, et al. Always Worth another Look? Thoracic ultrasonography before, during, and after pleural intervention. Ann Am Thorac Soc 2016;13:118–21.

40. Deutsch E, Beck S, Meer J, et al. Ultrasound guided chest tube placement for basilar pneumothorax. Intern Emerg Med 2016;11:483–5.

41. Salz TO, Wilson SR, Liebmann O, et al. An initial description of a sonographic sign that verifies intrathoracic chest tube placement. Am J Emerg Med 2010;28:626–30.

42. Nakitende D, Gottlieb M, Ruskis J, et al. Ultrasound for confirmation of thoracostomy tube placement by emergency medicine residents. Trauma 2016;19: 35–8.

43. Jenkins JA, Gharahbaghian L, Doniger SJ, et al. Sonographic identification of tube thoracostomy study (SITTS): confirmation of intrathoracic placement. West J Emerg Med 2012;13:305–11.

44. Zhang T, Wan B, Wang L, et al. The diagnostic yield of closed needle pleural biopsy in exudative pleural effusion: a retrospective 10-year study. Ann Transl Med 2020;8:491.

45. Wei Y, Shen K, Lv T, et al. Comparison between closed pleural biopsy and medical thoracoscopy for the diagnosis of undiagnosed exudative pleural effusions: a systematic review and meta-analysis. Transl Lung Cancer Res 2020;9:446–58.

46. Botana-Rial M, Leiro-Fernandez V, Represas-Represas C, et al. Thoracic ultrasound-assisted selection for pleural biopsy with Abrams needle. Respir Care 2013;58:1949–54.

47. Lin Z, Wu D, Wang J, et al. Diagnostic value of ultrasound-guided needle biopsy in undiagnosed pleural effusions: a systematic review and meta analysis. Medicine (Baltimore) 2020;99:e21076.

48. Hallifax RJ, Corcoran JP, Ahmed A, et al. Physician-based ultrasound-guided biopsy for diagnosing pleural disease. Chest 2014;146:1001–6.

49. Zhou X, Jiang P, Huan X, et al. Ultrasound-guided versus thoracoscopic pleural biopsy for diagnosing tuberculous pleurisy following Inconclusive thoracentesis: a randomized, controlled trial. Med Sci Monit 2018;24:7238–48.

50. Koegelenberg CF, Bolliger CT, Theron J, et al. Direct comparison of the diagnostic yield of ultrasound-assisted Abrams and Tru-Cut needle biopsies for pleural tuberculosis. Thorax 2010;65:857–62.

51. Psallidas I, Kanellakis NI, Bhatnagar R, et al. A pilot feasibility study in establishing the role of ultrasound-guided pleural biopsies in pleural infection (the AUDIO study). Chest 2018;154:766–72.

Pleural Fluid Analysis
Are Light's Criteria Still Relevant After Half a Century?

José M. Porcel, MD, FCCP, FACP, FERS[a],*, Richard W. Light, MD, FCCP[b],†

KEYWORDS

- Light's criteria • Pleural effusion • Exudate • Transudate

KEY POINTS

- Light's criteria were developed to discriminate between transudative and exudative pleural effusions, but should not be used with peritoneal or pericardial fluid for which they have no value.
- Light's criteria virtually identify all exudative pleural effusions and reveal many clinically unsuspected transudative effusions.
- The limited specificity of Light's criteria (ie, misclassification of transudates as exudates) can be overcome with the examination of the serum to pleural fluid protein gradient, the serum to pleural fluid albumin gradient, or the pleural fluid levels of N-terminal pro-brain natriuretic peptide.
- Because of their accuracy and simplicity, Light's criteria are the gold standard for separating pleural transudates from exudates in routine clinical practice and are expected to continue in this role for the foreseeable future.

INTRODUCTION

Pleural effusion (PE) is a key feature for a wide range of diseases. Although there are dozens of documented causes of PE, only a few are responsible for most of the cases in clinical practice.[1] Among 5625 consecutive patients who were subjected to a diagnostic thoracentesis over the last 25 years in a university hospital in Lleida (Spain), the most common diagnoses were heart failure (HF) (28.7%), cancer (26.3%), pneumonia (15.9%), tuberculosis (6.3%), postsurgery (4.4%), pericardial diseases (3.6%), and cirrhosis (2.6%) (update from one of the author's previous reporting).[2,3]

Because the differential diagnosis of PEs is wide, a systematic investigation is necessary. In addition to an accurate history and physical examination, which should include insonation (ie, ultrasonography),[4] pleural fluid (PF) aspiration for analyses remains the cornerstone in establishing the cause of a PE. Once PF is obtained, its classification as a transudate or exudate has long been considered the first pragmatic step in pursuing a diagnosis.[5]

WHY ESTABLISHING TRANSUDATE-EXUDATE DIFFERENTIATION IS IMPORTANT?

The categorization of PEs as transudates or exudates reflects the pathophysiological process causing the effusion.[1,5] A transudate is a plasma ultrafiltrate that occurs when the systemic factors influencing the formation of PF are altered (ie, increased hydrostatic pressure, decreased oncotic pressure, decreased pressure in the pleural space, movement of transudative fluid from the peritoneal cavity, or a combination thereof). Patients with transudates have normal pleural membranes and limited diagnostic possibilities. In contrast, an exudate mainly results from the increased microvascular permeability and/or impaired lymphatic drainage that is

[a] Pleural Medicine Unit, Department of Internal Medicine, Arnau de Vilanova University Hospital, IRBLleida, University of Lleida, Lleida, Spain; [b] Division of Allergy, Pulmonary and Critical Care, Vanderbilt University, Nashville, TN, USA

† Deceased.

* Corresponding author. C/Arquitecto Florensa 2, 25196 Lleida, Spain.
E-mail address: jporcelp@yahoo.es

Clin Chest Med 42 (2021) 599–609
https://doi.org/10.1016/j.ccm.2021.07.003
0272-5231/21/© 2021 Elsevier Inc. All rights reserved.

associated with the local pleural involvement by inflammatory or tumoral conditions and has a more extensive differential diagnosis. The differentiation between transudates and exudates is of great value because certain diseases produce exudates almost exclusively, whereas others are typically associated with transudates (**Table 1**).[6] Transudates are secondary to HF in more than 80% of the cases and, less commonly, to cirrhosis (8%).[2,3] Because both entities usually improve with diuretic therapy, it has been traditionally taught that the identification of a transudate simplifies the diagnostic pathway and makes further testing unnecessary.[7] The most common causes of exudates are cancer (40%), pneumonia (24%), and tuberculosis (10%): the diagnosis of which necessarily implies additional PF, imaging, and/or tissue biopsy evaluations.[2,3]

HOW WERE TRANSUDATES AND EXUDATES IDENTIFIED BEFORE LIGHT'S CRITERIA?

At the beginning of the 20th century, PEs were usually considered for practical purposes as either clear or thick.[8,9] Clear PEs were due to heart or renal diseases, inflammatory conditions (tuberculosis, other infections), and cancer, whereas thick PEs were subdivided into hemorrhagic (trauma) and purulent fluids (pyogenic, tuberculous, and lipid PEs). Thus, at that time, the macroscopic appearance was the starting point for the differential diagnosis of PEs. Over the years, some analytical parameters of PF became more relevant for suggesting an underlying cause. In particular, a PF commenced to be classified as an exudate when the protein levels exceeded 3 g/dL or its specific gravity was more than 1016.[10] Specific gravity is the ratio of the density of a substance (eg, PF) to that of a standard substance (ie, water, which has a specific gravity of 1000). Measurement of specific gravity, currently limited to urine samples, can be performed using instruments called hydrometers and refractometers or through reagent strip methods. Digital refractometers have replaced hydrometers for clinical applications. The rationale of measuring specific gravity is that it closely correlates with the protein content. A specific gravity of 1016 on a hydrometer and 1019 on

---

Table 1
Causes of pleural transudates and exudates

Transudates	Exudates
Common causes	Common causes
Heart failure	Malignancy
Cirrhosis	Pneumonia
	Tuberculosis
	Postsurgery (cardiothoracic, abdominal)
	Acute pericarditis and postcardiac injury syndrome
Less common causes	Less common causes
Hypoalbuminemia	Trauma (hemothorax)
Nephrotic syndrome	Idiopathic
Pulmonary arterial hypertension	Pulmonary embolism
Atelectasis	Abdominal diseases (eg, pancreatitis, abscesses)
Volume overload/hypervolemia	Autoimmune rheumatic diseases
Non-expansile lung[a]	Uremic pleural effusion
Peritoneal dialysis	
Rare causes	Rare causes
Superior vena cava syndrome[a]	Esophageal perforation
Constrictive pericarditis[a]	Chylothorax[b] and cholesterol effusions
Urinothorax[a]	Gynecologic (eg, OHS, endometriosis, Meigs syndrome)
Cerebrospinal fluid leak	Drugs (eg, dasatinib)
Non-cirrhotic portal hypertension	Benign asbestos pleural effusion
Extravascular migration of CVC	Viral pleuritis
	Sarcoidosis
	Amyloidosis[b]
	Chest radiation therapy

Abbreviations: CVC, central venous catheter; OH, ovarian hyperstimulation syndrome.
[a] They may also be exudates.
[b] They may also be transudates (eg, cirrhotic chylothorax, amyloid cardiomyopathy).

a refractometer corresponds to a protein level of 3 g/dL, and each deviation of 0.003 and 0.005, respectively, represents approximately 1 g/dL of protein.[11]

In an earlier study of 32 PFs due to HF and 137 due to cancer and tuberculosis, a specific gravity of 1016 or more had only 73% sensitivity and 72% specificity for an exudate diagnosis.[12] Six decades later, another study evaluated the specific gravity of 125 PFs (about half transudative) using both refractometric and dipstick methods.[13] At the best dividing point of 1022, the respective sensitivities and specificities for identifying exudates were 92.1% and 68.1% by a refractometer and 87.3% and 58.4% by a dipstick. The technique was abandoned due to inaccurate measurements and the logic of trying to measure PF proteins directly rather than indirectly.

A pioneering study noted that the concentration of PF protein was of greater value than specific gravity: 84% of 43 PFs attributable to HF had less than 3 g/dL, whereas 92.8% of 167 PFs due to cancer and all 20 tuberculous PFs had greater than 3 g/dL.[14] As a fast-screening test for protein, urinary reagent strips have also been used for testing PF samples. Overall, 69% of PFs were correctly classified by this method in a study of 286 exudates and 97 transudates, in which the finding of 3+ proteins was seen in 78% of the former and just 6% of the latter.[15] However, the pre-analytical step of diluting PFs with normal saline (1:10) was impractical but required due to the higher protein concentrations in PFs compared with urine.

It was later suggested that the lactate dehydrogenase (LDH) activity of the PF served better than proteins and specific gravity in differentiating transudates from exudates.[16] In a study of 80 patients with PEs, of which 27 were transudative, the respective sensitivity and specificity of different parameters for identifying exudates were as follows: PF LDH greater than 550 U/L (96% and 100%), PF-to-serum LDH ratio greater than 1 (91% and 78%), protein ≥ 3 g/dL (100% and 30%), and specific gravity ≥1016 (87% and 40%).[16]

LIGHT'S CRITERIA

These previous observations led to the combining of serum and PF protein and LDH measurements into the formulation of an original rule, which has been known as Light's criteria (**Box 1**).[17] The rationale for combining the PF to serum protein ratio and the PF LDH is that the former is an indication of the pleural microvascular permeability, whereas the latter reflects the degree of pleural inflammation. The rule was derived empirically by Dr.

> **Box 1**
> **Light's criteria for the discrimination between transudates and exudates**
>
> A pleural effusion is classified as exudative if it meets one or more of the following conditions, while a transudate meets none:
>
> - A pleural fluid/serum protein ratio greater than 0.5
> - A pleural fluid/serum LDH ratio greater than 0.6
> - A pleural LDH concentration > two-thirds (67%) of the normal upper limit for serum LDH
>
> *Abbreviation:* LDH, lactate dehydrogenase.

Richard Light while he was a pulmonary fellow at Johns Hopkins Hospital. In 1971, an abstract of his preliminary findings was submitted to the American Thoracic Society Conference in Los Angeles, and it was rejected. In 1972, data were presented orally at the American College of Physicians Annual Session held in Atlantic City, and the derived original article was published the same year in the *Annals of Internal Medicine*.[17] The landmark investigation prospectively enrolled 150 patients with PEs, and it was found that the new three-part rule was able to identify 102 of 103 exudates and 46 of 47 transudates, which resulted in a sensitivity of 99%, specificity of 98%, positive likelihood ratio (LR) of 49.5, and negative LR of 0.01 for exudates.[17]

Eight years after their description, an article accepted "Light's criteria" as the standard rule for transudate–exudate differentiation,[18] while they were first referred to as such in 1989.[19] Enthusiasm for the impressive diagnostic accuracy initially attributed to Light's criteria was slightly tempered in subsequent studies, especially regarding their specificity. Nonetheless, the vast majority of clinical observations have consistently supported them as the major reference test to assist in determining the transudative or exudative nature of a PE.[20,21] In our updated series, which is by far the largest one described in literature (n = 5299), Light's criteria yield the following operating characteristics for identifying exudates: a sensitivity of 98%, specificity of 72%, accuracy of 90%, positive LR of 3.5, negative LR of 0.03, and odds ratio of 142. The markedly low LR negativity indicates that an exudative PE is virtually excluded if Light's criteria are not met. It should be highlighted that Light's criteria aim to maximize the identification of exudates to avoid the misdiagnosis of serious conditions. Even so, caution and judicious clinical reasoning is mandatory because malignant PEs may rarely meet Light's transudative criteria.[22,23]

Light's criteria are also considered the standard diagnosis in veterinary science. Studies on a small number of dogs and cats carried out by the Italian vet Dr. Andrea Zoia show that Light's criteria have discriminatory properties similar to those observed in humans (ie, nearly 100% sensitivity and 78% specificity for labeling pleural exudates).[24–26]

APPLICATION OF LIGHT'S CRITERIA TO OTHER SEROUS FLUIDS

Light's criteria have been extrapolated to the study of the pathologic accumulation of fluid in other serous cavities of the body, such as the peritoneal and the pericardial cavities, in an initial attempt to uncover etiologic factors.

The initial approach used in the differential diagnosis of ascites consisted of separating transudates caused by liver diseases from exudates found in cancer, infectious and inflammatory diseases, based on the concentration of peritoneal fluid proteins; transudates being characterized by protein levels less than 2.5 g/dL (occasionally, 3 g/dL was used as the level of discrimination).[27] However, this criterion could not separate noncirrhotic transudative sources (eg, HF, constrictive pericarditis, Budd–Chiari syndrome, inferior vena cava obstruction, sinusoidal obstruction syndrome) from exudative ones. Moreover, about 20% to 25% of patients with cirrhosis have an ascitic total protein concentration greater than 2.5 g/dL, and a similar proportion of malignant ascites have a low protein concentration.[28] The application of Light's criteria appeared to only slightly improve the accuracy of protein as the single discriminating parameter. In a study of 62 cirrhosis and 37 non-hepatic causes of ascites, they yielded a sensitivity of 81%, a specificity of 76%, a positive LR of 3.38, and a negative LR of 0.25 for labeling exudates.[29] In 1981, Hoefs[30] described for the first time a good correlation between portal vein pressure and the calculation of the serum to ascites albumin gradient. It soon became apparent that a serum-ascites albumin difference greater than 1.1 g/dL offered better discrimination of the causes of ascites because it suggested the presence of portal hypertension not only in patients with a transudate type of ascites but also in cases of high protein concentration.[31] In a large prospective series of 901 ascites samples from 330 patients, an albumin gradient greater than 1.1 g/dL accurately identified portal hypertension 96.7% of the time, whereas the ascites fluid total protein

concentration did so only 55.6% of the time.[32] At that time, the albumin gradient was adopted and still remains in scientific guidelines as the initial step strategy to grouping the cause of ascites.[33]

With regard to pericardial effusions, a couple of earlier studies suggested that the individual three items which compose Light's criteria[34] or the full criteria themselves[35] were highly sensitive (98%) in detecting exudates but lacked enough specificity (72% in the most favorable series).[35] Both studies were limited by their small sample sizes (110[35] and 175 patients,[34] of whom only 16% and 27% had transudates, respectively) and the significant proportion of "transudates" that were obtained by open pericardial aspiration during heart surgery. Indeed, the utility of differentiating between pericardial transudates and exudates has been seriously questioned. Pericardial fluids, as compared with pleural or peritoneal, have greater levels of protein and LDH,[36–38] suggesting that they are not simply an ultrafiltrate of plasma. Therefore, most "normal pericardial fluids" are classified as exudates when adopting Light's criteria.[37,39] It seems that the infrequent finding of a pericardial "transudate" would only help to reliably rule out tuberculosis.

SEPARATING PLEURAL TRANSUDATES AND EXUDATES BY CRITERIA OTHER THAN LIGHT'S

After Light's criteria description, efforts to find new tests for categorizing PEs as transudates or exudates have been continuous. However, none of the numerous alternative proposed measures have been shown to be superior to Light's criteria.

Non-analytical Criteria

It may be mistakenly thought that the gross aspect of the PF yields useful diagnostic information concerning the transudative or exudative nature of a PE. The truth is that only 11 (13%) of 82 transudates exhibited a watery appearance in one study,[40] most of which were straw colored (67%) or had a reddish color (11%). In contrast, a watery fluid is not consistent with an exudate.

Two studies have evaluated whether clinical judgment before thoracentesis (ie, knowledge of clinical history, physical examination, basic laboratory studies, and chest radiograph) compares with Light's criteria in the identification of transudates and exudates. The first study, which involved 35 consecutive patients (16 transudates and 17 exudates), found that the physician's clinical judgment was accurate in 31 (93.9%) cases (87.2% for the exudative and 100% for the transudative processes), whereas Light's criteria correctly classified 29 (87.9%) PEs (88.2% of exudates and 87.5% of transudates), with no statistically significant differences between both approaches.[19] However, in a second study of 249 patients with PEs, the accuracy of Light's criteria was significantly superior to the initial clinical presumption for separating pleural transudates from exudates (93% vs 84%, $P<.01$).[41] Of note, while Light's criteria failed to correctly classify 25% of transudates, the clinical assessment did so 57% of the time. What is certain is that PF biochemical data should always be interpreted in the patient's clinical context and, therefore, clinical judgment should necessarily complement Light's criteria results.

A few studies comprising a small number of patients (<150) have evaluated whether computed tomography (CT) attenuation values in Hounsfield units (HUs) may characterize PFs as transudates or exudates.[42–45] Most of them, but not all,[43] have found that mean attenuation values of exudates are significantly higher than those of transudates. However, optimal cutoff values differed between studies, from ≥ 5[45] to ≥ 8.5[44] or ≥ 13.4 HU,[42] and their accuracy for labeling exudates was at most moderate (sensitivities of 72%–83% and specificities of 70%–86.7%). Interestingly, the use of intravenous contrast did not significantly affect the HU values of transudates and exudates. In conclusion, because of overlapping HU values in most PEs, CT has little clinical value in the characterization of PFs, in addition to being an impractical and expensive approach.

In the era of bedside ultrasonography, many experts believe that the sonographic appearance of the PE could predict the presence of an exudate. In one early series, echogenic effusions were invariably associated with exudates.[46] However, subsequent investigations have refuted this notion. In a retrospective series, 127 transudative PEs had an anechoic pattern in 45% of the cases but a complex non-septated pattern (ie, echogenic fluid without visualized loculations) in the remaining 55%.[47] A prospective study of 140 PEs showed that echogenicity on ultrasound had a poor sensitivity (65.1%) and specificity (57.1%) at identifying exudates.[48] In the same line, a recent retrospective evaluation of 300 PEs, of which 76% were exudates, reported that an anechoic appearance could be associated with either transudative (44%) or exudative (56%) PEs.[49] However, complex septated (ie, loculations present) and complex homogeneous effusions (ie, fluid with a hyperechoic echodensity similar to tissue) carried a 96% positive predictive value for exudates.[49] Therefore, in general, the echogenic qualities of the fluid are inaccurate for categorizing PEs as transudates or exudates. Finally, the measurement of pleural thickness using a linear probe also seems to be of no help. In a small prospective study of 73 patients, a pleural thickness less than 0.2 cm had 87.5% sensitivity and 56% specificity for the diagnosis of transudates.[50]

Analytical Criteria

Light's rule has been criticized for the requirement of serum samples to calculate ratios, the inclusion of two highly correlated criteria (PF LDH and PF to serum LDH ratio), and the application of dichotomous cutoff values to continuous variables (which implies that results close to the cutoff value are treated similarly to those in the extremes). To circumvent these aspects, different formulas have been described.[51] If the taking of a serum sample is to be avoided, it should be stressed that single PF tests (eg, protein, LDH, or cholesterol in isolation) are not accurate enough (**Table 2**), but, when combined, they adequately increase the discriminative value (**Table 3**). In particular, the combination of PF LDH greater than 67% of the normal upper limit of serum LDH and PF cholesterol greater than 40 to 55 mg/dL, using an "or" rule (wherein positivity of any of these tests represents a positive result), can equal Light's criteria for the identification of exudates.[52–54] In addition, dropping the PF to serum LDH ratio from Light's criteria (abbreviated Light's criteria) does not decrease their diagnostic accuracy (see **Table 3**). However, in our experience changing the cutoff level of PF LDH to greater than 45% (rather than the traditional >67%) of a laboratory's upper limit of normal for serum LDH values (known as modified Light's criteria), as suggested by Heffner and colleagues[55] in a meta-analysis, result in a significant decrease of specificity for a meaningless increase of sensitivity (see **Table 3**).[56] Finally, Bayesian strategies that derive continuous LRs for the common biochemical tests used in transudate–exudate differentiation are unfamiliar to most clinicians, require digital supporting platforms for calculations and knowledge of pre-test probabilities, and perform very similarly to Light's criteria.[57,58]

LIMITATIONS OF TRANSUDATE–EXUDATE STUDIES

In almost all transudate–exudate studies, there are usually a number of methodological biases.[51,59] No single gold standard exists to establish the transudative or exudative origin of a PE. This differentiation is based on the subjective interpretation of clinical data by the physician, who assumes that the patient has the type of effusion

Table 2
Diagnostic accuracy for individual tests that identify pleural exudates[a]

Test	No. of Transudates/exudates	Sensitivity, % (95% CI)	Specificity, % (95% CI)	Accuracy, % (95% CI)	LR + (95% CI)	LR - (95% CI)	OR (95% CI)
P-PF >3 g/dL	1923/3666	85 (84–86)	83 (82–85)	84 (83–85)	5.1 (4.6–5.7)	0.18 (0.17–0.20)	28 (24–33)
P-R >0.5	1841/3245	87 (86–88)	86 (84–87)	87 (86–87)	6.2 (5.5–6.9)	0.15 (0.14–0.17)	41 (34–48)
LDH-PF >250 U/L[b]	1921/3638	81 (79–82)	91 (89–92)	84 (83–85)	8.7 (7.6–10.1)	0.22 (0.20–0.23)	41 (34–48)
LDH-R >0.6	1694/2809	89 (88–90)	84 (82–86)	87 (86–88)	5.5 (4.9–6.1)	0.13 (0.12–0.15)	42 (35–50)
C-PF >45 mg/dL	1417/1084	81 (79–84)	88 (86–90)	85 (84–86)	6.8 (5.9–7.8)	0.21 (0.19–0.24)	32 (26–40)
C-PF >55 mg/dL	1417/1084	67 (64–70)	94 (93–95)	82 (81–84)	11.3 (9.2–14)	0.35 (0.32–0.38)	32 (25–42)
P-G ≤3.1 g/dL	1841/3245	87 (85–88)	80 (78–82)	84 (83–85)	4.4 (4.0–4.8)	0.17 (0.15–0.18)	26 (22–30)
P-G <2.5 g/dL	1841/3245	70 (68–71)	94 (93–95)	78 (77–80)	11.9 (9.9–14.3)	0.32 (0.31–0.34)	37 (30–45)
A-G ≤1.2 g/dL	1355/705	68 (64–71)	91 (90–93)	83 (81–85)	7.6 (6.4–9.1)	0.36 (0.32–0.40)	22 (17–28)

Abbreviations: A-G, pleural fluid to serum albumin gradient; CI, confidence interval; C-PF, pleural fluid cholesterol; LDH-PF, pleural fluid lactate dehydrogenase; LDH-R, pleural fluid to serum LDH ratio; LR +, likelihood ratio positive; LR -, likelihood ratio negative; OR, odds ratio; P-G, pleural fluid to serum protein gradient; PF, pleural fluid; P-PF, pleural fluid protein; P-R, pleural fluid to serum protein ratio.

[a] This is an update from one of the author's previous series (Refs. 2 and 3). Note that LR positive ≥3, LR negative ≤0.3, and OR ≥50 represent tests with good discriminative properties.

[b] This cutoff value represents two-thirds the upper limit of normal for serum LDH in our laboratory.

Table 3
Diagnostic accuracy for test combinations that identify pleural exudates[a]

Test[b]	No. of Transudates/exudates	Sensitivity, % (95% CI)	Specificity, % (95% CI)	Accuracy, % (95% CI)	LR + (95% CI)	LR −(95% CI)	OR (95% CI)
P-PF or LDH-PF	1921/3660	96 (95–97)	78 (76–80)	90 (89–91)	4.3 (4.0–4.7)	0.05 (0.04–0.06)	85 (70–103)
P-R or LDH-PF[c]	1845/3609	97 (96–97)	80 (78–81)	91 (90–92)	4.7 (4.3–5.2)	0.04 (0.04–0.05)	110 (89–136)
P-R or LDH-R[c]	1696/3226	97 (96–97)	76 (74–78)	89 (88–90)	4.0 (3.6–4.3)	0.05 (0.04–0.06)	86 (69–106)
LHD-PF or C-PF >55 mg/dL	1443/3183	97 (96–98)	84 (82–85)	93 (92–94)	5.9 (5.3–6.7)	0.04 (0.03–0.04)	168 (131–215)
LDH-PF >170 U/L or C-PF >45 mg/dL	1539/3497	99 (99–100)	54 (51–56)	85 (84–86)	2.2 (2.0–2.3)	0.01 (0.01–0.02)	193 (124–300)
P-PF or LDH-PF or C-PF >55 mg/dL	1516/3567	99 (98–99)	71 (69–73)	91 (90–91)	3.4 (3.2–3.7)	0.02 (0.01–0.02)	208 (150–287)
P-PF or LDH-PF >170 U/L or C-PF >45 mg/dL	1580/3615	100 (99–100)	50 (48–53)	85 (84–85)	2.0 (1.9–2.1)	0.008 (0.005–0.014)	241 (144–403)
P-R or LDH-R or LDH-PF >170 U/L[d]	1749/3638	99 (99–99)	56 (53–58)	85 (84–86)	2.2 (2.1–2.4)	0.02 (0.01–0.03)	114 (82–157)
Light's criteria (P-R or LDH-R or LDH-PF)	1706/3593	98 (98–99)	72 (70–74)	90 (89–91)	3.5 (3.3–3.8)	0.03 (0.02–0.03)	142 (109–186)

Abbreviations: A-G, pleural fluid to serum albumin gradient; CI, confidence interval; C-PF, pleural fluid cholesterol; LDH-PF, pleural fluid lactate dehydrogenase; LDH-R, pleural fluid to serum LDH ratio; LR +, likelihood ratio positive; LR −, likelihood ratio negative; OR, odds ratio; P-G, pleural fluid to serum protein gradient; PF, pleural fluid; P-PF, pleural fluid protein; P-R, pleural fluid to serum protein ratio.

[a] This is an update from one of the author's previous series (Refs. 2 and 3). Note that LR positive ≥3, LR negative ≤0.3, and OR ≥50 represent tests with good discriminative properties.

[b] With the use of cutoff values from the individual tests in **Table 3**, unless otherwise indicated.

[c] Also known as "abbreviated Light's criteria".

[d] Also known as "modified Light's criteria", whereby LDH-PF cutoff is set at greater than 45% of a laboratory's upper limit of normal for serum LDH values (ie, 170 U/L in our laboratory).

(transudate or exudate) which is typically associated with the underlying disease. In this clinical assessment, PF analyses are also integrated for achieving a final diagnosis (incorporation bias). More importantly, it should be recognized that more than one disease may potentially be responsible for a PE. For example, a prospective case series of 126 patients with unilateral PEs identified multiple etiologies underlying the accumulation of PF in 30% of the cases.[60] Transudate–exudate studies generally exclude patients with dual or uncertain causes of PEs (selection bias). For instance, the original study by Light and colleagues[17] excluded 18% of the initially recruited patients from the analysis because the precise cause of their PEs could not be determined. Similarly, about 14% of 982 PF samples had to be dismissed from a transudate–exudate study due to the coexistence of two or more disease processes that could explain the PF formation.[61] Both incorporation and selection biases may inflate the diagnostic properties of any test undergoing evaluation.

To add more complexity, some conditions may cause either a transudate or an exudate (eg, non-expansile lungs, chylothorax, urinothorax, superior vena cava syndrome, amyloidosis).[5,6] Notably, although previously thought to be transudates on occasion, PEs due to pulmonary embolism are invariably exudates when Light's criteria are used as the reference standard.[62] Moreover, some patients with bilateral PEs may have the so-called Contarini's syndrome, which is defined by the existence of a different cause of the PF for each side (eg, an exudative infectious PE on one side may trigger HF, which in turn produces a contralateral transudate).[63]

IMPROVING THE SPECIFICITY OF LIGHT'S CRITERIA

Light's criteria combine tests using an "either-or" rule in an attempt to maximize sensitivity for the identification of exudates, which invariably has an effect on decreasing specificity (ie, some transudates are misclassified as exudates). The positive LR of Light's criteria to diagnose exudates decreases in the presence of the so-called discordant exudates (ie, only the protein ratio [protein discordant] or the PF LDH [LDH discordant] are consistent with an exudate). In particular, a protein discordant exudate increases the risk of a false-positive exudate.[61] Overall, Light's criteria misclassify about 25% to 30% of transudates as exudates,[5,6] usually by a small margin (eg, median protein ratio of 0.51 and median LDH ratio of 0.63 in a series of 107 misclassified HF-related

effusions).[64] This miscategorization is especially frequent in patients who have received diuretic treatment or have bloody PFs (>10,000 erythrocytes/μL, which occurs in about 15% of transudates).[51,65] While diuresis remove more water than solutes (protein and LDH) from the pleural space, erythrocytes might raise pleural LDH levels.[65]

To address the decreased specificity of Light's criteria, it has been recommended that the gradient between the serum and the PF albumin levels (albumin gradient), the protein gradient or, in suspected misclassified PEs of cardiac origin, the PF levels of natriuretic peptides be examined.[51] When Light's criteria return results near cutoff points for exudate but the clinical probability of HF, cirrhosis, or other causes of transudate is at least moderate, an albumin gradient greater than 1.2 g/dL or a protein gradient exceeding 3.1 g/dL points to a true transudate.[51] The test which should be chosen is a matter of personal preference. However, we advocate that the protein gradient first be examined because it is already available from Light's criteria. The only caveat to bear in mind is that the threshold for the protein gradient is better when set at 2.5 mg/dL.[66] In a retrospective series of 276 HF-related PEs which met Light's exudative criteria, a serum PF protein gradient greater than 3.1 g/dL identified 46% correctly, a protein gradient greater than 2.5 g/dL identified 79% correctly, and an albumin gradient greater than 1.2 g/dL identified 78% correctly.[66] The same study suggested a scoring model to assist clinicians in accurately identifying false cardiac exudates, which consisted of age $\geq$75 years (3 points), albumin gradient greater than 1.2 g/dL (3 points), PF LDH less than 250 U/L (representing two-thirds of the laboratory's upper limit of normal for serum LDH; 2 points), bilateral effusions on chest radiograph (2 points), and protein gradient greater than 2.5 g/dL (1 point). At the best cutoff of $\geq$7 points, this scoring system yielded 92% diagnostic accuracy, a positive LR of 12.7, and a negative LR of 0.39 for labeling "false cardiac exudates".[66]

When PF meets the criteria for an exudative effusion by only a small margin and the clinical picture is consistent with HF, one can presume that the fluid is actually a transudate if high levels of the N-terminal pro-brain natriuretic peptide (NT-proBNP) are demonstrated, either in the PF or blood.[67] In a meta-analysis of 12 studies that included 599 PEs due to HF and 1055 non-cardiac PEs, NT-proBNP levels in PF had a sensitivity of 94%, a specificity of 91%, a positive LR of 10.9, and a negative LR of 0.07 in identifying PEs with a cardiac origin.[68] Respective figures for blood NT-proBNP extracted from 4 studies were 92%, 88%, 7.8, and 0.10.[68] The most widely used cutoff point is 1500 pg/mL,[69,70] though with the advent of more sensitive new generation tests this threshold needs to be reevaluated. NT-proBNP is a more useful biomarker of HF than BNP when measured in PF,[70] but it has similar discriminating capabilities as midregion pro-atrial natriuretic peptide.[71] In addition, NT-proBNP concentrations allow clinicians to correctly identify greater than 80% of those cardiac PEs misclassified as exudates by Light's criteria.[70] Furthermore, natriuretic peptides are optimal for differentiating between cardiac and hepatic transudates, as the pathophysiological mechanisms underlying PF formation differ in the two processes. Detection of elevated PF levels of NT-proBNP in patients with established non-cardiac causes of PE (eg, pneumonia, cancer, pericardial disease) is currently a frequent situation which may reflect some degree of underlying decompensated cardiac disease contributing partially to PF development.

WHY LIGHT'S CRITERIA HAVE STOOD THE TEST OF TIME

There are several reasons that explain the durability of Light's criteria among the most acclaimed clinical rules during the last half century.[72] First, they are simple and easy to remember. Second, they make use of readily accessible PF and serum parameters. Third, they are 90% accurate, which implies that demonstrating the superiority of any new alternative criteria over Light's criteria would require a sample size of greater than 9100 patients (α 0.05, β 0.1, margin of error/precision 0.01). Finally, highly specific biomarkers for the full spectrum of diseases that may produce PEs are either lacking or in development.[73,74] In the meantime, Light's criteria represent an important milepost in our diagnostic approach to PEs.

SUMMARY

Fifty years from their initial description, Light's criteria are still unhesitatingly accepted as the default reference test for separating pleural transudates and exudates. Efforts should be focused not so much on trying to find an even more reliable technique for categorizing PEs but on improving the misclassification rate of transudates that characterize Light's criteria. Despite their shortcomings, Light's criteria may well continue their reign for another 50 years. Long live the Light's criteria!

DISCLOSURE

The authors have nothing to disclose.

REFERENCES

1. Porcel JM, Light RW. Diagnostic approach to pleural effusion in adults. Am Fam Physician 2006;73(7): 1211–20.
2. Porcel JM. Pearls and myths in pleural fluid analysis. Respirology 2011;16(1):44–52.
3. Porcel JM, Esquerda A, Vives M, et al. Etiology of pleural effusions: analysis of more than 3,000 consecutive thoracenteses. Arch Bronconeumol 2014;50(5):161–5.
4. Porcel JM. Time to embrace POCUS as part of the bedside diagnosis of respiratory diseases. Respirology 2020;25(5):466–7.
5. Porcel JM, Light RW. Pleural effusions. Dis Mon 2013;59(2):29–57.
6. Porcel JM. Pleural fluid biochemistry: a first step towards an etiological diagnosis of pleural effusions. Span J Med 2021. https://doi.org/10.24875/SJMED. 21000006.
7. Peterman TA, Speicher CE. Evaluating pleural effusions. A two-stage laboratory approach. JAMA 1984;252(8):1051–3.
8. Dickson WA. Pleural effusions in general practice. Br Med J 1930;2(3650):1036–52.
9. Burrell LS. Pleural effusion. Br Med J 1931;1(3666): 619–21.
10. Carr DT, Soule EH, Ellis FH Jr. Management of pleural effusions. Med Clin North Am 1964;48:961–75.
11. Light RW. Falsely high refractometric readings for the specific gravity of pleural fluid. Chest 1979; 76(3):300–1.
12. Leaullen EC, Carr DT. Pleural effusion. A statistical study of 436 patients. N Engl J Med 1955;252(3): 79–83.
13. Abdollahi A, Nozarian Z. Diagnostic value of measurement specific gravity by refractometric and dipstick method in differentiation between transudate and exudate in pleural and peritoneal fluid. Iran J Pathol 2016;11(4):363–9.
14. Carr DT, Power MH. Clinical value of measurements of concentrations of protein in pleural fluid. N Engl J Med 1958;259(19):926–7.
15. Burgess LJ, Taljaard JJ, Maritz FJ. A rapid screening test for pleural exudates. S Afr Med J 1999;89(1):14.
16. Chandrasekhar AJ, Palatao A, Dubin A, et al. Pleural fluid lactic acid dehydrogenase activity and protein content. Value in diagnosis. Arch Intern Med 1969; 123(1):48–50.
17. Light RW, Macgregor MI, Luchsinger PC, et al. Pleural effusions: the diagnostic separation of transudates and exudates. Ann Intern Med 1972;77(4): 507–13.

18. Good JT Jr, Taryle DA, Maulitz RM, et al. The diagnostic value of pleural fluid pH. Chest 1980;78(1): 55–9.

19. Scheurich JW, Keuer SP, Graham DY. Pleural effusion: comparison of clinical judgment and Light's criteria in determining the cause. South Med J 1989;82(12):1487–91.

20. Vives M, Porcel JM, Vicente de Vera M, et al. A study of Light's criteria and possible modifications for distinguishing exudative from transudative pleural effusions. Chest 1996;109(6):1503–7.

21. Gázquez I, Porcel JM, Vives M, et al. Comparative analysis of Light's criteria and other biochemical parameters for distinguishing transudates from exudates. Respir Med 1998;92(5):762–5.

22. Porcel JM, Alvarez M, Salud A, et al. Should a cytologic study be ordered in transudative pleural effusions? Chest 1999;116(6):1836–7.

23. Ferreiro L, Gude F, Toubes ME, et al. Predictive models of malignant transudative pleural effusions. J Thorac Dis 2017;9(1):106–16.

24. Zoia A, Slater LA, Heller J, et al. A new approach to pleural effusion in cats: markers for distinguishing transudates from exudates. J Feline Med Surg 2009;11(10):847–55.

25. Zoia A, Drigo M. Diagnostic value of Light's criteria and albumin gradient in classifying the pathophysiology of pleural effusion formation in cats. J Feline Med Surg 2016;18(8):666–72.

26. Zoia A, Petini M, Righetti D, et al. Discriminating transudates and exudates in dogs with pleural effusion: diagnostic utility of simplified Light's criteria compared with traditional veterinary classification. Vet Rec 2020;187(1):e5.

27. Huang LL, Xia HH, Zhu SL. Ascitic fluid analysis in the differential diagnosis of ascites: focus on cirrhotic ascites. J Clin Transl Hepatol 2014;2(1): 58–64.

28. Paré P, Talbot J, Hoefs JC. Serum-ascites albumin concentration gradient: a physiologic approach to the differential diagnosis of ascites. Gastroenterology 1983;85(2):240–4.

29. Boyer TD, Kahn AM, Reynolds TB. Diagnostic value of ascitic fluid lactic dehydrogenase, protein, and WBC levels. Arch Intern Med 1978;138(7):1103–5.

30. Hoefs JC. Increase in ascites white blood cell and protein concentrations during diuresis in patients with chronic liver disease. Hepatology 1981;1(3): 249–54.

31. Rector WG Jr, Reynolds TB. Superiority of the serum-ascites albumin difference over the ascites total protein concentration in separation of "transudative" and "exudative" ascites. Am J Med 1984; 77(1):83–5.

32. Runyon BA, Montano AA, Akriviadis EA, et al. The serum-ascites albumin gradient is superior to the exudate-transudate concept in the differential diagnosis of ascites. Ann Intern Med 1992;117(3):215–20.

33. Aithal GP, Palaniyappan N, China L, et al. Guidelines on the management of ascites in cirrhosis. Gut 2021; 70(1):9–29.

34. Meyers DG, Meyers RE, Prendergast TW. The usefulness of diagnostic tests on pericardial fluid. Chest 1997;111(5):1213–21.

35. Burgess LJ, Reuter H, Taljaard JJ, et al. Role of biochemical tests in the diagnosis of large pericardial effusions. Chest 2002;121(2):495–9.

36. Akyuz S, Arugaslan E, Zengin A, et al. Differentiation between transudate and exudate in pericardial effusion has almost no diagnostic value in contemporary medicine. Clin Lab 2015;61(8):957–63.

37. Imazio M, Biondo A, Ricci D, et al. Contemporary biochemical analysis of normal pericardial fluid. Heart 2020;106(7):541–4.

38. Buoro S, Tombetti E, Ceriotti F, et al. What is the normal composition of pericardial fluid? Heart 2020. https://doi.org/10.1136/heartjnl-2020-317966. heartjnl-2020-317966.

39. Ben-Horin S, Bank I, Shinfeld A, et al. Diagnostic value of the biochemical composition of pericardial effusions in patients undergoing pericardiocentesis. Am J Cardiol 2007;99(9):1294–7.

40. Villena V, López-Encuentra A, García-Luján R, et al. Clinical implications of appearance of pleural fluid at thoracentesis. Chest 2004;125(1):156–9.

41. Romero-Candeira S, Hernández L, Romero-Brufao S, et al. Is it meaningful to use biochemical parameters to discriminate between transudative and exudative pleural effusions? Chest 2002; 122(5):1524–9.

42. Nandalur KR, Hardie AH, Bollampally SR, et al. Accuracy of computed tomography attenuation values in the characterization of pleural fluid: an ROC study. Acad Radiol 2005;12(8):987–91.

43. Abramowitz Y, Simanovsky N, Goldstein MS, et al. Pleural effusion: characterization with CT attenuation values and CT appearance. AJR Am J Roentgenol 2009;192(3):618–23.

44. Çullu N, Kalemci S, Karakaş Ö, et al. Efficacy of CT in diagnosis of transudates and exudates in patients with pleural effusion. Diagn Interv Radiol 2014;20(2): 116–20.

45. Yalçin-Şafak K, Umarusman-Tanju N, Ayyıldız M, et al. Efficacy of computed tomography (CT) attenuation values and CT findings in the differentiation of pleural effusion. Pol J Radiol 2017;82:100–5.

46. Yang PC, Luh KT, Chang DB, et al. Value of sonography in determining the nature of pleural effusion: analysis of 320 cases. AJR Am J Roentgenol 1992; 159(1):29–33.

47. Chen HJ, Tu CY, Ling SJ, et al. Sonographic appearances in transudative pleural effusions: not always

an anechoic pattern. Ultrasound Med Biol 2008; 34(3):362–9.

48. Asciak R, Hassan M, Mercer RM, et al. Prospective analysis of the predictive value of sonographic pleural fluid echogenicity for the diagnosis of exudative effusion. Respiration 2019;97(5):451–6.

49. Shkolnik B, Judson MA, Austin A, et al. Diagnostic accuracy of thoracic ultrasonography to differentiate transudative from exudative pleural effusion. Chest 2020;158(2):692–7.

50. Doğan C, Demirer E. Efficacy of ultrasonography in the diagnosis of transudative pleural fluids. J Bronchology Interv Pulmonol 2021;28(2):143–9.

51. Porcel JM. Identifying transudates misclassified by Light's criteria. Curr Opin Pulm Med 2013;19(4): 362–7.

52. Porcel JM, Vives M, Vicente de Vera MC, et al. Useful tests on pleural fluid that distinguish transudates from exudates. Ann Clin Biochem 2001;38(Pt 6): 671–5.

53. Wilcox ME, Chong CA, Stanbrook MB, et al. Does this patient have an exudative pleural effusion? The Rational Clinical Examination systematic review. JAMA 2014;311(23):2422–31.

54. Lépine PA, Thomas R, Nguyen S, et al. Simplified criteria using pleural fluid cholesterol and lactate dehydrogenase to distinguish between exudative and transudative pleural effusions. Respiration 2019; 98(1):48–54.

55. Heffner JE, Brown LK, Barbieri CA. Diagnostic value of tests that discriminate between exudative and transudative pleural effusions. Chest 1997;111(4): 970–80.

56. Porcel JM, Vives M. Classic, abbreviated, and modified Light's criteria: the end of the story? Chest 1999; 116(6):1833–6.

57. Heffner JE, Highland K, Brown LK. A meta-analysis derivation of continuous likelihood ratios for diagnosing pleural fluid exudates. Am J Respir Crit Care Med 2003;167(12):1591–9.

58. Porcel JM, Peña JM, Vicente de Vera C, et al. Bayesian analysis using continuous likelihood ratios for identifying pleural exudates. Respir Med 2006; 100(11):1960–5.

59. Heffner JE. Evaluating diagnostic tests in the pleural space. Differentiating transudates from exudates as a model. Clin Chest Med 1998;19(2):277–93.

60. Bintcliffe OJ, Hooper CE, Rider IJ, et al. Unilateral pleural effusions with more than one apparent etiology. A prospective observational study. Ann Am Thorac Soc 2016;13(7):1050–6.

61. Ferreiro L, Sánchez-Sánchez R, Valdés L, et al. Concordant and discordant exudates and their

effect on the accuracy of Light's criteria to diagnose exudative pleural effusions. Am J Med Sci 2016; 352(6):549–56.

62. Porcel JM, Esquerda A, Porcel L, et al. Is pulmonary embolism associated with pleural transudates, exudates, or both? Span J Med 2021;1(1):21–5.

63. Porcel JM, Civit MC, Bielsa S, et al. Contarini's syndrome: bilateral pleural effusion, each side from different causes. J Hosp Med 2012;7(2):164–5.

64. Bielsa S, Porcel JM, Castellote J, et al. Solving the Light's criteria misclassification rate of cardiac and hepatic transudates. Respirology 2012;17(4):721–6.

65. Porcel JM, Esquerda A, Martínez M, et al. Influence of pleural fluid red blood cell count on the misidentification of transudates. Med Clin (Barc) 2008; 131(20):770–2.

66. Porcel JM, Ferreiro L, Civit C, et al. Development and validation of a scoring system for the identification of pleural exudates of cardiac origin. Eur J Intern Med 2018;50:60–4.

67. Porcel JM. Utilization of B-type natriuretic peptide and NT-proBNP in the diagnosis of pleural effusions due to heart failure. Curr Opin Pulm Med 2011;17(4): 215–9.

68. Han ZJ, Wu XD, Cheng JJ, et al. Diagnostic accuracy of natriuretic peptides for heart failure in patients with pleural effusion: a systematic review and updated meta-analysis. PLoS One 2015;10(8): e0134376.

69. Porcel JM, Vives M, Cao G, et al. Measurement of pro-brain natriuretic peptide in pleural fluid for the diagnosis of pleural effusions due to heart failure. Am J Med 2004;116(6):417–20.

70. Porcel JM, Martínez-Alonso M, Cao G, et al. Biomarkers of heart failure in pleural fluid. Chest 2009; 136(3):671–7.

71. Porcel JM, Bielsa S, Morales-Rull JL, et al. Comparison of pleural N-terminal pro-B-type natriuretic peptide, midregion pro-atrial natriuretic peptide and mid-region pro-adrenomedullin for the diagnosis of pleural effusions associated with cardiac failure. Respirology 2013;18(3):540–5.

72. Light RW. The Light criteria: the beginning and why they are useful 40 years later. Clin Chest Med 2013; 34(1):21–6.

73. Porcel JM. Biomarkers in the diagnosis of pleural diseases: a 2018 update. Ther Adv Respir Dis 2018;12. 1753466618808660.

74. Mercer RM, Corcoran JP, Porcel JM, et al. Interpreting pleural fluid results. Clin Med (Lond) 2019;19(3): 213–7.

Setting up a Pleural Disease Service

Helen McDill, MBBS, BSc[a],*, Nick Maskell, MD[a,b]

KEYWORDS

- Pleural • Service • Team • Effusion • Management

KEY POINTS

- Pleural disease is becoming more frequent and complex requiring specialist management.
- A pleural unit requires an MDT approach with different specialties closely working together to deliver a cohesive care.
- Although there are challenges, using local resources and adapting as needed and promoting the development of new ideas, most hospitals should be able to deliver a specialized pleural disease service.

INTRODUCTION—THE NEED FOR A SPECIALIST PLEURAL SERVICE

Diagnosing and managing pleural disease can be complex and challenging. Pleural effusions are common with an estimated 1.5 million new pleural effusions identified every year in the United States[1] and complex with more than 60 known conditions affecting the pleura.[2] The burden of pleural disease is growing with approximately 15% of all patients diagnosed with malignancy developing a malignant pleural effusion (MPE).[3] The estimated annual incidence in the United States is greater than 150,000 cases[3] with evidence cancer incidence and prevalence is globally increasing.[4] There is also evidence pleural infection is increasing with one specific North American study estimating the incidence is rising on average 2.8% per year[5] and a subsequent further study in Utah confirming a 2 to 3 fold increase in incidence.[6] Given the increasing complexity and incidence of pleural disease, there is a growing view that dedicated pleural services will improve the standard of care and reduce the length of stay by providing more ambulatory services.[7–10]

Alongside our growing understanding of pleural pathology, there have also been significant advances in both diagnostic and therapeutic options. Pulmonologists' procedural skills are ever-expanding and frequently include IPC (indwelling pleural catheter) insertion, pleuroscopy and image-guided pleural biopsies. Hence the development of the "interventional pulmonologist." The widespread use of thoracic ultrasound (TUS) has made procedures safer,[11–13] the detection of small volume effusions easier[9] but also allows US-guided procedures and image-guided biopsies to be performed as out-patients, allowing for ambulatory and individualized care.[14] Few general pulmonologists will be competent in all these procedures, leading to the setting up of specialist pleural services to allow greater patient access to these skills.[7–10] These services lend themselves to robust training for doctors and other health care professionals. This is a vital part of the service to help minimize the risks of iatrogenic injury.[11–13,15]

The increasing complexity and frequency of pleural disease and the increasing use of TUS for procedural safety and to guide diagnostic management, as well as the increasing repertoire of procedures, mean a dedicated specialist pleural service is essential to provide optimal and timely pleural care.

Funding: The article was not funded.
[a] Bristol Academic Respiratory Unit, North Bristol NHS Trust, England; [b] University of Bristol, Bristol, England
* Corresponding author.
E-mail address: h.mcdill@nhs.net

chestmed.theclinics.com

Optimizing the Current Pleural Pathway

Traditionally, any patient with any type of pleural collection resulted in hospital admission for intercostal drainage, with a prolonged admission for those with MPE requiring histologic confirmation and longer for those with pleural infection or those with persistent air leaks.[8] The resultant hospital inpatient stay was both inconvenient and costly for patients. Driven by this there has been a move toward ambulatory pathways provided by a specialist pleural service with increasing use of IPC's, Heimlich valves, day case pleuroscopy, and ambulatory TUS and cutting needle pleural biopsies.[16,17]

Emergency admission for pleural effusions are now seen as a marker of an inefficient health care[10] and for most patients, excluding pleural infection, outpatient management is possible[11] and has shown to be effective, cost-effective, and preferred by patients.[16,18]

By providing early specialist pleural care, the aim is to minimize the number of procedures performed, avoid unnecessary hospital admissions and limit the time spent at hospital whilst allowing both ambulatory therapeutic and diagnostic management, which has additional cost benefits.[7] However, patients on these ambulatory pathways, especially with "devices in situ" may require high levels of support from rapid access pleural clinics, phone and home visit support from specialist nurses, and community teams.[8,10]

Skills and Procedures Within the Pleural Pathway

The population referred, referral pathways in your area, the skillset of your team, and access to other services (interventional radiology, thoracic surgery) will determine the number and type of pleural procedures performed. Ideally, all pleural services should be able to perform TUS, pleural aspiration and intercostal drainage, IPC insertion, ultrasound-guided image biopsies, and pleuroscopy. They also require good access to thoracic surgery and interventional radiology.[10,11,17]

Thoracic Ultrasound

Over the past 2 decades, TUS has become a vital tool in the diagnosis and management of pleural disease. Studies have shown that the rate of complications can be significantly reduced by the introduction of point-of-care ultrasound for all pleural procedures.[12,13,18,19] It is incorporated into international guidelines in the United Kingdom and United States and is the standard of care for drainage of pleural fluid.[20,21] More advanced techniques can be used with TUS including real-time guidance of any pleural intervention (aspiration or biopsy) and identification of the intercostal vessels before intervention minimizing the likelihood of vascular injury and the ability to identify iatrogenic complications including bleeding from the parietal pleura or the rapid collection of highly echogenic fluid in the pleural space.[14,22–24]

TUS is the pivotal tool for pulmonologists in the management of pleural effusions, not only it is more sensitive than a chest radiograph for the diagnosis,[25] it also provides much more information about the size, depth, pleural thickening, septations and complexity of the effusion, and diaphragm movement and helps assess an underlying cause. Various studies have demonstrated the sensitivity and specificity of TUS to diagnosis malignant pleural disease in the presence of pleural or diaphragmatic nodules, pleural thickening >1 cm, and echogenic swirling sign[26,27] (**Fig. 1**).

TUS also plays an important part in pleural infection. Complex parapneumonic effusions are often septated and loculated[28] and TUS is superior at diagnosing septations compared with computerized tomography (CT).[29] TUS can be used in pneumothorax but is not routine practice. Pneumothorax shows loss of lung sliding in B-Mode[30] and M-Mode shows the classical pattern of horizontal lines above the pleural line and granular pattern below the pleural line (seashore pattern). Care must be taken interpreting these features as they can also be mimicked by severe emphysema or pleurodesis.[31]

Thoracocentesis

In 2008, the National Patient Safety Agency (NPSA) produced a report in the United Kingdom that highlighted increased harm when performing non–ultrasound-guided pleural procedures.[15] This report recommended that TUS should be used for all pleural procedures. Multiple further papers have reinforced the conclusions of the NPSA report. A study of 67 patients, prospectively identified site of puncture either using clinical decision making alone or TUS, showed 15% of the sites identified without TUS were "inaccurate" and likely to cause organ damage.[32] Other studies have shown a significantly lower rate of pneumothorax when TUS is used.[33]

TUS can either guide the marking of a safe site at which a pleural procedure is performed or can be used to guide procedures real-time where the needle is visualized throughout. Realtime TUS guidance is advised for a select group including pleural biopsies, small or complex effusions, and

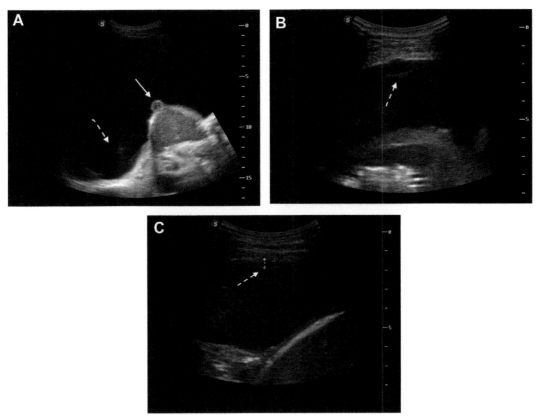

Fig. 1. TUS images demonstrating features that help predict the sensitivity of malignant pleural disease. (*A*) TUS demonstrating MPE with echogenic fluid (*dashed arrow*) and metastatic diaphragmatic nodule (*solid arrow*). (*B*) TUS demonstrating MPE with frank pleural nodularity (*dashed arrow*). (*C*) TUS demonstrating pleural thickening (*dashed arrow*). (*Courtesy of* Dr Maged Hassan, Alexandria University Faculty of Medicine, Egypt.)

pneumothorax-induced pleuroscopy.[31] Realtime TUS requires a greater level of skill and experience and this has been reflected in the United Kingdom training curriculum recently.[11,34]

Pleuroscopy/Local Anesthetic Thoracoscopy

Day-case pleuroscopy can be performed in the vast majority of patients and is widely performed and provides utility where patients are too frail for a VATS or timely access to thoracic surgery cannot be accessed.[35,36] It allows the interventionist to gain biopsies under direct vision, leading to a sensitivity greater than 90% in malignancy and therapeutic management of pleural fluid at the same time via drainage and possible IPC insertion and/or talc poudrage.[37]

Prethoracoscopic TUS helps the operator choose the optimal entry site to the pleural cavity and can help plan the procedure according to pleural adhesions seen on TUS.[31] In the presence of no pleural effusion, TUS can identify pleural adhesions that may complicate entry and reduced the size of pleural cavity in the case of tethered

lung by identifying the absence of sliding visceral pleura.[38] If a pneumothorax is induced with a Boutin needle, real-time TUS guides the initial pleural puncture.[31]

Image-Guided Pleural Biopsies

The gold standard test for diagnosing the etiologies of pleural effusions is pleuroscopy, but in some cases, the patients may not be fit enough to undergo this or it may not be feasible due to lung tethering or adhesions.[39] In these circumstances, real-time TUS guidance is particularly helpful for performing percutaneous biopsies of the parietal pleura.[31] The optimal site is where there is a pleural mass or thickening but biopsies can also be obtained from normal-looking pleura. Visceral organs and intercostal vessels should ideally be identified on TUS and avoided.[31] The most common needle used is a core cutting needle depending on operator familiarity and experience. After creating a small incision in the skin, the needle is advanced at a shallow angle under real-time. Once the pleural thickening is reached, the cutting portion of the needle is advanced to include the parietal pleura and the adjacent chest wall structures.[40] It is suggested taking 8 to 10 core biopsies, potentially across 2 different sites, is advisable to ensure sufficient tissue for diagnosis and molecular profiling.[41] **Fig. 2**.

Core-cutting biopsy needles have good diagnostic yield, which is similar whether CT or TUS is used.[42] The reported sensitivity of pleural biopsies with this type of needle ranges 70% to 90%.[42,43] Traditionally, image-guided biopsies have been performed by radiologists, but in the United Kingdom, owing to the widespread use of point-of-care TUS, many specialist pleural centers are now able to offer TUS-guided pleural biopsies as day cases. These are performed by physicians and can reduce the load on radiologists with improved diagnostic pathway times whilst maintaining diagnostic accuracy.[39,44,45]

One advance of pulmonologists becoming competent in TUS-guided biopsies is the option of performing a combination pleural aspiration and biopsy at their first out-patient appointment becomes achievable in a "one-stop shop" pleural clinic.[40] It has been shown combination in these procedures with TUS evidence of pleural thickening improves diagnostic sensitivity from 38% to 83% in comparison with aspiration alone, and in patients eventually diagnosed with malignancy from 30% to 90%.[46] However, we have to bear in mind whilst this approach has the benefit to streamline outpatient pathways and waiting times with a cost reduction, it does not offer definitive management of MPE and the diagnostic yield is not as high as that obtained with pleuroscopy.[40,41]

Outside of malignancy, a pilot study has shown in bacterial infection, cultures of pleural biopsies performed under TUS at the time of chest tube insertion lead to an improvement of microbiological yield by 25% in comparison to standard plain and blood culture bottle pleural fluid cultures alone.[47]

The Modern Diagnostic Pleural Pathway

For patients with possible thoracic malignancy, health care models are increasingly using rapid access clinics; patients presenting with nonacute dyspnea, chest pain, or a pleural effusion on a chest radiograph via these pathways will often go on have undergone a contrast-enhanced CT before referral to a specialist pleural clinic particularly in the United Kingdom as part of the NOLCP (National Optimal Lung cancer pathway). When assessing patients in a dedicated pleural clinic, TUS in experienced hands will often detect abnormalities increasing the preintervention likelihood of

malignancy. Given the low overall diagnostic yield of malignancy from pleural fluid cytology, as shown in **Fig. 3**,[48] it may be appropriate to consider a combined pleural aspiration and pleural biopsy to increase diagnostic yield as part of rapid diagnostic pathway.[40] Some pleural centers are now bypassing cytology and going straight to pleuroscopy, when there is a high clinical possibility of mesothelioma, due to low cytology yields.[48,49]

IPC (Indwelling Pleural Catheter) and Out-Patient Pleurodesis

Over the last 2 decades, IPCs have revolutionized the management of MPE. Previously, management was confirmed to inpatient approaches such as talc pleurodesis via chest tube. However, 2 large randomized control trials (RCTs), TIME2 (Second Therapeutic Intervention in Malignant Effusion) and AMPLE (Australasian Malignant Pleural Effusion), reported the suitability of IPCs as a first-line therapeutic approach for MPE.[50,51] IPCs can be inserted as a day case in theatre or a procedural suite and are associated with significantly shorter hospital stays compared with chest drain and talc pleurodesis, improved patient-reported dyspnea and the reduction in further pleural procedures. However, their successful use is dependent on adequate community follow-up and support. Rates of non-serious complications are high in most IPC studies and a dedicated pleural team is required to educate patients and carers, support community teams, and provide regular and ad-hoc advice.[52]

IPC management can be optimized in expansile lung to try and achieve pleurodesis and IPC removal in an out-patient setting. ASAP (Randomized Trial of Pleural Fluid Drainage Frequency in Patients with Malignant Pleural Effusions) and AMPLE-2 (Aggressive vs symptom-guided drainage of malignant pleural effusion via indwelling pleural catheters) studies looked at conditions leading to quicker autopleurodesis.[53,54] Aggressive or daily drainage in both studies increased autopleurodesis (24% to 47% in ASAP and 11.4% to 37.2% in AMPLE-2). Costs of increased bottle use may be offset by longer-term IPC community management. IPC-PLUS was the first RCT looking at IPC-delivered talc pleurodesis as an out-patient,[55] demonstrating it could be delivered efficaciously with successful pleurodesis at day 35 in 43% of patients compared with 23% in the autopleurodesis group.

The treatment of MPE has rapidly evolved, with a large volume of high-quality research on both chemical pleurodesis and IPC management over

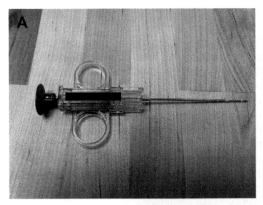
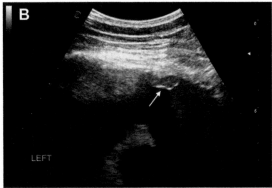
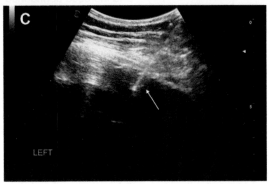

Fig. 2. *A)* An example of a core-cutting needle used for percutaneous biopsy. (*B*) TUS image of pleural nodularity (*solid arrow*). (*C*) Real-time ultrasound-guided core-cutting needle biopsy, visualizing the needle passing through the pleural nodularity (*solid arrow*). (*Courtesy of* Dr Maged Hassan, Alexandria University Faculty of Medicine, Egypt.)

the last decade. This has allowed us to focus on patient preferences and an individualized approach to management of their MPE,[56] which should be central to any dedicated pleural service.

Ambulatory Pneumothorax Management

Patients with pneumothorax have historically been managed in the inpatient setting, for many young patients, this is inconvenient as they are systemically well and hindered being attached to a chest drain bottle. Recently following RCT evidence in a select cohort of patients with minimal symptoms, there is an increasing trend of managing primary spontaneous pneumothorax (PSP) conservatively, in light of modest evidence conservative management was noninferior to interventional management.[57] Though this less invasive approach is welcome by patients, it does come with a risk within your pleural service and the ambulatory pleural service needs to be set up, so it can see these patients at short notice in an out-patient setting to monitor their progress and ensure they are improving. Also, with the introduction of new ambulatory technology, we are able to undertake ambulatory management of patients not suitable

for conservative management, within a dedicated pleural out-patient setting. The Heimlich Valve is a plastic cylinder with a rubber valve that allows unidirectional flow, allowing the proximal end to be connected to a chest drain and the distal end to allow air to pass out but not be entrained. Newer devices (Pleural Vent) have been created to include an insertion catheter and valve in one device (picture) and can be directly attached to the skin[58] (**Fig. 4**).

Although the 2016 BTS guidelines only advocate the use of Heimlich valves in secondary spontaneous pneumothorax to allow ambulation,[59] a recent large RCT has recently been published advocating their use within an ambulatory pathway by a dedicated pleural service. RAMPP (randomized ambulatory management of primary pneumothorax), randomized patients with symptomatic PSP to an ambulatory device or standard treatment (pleural aspiration, chest tube insertion, or both) and found ambulatory management significantly reduced the duration of hospitalizations including readmission in the first 30 days but at the expense of increased adverse events.[60] These findings will be reflected in the next BTS guidelines due to be published in late 2021.

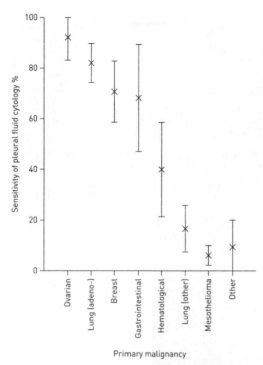

Fig. 3. Scatter plot of sensitivity of pleural fluid cytology by malignancy (error bars represent 95% confidence intervals). (*From* Arnold DT, de Fonseka D, Perry S, et al. Investigating unilateral pleural effusions: the role of cytology. Eur Respir J 2018. Reproduced with permission of the © ERS 2021: European Respiratory Journal 52 (5) 1801254; DOI: 10.1183/13993003.01254-2018 Published 8 November 2018.)

More caution is required when managing patients with secondary pneumothorax. These usually require a period of hospitalization but can be ambulated early using a pneumostat or Heimlich valve. The Hi-SPEC (Heimlich Valves in Secondary Spontaneous Pneumothorax: Enhancing Care) study showed the pleural vents tended to block or become dislodged and should be avoided in this setting. This is likely to be because of the longer periods they were required to be in-situ due to bigger air leaks that took longer to settle.[61]

In summary, the results of these recent RCTs have shifted the paradigm of how we can manage particularly PSP as an outpatient through a dedicated pleural service working in conjunction with the front door of the hospital and allowing a patient-centric approach.

The Value of a Specialist Pleural Unit

Safety

As well as the development of specialist knowledge and technical skills with TUS, basic and more advanced pleural procedures forming a subset of specialist skills improving patient care; the recognition following the NPSA advice for "pleural safety" has also added to the drive for specialist pleural care.[15] As already discussed TUS underpins the push for safety and is formalized in guidelines worldwide for all pleural procedures. In the United Kingdom, TUS proficiency is a core component of current registrar training, not only in respiratory but also in other areas of acute medicine.[11,34] One important role of any pleural service is the ongoing TUS training of trainees. Their attendance at dedicated pleural lists and clinics will allow them to develop proficiencies and increase confidence when undertaking emergency procedures out of hours.[9] Delivering this training and evaluating competency in TUS is a key component of a tertiary led-pleural service.[11]

As our understanding of pleural disease and procedures and adverse events associated with mortality and morbidity, there is a growing realization these interventions should be performed by experienced interventionists within a pleural unit.[11] Early expert opinion reduces the number of procedures and subsequently the number of complications.

Education and training

There is growing recognition for the need to formalize training pathways for TUS acquisition skills and procedural competency not only for pulmonologists but also for clinicians providing cover out of hours to this group of patients.[11] Surveys of residents in the United States have shown low levels of confidence in their pleural procedures and lack of ability to manage complications.[52]

An essential component of running a safe pleural unit is the recognition of trainees who will be required to perform basic emergency pleural procedures such as intercostal drainage and large volume aspiration.[10] This standard can be achieved within a relatively short period, with a dedicated pleural service leading the delivery to residents in acute specialties who might be faced with emergency pleural procedures. There is a move from the traditional early training on patients to more focus on theoretic knowledge, stimulation-based manikin training, and competency-led assessments.[11,52] Increasingly in postgraduate education, "Entrustable Professional Activities" (EPAs) are being used as an assessment tool to recognize procedural independence.[34] They are widely used in pulmonary and critical care programs in the United States.[62] TUS and pleural procedural competency are well suited to have an EPA approach underpinning training and competence assessments. The UK has recently adopted this approach progressing

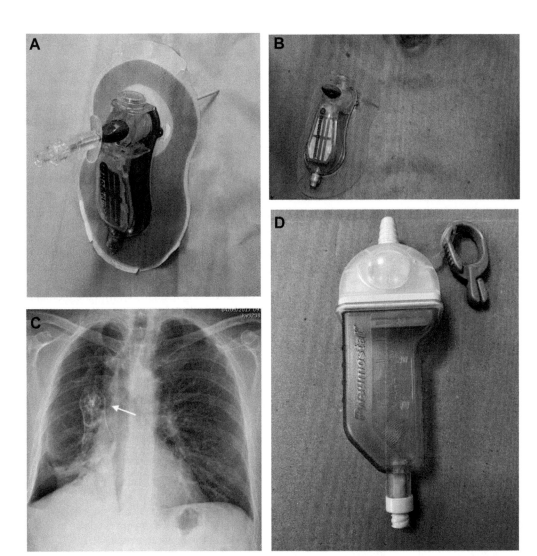

Fig. 4. Devices to allow ambulation in pneumothorax (*A*) Pleural Vent with needle for insertion (*B*) Pleural Vent in situ on the skin (*C*) Pleural vent in situ on chest radiograph (*arrow*) (*D*) Image of Pneumostat. (*Images courtesy* of Dr Steven Walker, University of Bristol, UK.)

from level 1, observing only to level 4, independent practice within the 4 operator pathways (emergency, basic, advanced, or expert).[11,34] Specialist pleural units can foster this training and supervision of competencies.

Specialist units are also the best environment to develop training in advanced ultrasound and complex procedural skills. Training can be delivered whilst working in the unit to research and clinical fellows, as well as rotational pulmonologists developing further subspecialists in this area.[7,8]

Research and audit
Historically, there has been a lack of good-quality, large RCTs in pleural disease and previously patients have been managed by many different specialties.[63] However, this has changed over the last decade and a specialist pleural unit provides the opportunity to participate in research by collecting data and tissue, and enroll patients in growing number of RCTs assessing new management strategies and therapies.[7,8] Similarly this also allows data collection and monitoring for audit and improvement, a key component of a specialist unit that will address problems, innovate, and improve efficiency.[7]

The pleural multidisciplinary team
There is no strict template for setting up a pleural service but core members of the pleural team are

typically multidisciplinary. This will vary greatly between different centers and is largely based on the services that exist locally and how well they are established.[8] The fundamental aim should be to work together to provide streamlined diagnostic and management outpatient pathways, focusing on patient care, timely and safe procedures, minimizing admissions and safe ambulatory pathways.[7–10] The below figure suggests the specialties, the departments, and the staff roles that should be central in any comprehensive pleural service. Although it is convenient to have all resources on one site, it is not necessary and relies on teamwork and adaptability of existing referral pathways. Some of the responsibilities are interchangeable between specialities[8] (**Fig. 5**).

The medical team

In most circumstances, a pulmonologist with experience and interest in pleural disease will be the nominated "pleural lead" and be the fulcrum around which the pleural team operates. They will typically take an overview of the service and determine its structure and the overall long-term direction. This role will involve education and teaching of pleural skills across the department, as well as also ensuring safe pleural pathways are followed in and out of hours.[8,10] Although advanced TUS and procedural skills are desirable, they are not essential and can be bridged by close working relationships with thoracic surgery and interventional radiology teams.[8]

A dedicated pleural fellow, although not essential, can be of significant benefit to the efficiency of a pleural service. This role could be filled by a research fellow or a rotating pulmonology trainee. They will have the time and knowledge to offer increased flexibility with reviews and procedural skills,[8] whilst also helping develop training for other trainees.[10]

Radiology services

Specialist thoracic radiology services are an integral part of any pleural service, they will have expertise in pleural imaging and can help provide training and mentorship for pulmonologists in TUS and image-guided procedural skills.[7–10] Interventional radiologists will be able to help with complex cases when expert TUS or image-guided skills are required. In addition to TUS, CT, PET, and MRI are all used increasingly in pleural medicine, often with more than one modality used in an individual patient, and expert thoracic radiological interpretation is essential, as well as providing a service for CT-guided biopsy.[8,52] A thoracic radiologist will also be invaluable when interpreting CT

with specific pleura protocols, enhancing the diagnosis accuracy in pleural malignancy.[64]

Thoracic surgery services

The advances in pleural medicine over the last few years have limited the role of the thoracic surgeon by pulmonologists acquiring skills in pleuroscopy for tissue diagnosis and intrapleural fibrinolytic use in pleural infection.[8] Despite this there is still a vital role for the thoracic surgeon in cases of pleural infection that have failed medical management, those with persistent pneumothoraces and ongoing air leaks, and those requiring diagnostic VATS or decortication.[8,10] With the rise of pulmonology-guided interventions, urgent surgical thoracic assistance may also be required to manage complications that arise with visceral puncture or laceration of the intercostal artery.[10] A close working relationship with the thoracic surgical team is therefore essential if you want to run an effective pleural service.[52]

Pathology services

Rapid and accurate cell, tissue, biochemical and molecular analysis is crucial in pleural medicine more than ever, with the rapid rise of treatment options for pleural malignancies.[8,11] Given the low sensitivity of cytology in mesothelioma and the difficulties in diagnosing some cases histologically, a specialist pathologist with access to molecular markers such as BAP-1 (BRAC associated protein 1) and p16 FISH is vital. Some pleural services will offer a regional mesothelioma multidisciplinary team (MDT) service to ensure mesothelioma diagnoses are robust, where pathologist is a pivotal member of this mesothelioma MDT.

Cancer and palliative care services

Specialist thoracic oncologists are a key component of any thoracic MDT and many have a specialist interest in pleural malignancy. Also given over half of the pleural presentations generally seen within a pleural unit are MPE, it is essential there are easy, quick pathways for referrals after diagnosis and the ability to support with ongoing management of an MPE and symptom control with palliative care support.[8,10] Thoracic oncologists are also in a prime position to offer patients entry into key clinical trials.[8]

Nursing staff

A specialist pleural nurse is a key asset to any pleural unit, they will often help provide support to ambulatory outpatients with IPCs or Heimlich valves and help support the community teams with ongoing future management and problems. They can also help provide education to respiratory ward nursing staff and teach them how to

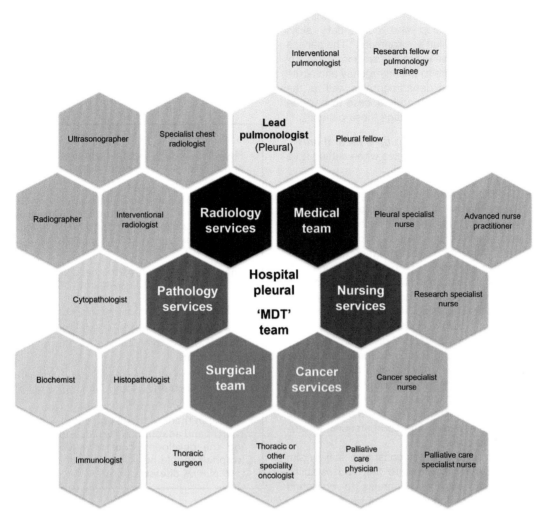

Fig. 5. The core hospital services and teams required by a pleural team and the hospital staff who will form the pleural MDT. (*Modified from* Bhatnagar R, Maskell N. Developing a 'pleural team' to run a reactive pleural service. Clin Med 2013; 13: 452–456.)

manage intercostal drains, IPCs, and suction devices, they can also help with the procedures and procedural checklists, implement care bundles and quality improvement projects and actively help promote and recruit to clinical trials.[8,10] In many institutions, advanced nurse practitioners have acquired TUS skills and can perform pleural procedures and teach and supervise other trainee's.[52]

The pleural team day-to-day running

There are many different ways a pleural service could be run based on your local resources and infrastructure. A pleural service could be run from an emergency admission ward, a day case ward, or pulmonology outpatients.[8] The key, in addition to adequate staff and MDT support, is the basic infrastructure to function efficiently.[10] Dedicated pleural clinic or dedicated clinic "hot" slots are extremely useful to ensure patients can be seen quickly following a community referral,[7] especially in the context of suspected pleural malignancy.[41] This may allow the adoption of the pleural "one-stop shop" facilitating a clinical assessment and an initial diagnostic procedure (usually pleural aspiration but also be an image-guided biopsy) and a therapeutic option, all in a single outpatient visit.[40] Interventional pleural lists are also becoming increasingly more common, with guidelines advocating procedures are performed away from bed spaces and the ward environment. As a result, it is essential as a pleural service you have access to a dedicated procedure room, endoscopy suite, or theater space with adequate staff and dedicated equipment.[10] Pleural lists will also help trainees develop and consolidate skills learned in a controlled environment.[8] The service also needs to be able to provide ad-hoc and emergency in-patient care to the emergency and acute medical admissions department, as well as the pulmonology ward with ready access to bedside TUS and equipment to manage these patients.

Key challenges of a setting up a pleural unit
There can be several obstacles when setting up a pleural unit:

- Deskilling general pulmonologists without a subspecialist interest in pleural disease, emergency and acute medical colleagues and trainees by taking procedures away from them and setting higher goalpost to achieve procedure competency through TUS skills.[10,11] But this can be overcome by ongoing education, supporting development of those interested in pleural disease by involving them in service delivery and ensuring a 2-way referral process.[7]
- The delivery of a safe and timely pleural service, particularly out of hours and in remote regions. An integral and wider component of the pleural service is the identification of individuals who perform 24/7 cover and ensuring they have training and competencies to provide that cover.[10,11]
- Funding can be a key constraint. Initially aim for a basic infrastructure that you establish gradually, with a willingness to challenge traditional methods and enthusiasm for innovation. This core work can be supported by business cases for future development. It is essential to have accurate documentation and coding to allow remuneration and future investment.[8,10,11]

SUMMARY

Given the frequency and complexity of pleural disease today, combined with an expanding array of pleural procedures and the need for TUS proficiency, a specialist pleural service is essential for the management of pleural diseases Early specialist intervention has led to ambulatory pathways, improved patient care and safety, reduced waiting times, improved admission duration and overall costs.[10,65] Pleural services are also ideal for the development of nurses and doctors interested in pleural medicine, and the continued support of large-scale research trials in the pleural community.[9] Using local resources and adapting as needed, or developing and promoting new services, it should be possible to deliver standardized, high-quality pleural care in any hospital environment.

CLINICS CARE POINTS

- Pleural disease is becoming more frequent and complex requiring specialist management.
- Pleural procedural skills are becoming more specialist with the need for TUS proficiency and the ability to perform TUS image-guided procedures within a specialist pleural service.
- There is recognition of the need for formal TUS teaching and assessment of competencies maintained by a specialist service following procedural safety concerns.
- The development of a specialist pleural unit allows active recruitment to large-scale pleural trials
- A pleural unit requires an MDT approach with different specialties closely working together to deliver a cohesive care.
- Although there are challenges, using local resources and adapting as needed and promoting the development of new ideas, most hospitals should be able to deliver a specialized pleural disease service.

AUTHOR CONTRIBUTIONS

N. Maskell conceived the article; H. McDill drafted the article; NM critically revised the draft; and all authors reviewed and approved the final article.

ACKNOWLEDGMENTS

The authors thank Dr Maged Hassan (University of Alexandria) and Dr John Corcoran (Plymouth NHS Trust) for providing the thoracic ultrasound images and thoracic ultrasound-guided biopsy images. They also thank Dr Steven Walker (University of Bristol) for providing the pleural vent images.

DISCLOSURE

The authors have nothing to disclose.

REFERENCES

1. Maldonado F, Lentz RJ, Light RW. Diagnostic approach to pleural diseases: new tricks for an old trade. F1000Res 2017;6:1–6.

2. Sahn SA, Heffner JH. Pleural fluid analysis. In: Light RW, Lee YCG, editors. Textbook of pleural diseases. London: Arnold Press; 2008. p. 209–26.

3. American Thoracic Society. Management of malignant pleural effusions. Am J Respir Crit Care Med 2000;162:1987–2001.

4. Bray F, Ferlay J, Soerjomataram I, et al. Global cancer statistics 2018: GLOBOCAN estimates of incidence and mortality worldwide for 36 cancers in 185 countries. CA Cancer J Clin 2018;68: 394–424.

5. Grijalva CG, Zhu Y, Nuorti JP, et al. Emergence of parapneumonic empyema in the USA. Thorax 2011;66:663–8.

6. Bender JM, Ampofo K, Shang X, et al. Parapneumonic empyema deaths during past century, Utah. Emerg Infect Dis 2009;15:44–8.

7. Hooper CE, Lee YG, Maskell NA. Invited review series: how to set up pulmonary subspeciality services. Respirology 2010;15:1028–36.

8. Bhatnagar R, Maskell N. Developing a 'pleural team' to run a reactive pleural service. Clin Med 2013;13: 452–6.

9. Bhatnagar R, Maskell N. Setting up a pleural practice. In: Light RW, Lee GC, editors. 3. Textbook of pleural disease. Roca Raton: CRC Press; 2016. p. 620–5.

10. George V, Evison M. The specialist pleural service: when, why and who?. In: Maskell NA, Laursen CB, Lee YCG, et al, editors. Pleural disease (ERS Monograph). Sheffield: European Respiratory Society; 2020. p. 282–94.

11. Evison M, Blyth KG, Bhatnagar R, et al. Providing safe and effective pleural medicine services in the UK: an aspirational statement from UK pleural physicians. BMJ Open Respir Res 2018;5:e000307.

12. Mercaldi CJ, Lanes SF. Ultrasound guidance decreases complications and improves the cost of care among patients undergoing thoracentesis and paracentesis. Chest 2013;143:532–8.

13. Gordon CE, Feller-Kopman D, Balk EM, et al. Pneumothorax following thoracentesis: a systematic review and meta-analysis. Arch Intern Med 2010; 170:332–9.

14. Corcoran JP, Tazi-Mezalek R, Maldonado F, et al. State of the art thoracic ultrasound: intervention and therapeutics. Thorax 2017;72:840–9.

15. National Patient Safety Agency (NPSA). Rapid response report: risk of chest drain insertion. 2008. NPSA/2008/RRR03. Available at: http://www.12 npsa.nhs.uk/nrls/alerts-and-directives/rapidrr/risks-of-chest-drain-insertion/.

16. Young RL, Bhatnagar R, Mason ZD, et al. Evaluation of an ambulatory pleural service: costs and benefits. Thorax 2013;68(Suppl. 3):A42.

17. Hooper C, Lee YCG, Maskell N. Investigation of a unilateral pleural effusion in adults: British thoracic society pleural disease guideline 2010. Thorax 2010;65(Suppl. 2). ii4–ii17.

18. Mummadi S, Hahn P. Outcomes of a clinical pathway for pleural disease management: "pleural pathway". PulmMed 2018;2018:1–6.

19. Mercer RM, Psallidas I, Rahman NM. Ultrasound in the management of pleural disease. Exp Rev Respir Med 2017;11:323–31.

20. Havelock T, Teoh R, Laws D, et al. Pleural procedures and thoracic ultrasound: British thoracic society pleural disease guideline 2010. Thorax 2010; 65(Suppl. 2):ii61–76.

21. Feller-Kopman D, Reddy C, DeCamp M, et al. Management of Malignant pleural effusion. An official ATS/STS/STR clinical practice guideline 2018. Am J Respir Crit Care Med 2018;198:7.

22. Salamonsen M, Dobeli K, McGrath D, et al. Physician-performed ultrasound can accurately screen for a vulnerable intercostal artery prior to chest drainage procedures. Respirology 2013; 18:942–7.

23. Corcoran JP, Psallidas I, Ross CL, et al. Always worth another look? Thoracic ultrasonography before, during, and after pleural intervention. Ann Am Thorac Soc 2016;13:118–21.

24. Wiesen J, Raman D, Adams J, et al. A patient with lung cancer presenting with respiratory failure and shock. Chest 2013;144:e1–4.

25. Gryminski J, Krakowka P, Lypacewicz G. The diagnosis of pleural effusion by ultrasonic and radiologic techniques. Chest 1976;70:33–7.

26. Qureshi NR, Rahman NM, Gleeson FV. Thoracic ultrasound in the diagnosis of malignant pleural effusion. Thorax 2009;64:139–43.

27. Bugalho A, Ferreira D, Dias SS, et al. The diagnostic value of transthoracic ultrasonographic features in predicting malignancy in undiagnosed pleural effusions: a prospective observational study. Respiration 2014;87:270–8.

28. Light RW. Parapneumonic effusions and empyema. Proc Am Thorac Soc 2006;3:75–80.

29. McLoud TC, Flower CD. Imaging the pleura: sonography, CT, and MR imaging. AJR Am J Roentgenol 1991;156:1145–53.

30. Lichtenstein DA, Menu Y. A bedside ultrasound sign ruling out pneumothorax in the critically ill. Lung sliding. Chest 1995;108:1345–8.

31. Banka RA, Skaarup SH, Mercer RM, et al. Thoracic ultrasound: a key tool beyond procedure guidance. In: Maskell NA, Laursen CB, Lee YCG, et al, editors. Pleural disease (ERS Monograph). Sheffield: European Respiratory Society; 2020. p. 73–89.

32. Diacon AH, Brutsche MH, Soler M. Accuracy of pleural puncture sites: a prospective comparison of clinical examination with ultrasound. Chest 2003; 123:436–41.

33. Jones PW, Moyers JP, Rogers JT, et al. Ultrasound-guided thoracentesis: is it a safer method? Chest 2003;123:418–23.

34. Stanton A, Edey A, Evison M, et al. BTS Training standards for thoracic ultrasound. BMJ Open Respir Res 2020;7:e000552.

35. Rahman NM, Ali NJ, Brown G, et al. Local anaesthetic thoracoscopy: British Thoracic society pleural disease guideline 2010. Thorax 2010;65(Suppl. 2): ii54–60.

36. Psallidas I, Corcoran JP, Fallon J, et al. Provision of day-case local anesthetic thoracoscopy: a multi-center review of practice. Chest 2017;151:511–2.

37. Bibby AC, Dorn P, Psallidas I, et al. ERS/EACTS statement on the management of malignant pleural effusions. Eur J Cardiothorac Surg 2019;55: 116–32.

38. Marchetti G, Valsecchi A, Indellicati D, et al. Ultrasound-guided medical thoracoscopy in the absence of pleural effusion. Chest 2015;147:1008–12.

39. Hallifax RJ, Corcoran JP, Ahmed A, et al. Physician-based ultrasound-guided biopsy for diagnosing pleural disease. Chest 2014;146:1001–6.

40. Hassan M, Munavvar M, Corcoran JP. Pleural interventions: less is more?. In: Maskell NA, Laursen CB, Lee YCG, et al, editors. Pleural disease (ERS Monograph). Sheffield: European Respiratory Society; 2020. p. 90–104.

41. Bhatnagar R, Corcoran JP, Maldonado F, et al. Advanced medical interventions in pleural disease. Eur Respir Rev 2016;25:199–213.

42. Qureshi NR, Gleeson FV. Imaging of pleural disease. Clin Chest Med 2006;27:193–213.

43. Maskell N, Gleeson F, Davies R. Standard pleural biopsy versus CT-guided cutting-needle biopsy for diagnosis of malignant disease in pleural effusions: a randomised controlled trial. Lancet 2003;361: 1326–30.

44. Christiansen IS, Clementsen PF, Bodtger U, et al. Transthoracic ultrasound-guided biopsy in the hands of chest physicians – a stepwise approach. Eur Clin Respir J 2019;6:1579632.

45. Diacon AH, Schuurmans MM, Theron J, et al. Safety and yield of ultrasound-assisted transthoracic biopsy performed by pulmonologists. Respir Int Rev Thorac Dis 2004;71:519–22.

46. Koegelenberg CFN, Irusen EM, von Groote-Bidlingmaier F, et al. The utility of ultrasound-guided thoracentesis and pleural biopsy in undiagnosed pleural exudates. Thorax 2015;70:995–7.

47. Psallidas I, Kanellakis NI, Bhatnagar R, et al. A pilot feasibility study in establishing the role of ultrasound-guided pleural biopsies in pleural infection (The AUDIO Study). Chest 2018;154: 766–72.

48. Arnold DT, de Fonseka D, Perry S, et al. Investigating unilateral pleural effusions: the role of cytology. Eur Respir J 2018;52:1–9.

49. Tsim S, Paterson S, Cartwright D, et al. Baseline predictors of negative and incomplete pleural cytology in patients with suspected pleural malignancy - data supporting 'Direct to LAT' in selected groups. Lung Cancer 2019;133:123–9.

50. Davies HE, Mishra EK, Kahan BC, et al. Effect of an indwelling pleural catheter vs chest tube and talc pleurodesis for relieving dyspnea in patients with malignant pleural effusion: the TIME2 randomized controlled trial. J Am Med Assoc 2012;307:2383–9.

51. Thomas R, Fysh ETH, Smith NA, et al. Effect of an indwelling pleural catheter vs talc pleurodesis on hospitalization days in patients with malignant pleural effusion: the AMPLE randomized clinical trial. J Am Med Assoc 2017;318:1903–12.

52. Cameron K, Teodoro D, Kasis A, et al. Development and maintenance of a pleural disease service: role of the "pleurologist". Semin Respir Crit Care Med 2019;40:297–304.

53. Muruganandan S, Azzopardi M, Fitzgerald DB, et al. Aggressive versus symptom-guided drainage of malignant pleural effusion via indwelling pleural catheters (AMPLE-2): an open-label randomised trial. Lancet Respir Med 2018;6:671–80.

54. Wahidi MM, Reddy C, Yarmus L, et al. Randomized trial of pleural fluid drainage frequency in patients with malignant pleural effusions. The ASAP Trial. Am J Respir Crit Care Med 2017;195:1050–7.

55. Bhatnagar R, Keenan EK, Morley AJ, et al. Outpatient talc administration by indwelling pleural catheter for malignant effusion. N Engl J Med 2018; 378:1313–22.

56. Arnold DT, Roberts M, Wahidi M, et al. Optimal diagnosis and treatment of malignant disease: challenging the guidelines. In: Maskell NA, Laursen CB, Lee YCG, et al, editors. Pleural diseases (ERS Monograph). Sheffield: European Respiratory Society; 2020. p. 138–54.

57. Brown S, Ball E, Perrin K, et al. Conservative versus interventional treatment for spontaneous pneumothorax. N Engl J Med 2020;382:405–15.

58. Mercer RM, Hallifax RJ, Maskell NA. Novel technology: more than just indwelling pleural catheters. In: Maskell NA, Laursen CB, Lee YCG, et al, editors. Pleural disease (ERS Monograph). Sheffield: European Respiratory Society; 2020. p. 250–62.

59. MacDuff A, Arnold A, Harvey J. Management of spontaneous pneumothorax: British thoracic society pleural disease guideline 2010. Thorax 2010; 65(Suppl. 2):ii18–31.

60. Halifax R, McKeown SP, Sivakumar P, et al. Ambulatory management of primary spontaneous

pneumothorax: an open-label, randomised control trial. Lancet 2020;396:39–49.

61. Walker SP, Keenan E, Bintcliffe O, et al. Ambulatory management of secondary spontaneous pneumothorax: a randomised controlled trial. Eur Respir J 2021. https://doi.org/10.1183/13993003.03375-2020.

62. Fessler HE, Addrizzo-Harris D, Beck JM, et al. Entrustable professional activities and curricular milestones for fellowship training in pulmonary and critical care medicine: report of a multisociety Working group. Chest 2014;146:813–34.

63. Feller-Kopman D, Light R. Pleural Disease review article. N Engl J Med 2018;378:740–51.

64. Raj V, Kirke R, Bankart MJ, et al. Multidetector CT imaging of pleura: comparison of two contrast infusion protocols. Br J Radiol 2011;84:796–9.

65. Sura P, Hyde E, Afify E, et al. Ambulatory and inpatient pleural service — the way forward. Thorax 2012;67:A113.

Section 2: Non-Malignant Pleural Disease

Hepatic Hydrothorax and Congestive Heart Failure Induced Pleural Effusion

Shaikh M. Noor Husnain, MD[a], Samira Shojaee, MD, MPH[b],*

KEYWORDS

- Congestive heart failure • Hepatic hydrothorax • Indwelling tunneled pleural catheters
- Pleural effusion • Non-malignant effusion

KEY POINTS

- Non-malignant recurrent pleural effusions such as refractory cardiac-induced pleural effusion and hepatic hydrothorax carry poor prognosis and indicate high 1-year mortality.
- The management of recurrent cardiac-induced pleural effusion and hepatic hydrothorax should always initiate with optimizing medical management.
- Management of hepatic hydrothorax that is refractory to medical management requires multidisciplinary discussion, a personalized approach and consideration of patient's TIPS and transplant candidacy.
- Management of cardiac-induced pleural effusion that is refractory to medical management requires multidisciplinary discussion, a personalized approach and consideration of patient's transplant candidacy and lung expandability.

INTRODUCTION

Pleural effusions (PEs) are frequently encountered in routine clinical practice, affecting more than 3000 people per million population every year. Transudative effusions are more common than exudative effusions and have varying diagnostic workup and prognostic and therapeutic implications.[1] Heart and liver failures are two of the most common causes of transudative PE. Because these effusions have nonmalignant etiologies, they are commonly referred to as benign effusions despite of the poor prognosis they foretell in their refractory stages. Like malignant effusions, symptom management is important and plays a significant role in palliation when these effusions become refractory to medical therapy. Herein, we review the pathophysiology and diagnosis of PE development in heart and liver failure and examine the existing evidence with particular focus on management and palliation.

LIVER FAILURE AND HEPATIC HYDROTHORAX

Chronic liver disease is the 5th leading cause of mortality worldwide.[2] PE in a patient with liver cirrhosis and portal hypertension in absence of cardiopulmonary disease is defined as hepatic hydrothorax (HH) and is seen in 5% to 15% of patients with end-stage liver disease (ESLD). Up to 25% of these patients have poor response to medical therapy (diuretics and salt restriction) with rapid recurrence of symptomatic effusion and are known as refractory HH.[3,4].

Pathophysiology

The exact mechanism by which HH develops is not completely understood. Proposed mechanisms described in literature are azygous vein hypertension causing formation of collateral anastomosis between portal and azygous system, transfer of peritoneal fluid through diaphragmatic

a Division of Pulmonary and Critical, Henry Ford Hospital, Detroit, MI, USA; b Department of Pulmonary and Critical Care Medicine, Section of Interventional Pulmonology, Virginia Commonwealth University Health System, 1200 East Broad Street, PO Box 980050, Richmond, VA 23298, USA
* Corresponding author.
E-mail address: sshojaee@mcvh-vcu.edu

Clin Chest Med 42 (2021) 625–635
https://doi.org/10.1016/j.ccm.2021.07.005
0272-5231/21/© 2021 Elsevier Inc. All rights reserved.

chestmed.theclinics.com

defects,[5] passage of fluid from peritoneal to pleural surface via transdiaphragmatic lymphatics,[6] hypoalbuminemia resulting in decreased colloid pressure, and lymphatic leakage from the thoracic duct.[7] Among these, the most widely accepted theory is the passage of ascitic fluid through diaphragmatic defects.[5]

Cirrhosis and portal hypertension, vasodilation of splanchnic and systemic arteries, and neurohormonal activation result in decreased sodium and water excretion, leading to ascites in the peritoneal space.[8] It is hypothesized that due to pressure gradient (positive intraabdominal pressure and negative intrathoracic pressure), fluid shifts through diaphragmatic defects known as pleuroperitoneal communications, resulting in HH. There are 4 types of pleuroperitoneal communications described in literature, ranging from no obvious defect (type 1), blebs on the diaphragm (type 2), defects or fenestration of the diaphragm (type 3, most common), and multiple gaps in the diaphragm (type 4).[9] These defects and blebs tend to occur more commonly in the right hemidiaphragm (59%-80%) compared with the more muscular and thicker left hemidiaphragm.[9]

Diagnostic Workup

Effusion in the setting of ascites and ESLD should raise suspicion of HH. A systematic approach is necessary for efficient diagnosis and management. Detailed clinical history and examination, radiographic/ultrasonographic assessment, and pleural fluid analysis are required in order to exclude cardiac, renal, and malignant causes of PE.[10,11] Paracentesis and thoracentesis in those with mild coagulation abnormalities are generally safe, although caution is warranted in the presence of anticoagulation or a bleeding diathesis, thrombocytopenia, and renal failure.[10,11]

Although HH is usually a transudative effusion, in cases where the effusion is mischaracterized, pleural fluid/serum bilirubin ratio less than 0.6 can be helpful.[12] Additionally, similar to serum–ascites albumin gradient, serum pleural fluid albumin gradient of greater than 1.1 g/dL is consistent with a transudative process[13] and tends to perform significantly better than just protein gradient of greater than 3.1 g/dL. On occasion, patients with cirrhosis have high liver capillary pressure, with a commensurate increase in lymphatic flow in the liver and the thoracic duct,[14] resulting in formation of chylous ascites, and triglyceride levels can help in their diagnosis.

For atypical presentation of hydrothorax and uncertain diagnosis, nuclear scans using intraperitoneal instillation of 99mTc-human serum albumin or 99mTc-sulfur-colloid[15] and scintigraphy are effective diagnostic tools which can help identify pleuroperitoneal communication even in the absence of ascites.[16,17]

Management of Hepatic Hydrothorax/ Refractory Hepatic Hydrothorax

Management of HH should be multidisciplinary and start with medical therapy. Once refractory HH is diagnosed, it is pivotal to assess for potentially curative liver transplantation. However, therapies like liver transplantation or other options such as transjugular intrahepatic portosystemic shunt (TIPS) do not follow a straightforward path as many patients do not qualify for either. In such patients, more personalized treatment strategies should be selected in a multidisciplinary fashion.

Management of excess fluid production

The sirst step in medical management is obtaining a negative sodium balance[18] to decrease ascitic fluid production and ultimately reduce fluid shift. Patients with ESLD and moderate ascites generally have weak sodium excretion and require sodium restriction.[19] Morando and colleagues[20] observed dietary sodium compliance in only 30% of patient.

However, in most cases, dietary restrictions are not sufficient, and diuretics are required. Treatment with distally acting aldosterone receptor antagonists and loop diuretics is the preferred regimen.[21] Medication titration is often required to achieve expected goals and require close monitoring of renal function, serum electrolytes, blood pressure, and orthostatic vitals.

An estimated 20% to 30% of patients who tolerate large doses of diuretics have lack of clinical response and continue to have recurrent HH (diuretic-resistant HH).[22] About 5% to 10% of patients cannot tolerate diuresis and experience diuretic induced hyponatremia and encephalopathy (diuretic-intractable HH).

Splanchnic and peripheral vasoconstrictors including octreotide, midodrine, and terlipressin have also been used to aid sodium excretion by decreasing the activation of renin–angiotensin–aldosterone system and increasing effective arterial volume causing sodium excretion.[23–25] More data are required to examine the role of these agents in management of HH.

Transjugular intrahepatic portosystemic shunt

Portal hypertension leads to fluid accumulation by increasing the portosystemic gradient (pressure between portal vein and hepatic vein/inferior vena cava [IVC]). Normal gradient is ≤ 5 mm

Hg,[26] and ascites rarely develop if postsinusoidal pressure gradient is $\leq$ 12 mm Hg.[27]

TIPS is a low resistance side-to-side shunt created between the intrahepatic branch of the portal vein and hepatic artery using a stent to decrease portal hypertension.[25]

A multidisciplinary team approach is necessary to evaluate a patient's candidacy for TIPS. Up to 50% of patients with refractory HH do not meet candidacy criteria.[28] Although TIPS has shown to reduce mortality in patients with variceal bleeding, no significant mortality benefit is seen for other conditions including HH.[29] In another study, TIPS performed for refractory HH versus refractory ascites did not show any survival benefit and response rate, and fluid accumulation was not different in either group.[30] A meta-analysis including 332 patients who received TIPS for HH showed 74% overall success (56% complete and 25% partial response). Hepatic encephalopathy occurred in 27% of patients, and 1-month and 1-year mortality rates were 19% and 48%, respectively.[31] Earlier studies used bare metal or uncovered stent; however, stent evolution has led to modern stent grafts that have superior patency and improved symptom control with less need for revision.[32–34]

Other means of bridge to transplant or palliation

Repeat thoracentesis Repeat thoracentesis is an effective and safe way to remove large fluid volumes and a standard procedure for symptom management in patients who are not TIPS or transplant candidates, although drainage of ascites before accessing the thoracic cavity is recommended.[3]

Coagulopathy, elevated international normalized ratio (INR), and thrombocytopenia are usual findings in patients with ESLD; however, the role of pre-thoracentesis plasma and platelet transfusion has not been studied.[35,36] Although thoracentesis is a safe procedure, most existing studies have not evaluated its safety within specific etiologies of PE.

In a single-center retrospective study, repeat thoracentesis in HH was safe although when compared with repeat thoracentesis in the non-HH group, the cumulative rate of complications increased with the increased number of thoracenteses.[37] The HH group (n = 82) required a higher median number of thoracentesis (5 vs 2) at shorter intervals (14 vs 35 days) compared with the non-HH group (n = 100). Within the HH group, higher Model For End-Stage Liver Disease (MELD) scores (odds ratio (OR) = 1.19, 95% confidence interval (CI) = 1.03–1.36, P = .012) and platelet count less than $50 \times 10^3/\mu L$ (OR = 9.67, 95% CI = 1.16–80.42, P = .035) were associated with higher hemothorax rates in multivariable analysis. Intercostal varicose

veins leading to spontaneous hemothorax are reported in patients with ESLD.[38] Although not studied specifically in patients with HH, we recommend ultrasound examination of the intercostal space with a linear/vascular ultrasound probe before thoracentesis in patients with HH, particularly those with thrombocytopenia and higher MELD scores.

Conventional chest tubes Conventional chest tubes often placed with the goal of pleural space evacuation lead to large volume, electrolyte, and protein loss in patients with HH. Guidelines from the American Association for the Study of Liver Diseases recommend against conventional chest tubes in HH.[39,40] High complication rates and increased mortality have been observed in multiple case series.[41,42] In a retrospective study of 55 patients with HH, 88% developed infectious complications, renal failure, or electrolyte imbalance and reported mortality rate at 33%[43] due to empyema and sepsis following chest tubes placement. In a retrospective study of 140,573 patients with liver cirrhosis, 205 patients with chest tubes were compared with 1776 who underwent thoracentesis only and showed that mortality was twice as high in the chest tube subgroup.[44]

Indwelling tunneled pleural catheters Indwelling tunneled pleural catheters (IPCs) have shown great palliative benefit for malignant PEs (MPEs), but it was not until 2017 when they were approved by the FDA for non-MPEs.[45].

Single-center retrospective and prospective data on IPCs in HH show a spontaneous pleurodesis rate of 15% to 33% with a pleural space infection rate of 15% to 33% (**Table 1**).[46–52] In one multicenter retrospective study[50] of 79 patients who underwent IPC placement, pleural space infection occurred in 10% of the population with 2.5% mortality secondary to sepsis due to empyema. Importantly, only 2 cases of electrolyte imbalance or renal failure related to IPC placement were reported, which may suggest a superior safety profile compared with reported complications of conventional chest tubes. This difference may be related to the volume/day drained. While most conventional chest tubes are placed with purpose of complete evacuation of the pleural space, IPCs are drained at maximum of 1 L/every other day schedule or no more than 1 L/d on symptomatic days. The primary goal of an IPC is symptom palliation and not pleural space evacuation.

Spontaneous pleurodesis rate of 28% to 33% with IPCs may represent an overestimated number because many of the patients who have achieved "pleurodesis" in these studies have done so after receiving liver transplant.

Table 1
Indwelling pleural catheters in hepatic hydrothorax

Study/HH Ones	Study Design	Sample Size	Palliative vs Bridge to Transplant	Patient-Centric Outcomes	Complications (%)	Pleurodesis (%)/Time to Pleurodesis
Chalhoub et al,[46] 2011	Single-center retrospective	8	Palliative	3.8 + 0.4/4 procedure satisfaction score	Exit site infection (12.5%)	Not recorded/ 73.6 ± 9 (mean, SD)
Bhatnagar et al,[47] 2014	Multicenter retrospective	19	Palliative	Not reported	• Pleural infection (5.3%) • Renal failure (5.3%) • Loculation (5.3%) • IPC dislodgement (5.3%)	11%/median of 222 d
Chen et al,[48] 2016	Single-center prospective	24	• Bridge to transplant (20%)	Not reported	• Pleural infection (16.7%)	33%/131.8 d (range, 14–287 d)
Kniese et al,[49] 2018	Single-center retrospective	62	• Bridge to transplant (53.2%)	Not reported	• Overall (35%) • Empyema (16%) • Death due to infection (5%) • Cellulitis (2%) • IPC dislodgement (10%)	14.5%/118, ±139.6 d (mean, SD)
Shojaee et al,[50] 2018	Multicenter rerrospective	79	• Palliative (73%) • Bridge to transplant (27%)	Not reported	• Pleural infection (10%) • Death due to infection (2.5%) • Renal failure (2.5%) • Pleural fluid leakage (5%) • Seroma (6%)	28%/median of 55 d (range, 10–370)
Frost et al,[51] 2020	Single-center Retrospective	27	Palliative	No additional intervention needed in 93% of total population	37.3% (cellulitis, IPC malfunction)	21%/etiology-specific time not available
Li et al,[52] 2019	Single-center retrospective	42	Palliative	Not reported	Pleural infection (7.1%)	51%/median of 115 d (interquartile range (IQR): 57–191 d)

Future studies need to focus on the role of IPC in patient-centric outcomes. In patients, who are liver transplant candidates and require frequent thoracentesis, multidisciplinary discussion is of paramount importance, and IPC should be only considered after careful examination of other options and disclosure of high infection complication rates and mortality to patients.[53]

Surgical management
Thoracoscopy, pleurodesis, and diaphragmatic defect repair Chemical pleurodesis and talc poudrage during video-assisted thoracoscopic surgery (VATS) for management of HH have been reported in case reports and small case series. Pooled data from 20 case reports and 13 case series (180 patients) showed pleurodesis success rate of 72% and pooled complication rate of 82%. Report of recurrence or partial response was not available due to varying follow-up intervals.[54]

Baseline disease severity assessed by Child–Turcotte–Pugh (CTP) classification is an important predictor of success. Patients with CTP C are shown to have a lower survival compared with CTP B (22% vs 50%) in a series of 11 patients with a median follow-up interval of 16 weeks.

Preoperative and postoperative optimization has been used in a surgical therapeutic modality known as the "4-step approach":(1) pneumoperitoneum induction for localization of diaphragmatic defects, (2) thoracoscopic pleurodesis, (3) postoperative continuous positive airway pressure (CPAP), and (4) drainage of ascites for abdominal decompression.[55,56]

Most retrospective case series in the literature include a small number of patients sampled over years to decades suggesting significant selection bias. This may also suggest that in carefully examined cases after multidisciplinary discussion, select patients benefit from surgical approaches to refractory HH.

Diaphragmatic defect surgical closure is associated with high mortality and has shown success in carefully selected population, primarily patients with CTP A class who do not meet criteria for other treatment options.[9] This treatment could have a high failure rate due to poor visualization of diaphragmatic defects (12%) during VATS.[57]

Liver transplant Liver transplantation is a definitive treatment of choice for decompensated cirrhosis. A referral for transplant evaluation should be made for patients with HH who are not already evaluated. Posttransplant outcomes are comparable for patients with HH with patients without HH.[58]

A retrospective study of 3487 patients with cirrhosis and PE showed that the most important determinant of the 3-year survival was liver transplantation. One- to 3-year mortality was 21.7% in patients who underwent liver transplantation compared with 77.5% in the nonliver transplant group.

Multidisciplinary discussion-based management

The overall short- and long-term outcome of a patient with HH is directly related to their candidacy for liver transplantation. Management of refractory HH needs multidisciplinary discussion among hepatology, pulmonary, transplant surgery, and interventional radiology. Despite the retrospective, single-center nature of most existing studies in the management of HH and significant selection bias in different therapeutic options, the literature has consistently shown that some of these management strategies carry significant morbidity and mortality.

Additionally, most of the studied palliative and therapeutic interventions of HH have not examined patient-centric outcomes. For these reasons, the palliative benefit of interventions should be balanced against potential risks and their downstream ramifications, such as exclusion from the transplant list. These interventions should also take into account patients' MELD score, history of prior hepatic encephalopathy, and numerous other predictive factors of outcomes in various interventions. As such, the care of a patient with cirrhosis and HH is one that should be highly personalized.

HEART FAILURE AND CARDIAC-INDUCED EFFUSION

Congestive heart failure (CHF) is the most common cause of transudative PE with an estimated 500,000 cases reported annually in the United States.[59] An estimated 87% of patients presenting with decompensated heart failure have PE on presentation.[60]

Presence of refractory PE in the setting of decompensated CHF has a 1-year mortality of 50%.[61] Most common presentation of CHF-induced PE is bilateral (70%), although unilateral right-sided (21%) and left-sided (9%) effusion can be seen.[62]

Pathophysiology

Primary mechanism for cardiac induced effusion is fluid entry from the lung interstitium into the pleural space.[63] The buildup of hydrostatic pressure in alveolar capillaries as a result of increased end diastolic left ventricular and left atrial pressure leads to increase in interstitial fluid. The fluid then moves to the pleural space form interstitial space due to pressure gradient. Additionally, due to increased downstream venous pressure, lymphatic flow is reduced and leads to fluid accumulation. Additionally, increased left atrial pressure or isolated right heart failure can result in elevated systemic venous pressure and enhanced fluid production and filtration from the parietal pleura and decreased lymphatic drainage due to pressure gradient.

Diagnostic Workup

CHF is the most common cause of bilateral PE. When the clinical presentation is that of decompensated heart failure, cardiomegaly, and bilateral PE, a clinical diagnosis can be made without thoracentesis and fluid analysis. If there are clinical suspicions of infection or presence of an underlying malignancy, diagnostic thoracentesis may be necessary.

A similar approach can be applied to unilateral effusions in the absence of other suspicious etiologies and clinical presentation of heart failure with N-Terminal Pro-B-Type Natriuretic Peptide (NT-proBNP) levels greater than 1500 pg. In response to ventricular distention, natriuretic peptides are released, and serum levels of NT-proBNP are greatly valuable in the diagnosis of CHF-induced PE. A pleural fluid NT-proBNP level greater than 1500 pg is shown to have a sensitivity of 94% and specificity of 91%, for diagnosing CHF-induced PE in a meta-analysis, although serum levels of NT-proBNP were also comparable with similar results.[64] A serum NT-proBNP level greater than 1500 pg^{ml-1} is diagnostic of cardiac-induced PE.[65,66] However, unilateral effusion with atypical features, such as large unilateral effusions (occupying 2/3 of hemithorax) or presence of pleuritic chest pain or fever, warrants fluid analysis including microbiology and cytology.

Although CHF is the most common cause of transudative PE, many CHF-induced effusions in patients treated with diuretics are pseudoexudates by Light's criteria. Serum albumin-PF gradient greater than 1.2 g/dl or a serum pleural fluid protein gradient of more than 3.1 g/dL can recategorize these effusions as transudates.

When the patient continues to be symptomatic despite optimization of medical therapy, therapeutic thoracentesis is indicated for symptom management.[67]

In summary, diagnosis of CHF-induced PE is usually established clinically in bilateral effusions and does not require pleural fluid analysis. However, in select cases where infection or malignancy is suspected, diagnostic and therapeutic thoracentesis should be performed.

Ultrasound examination of the pleural space is helpful in diagnosis and typically shows an unechoic nonseptated simple effusion.[68]

Management of Pleural Effusion Secondary to Heart Failure

Management of excess fluid production

Medical management with focus on cardiac function optimization is the mainstay of therapy. Most cardiac-induced PEs will resolve with diuresis. In a prospective study of patients with decompensated heart failure, optimization of cardiac function with oxygen, digoxin, nitrates, sympathomimetic agents, synthetic α natriuretic peptides, and diuretics lead to resolution of effusion in 89% of patients. Loop diuretics are mainstay of therapy,[69] as well as maintaining a negative sodium balance with minimal activation of neurohormonal pathways.

Unfortunately, 30% to 50% of patients with decompensated heart failure become refractory to medical therapy annually due to adverse events such as renal failure and electrolyte imbalance, hypotension, and syncope.[61]

Thoracentesis

Thoracentesis is the primary method in the management of refractory cardiac-induced effusion. Frequent thoracentesis may be necessary for symptom management and can be complex due to the combination of dual antiplatelets and anticoagulation therapy in many patients with decompensated heart failure. Although the risk of pleural procedures on these medications has not been specifically assessed in the population with CHF, Dangers and colleagues[70] noted that among 182 patient who were on antiplatelet therapy compared with 942 who were not, the 24-h incidence of bleeding was 3.23% (95% CI, 1.08%-5.91%) in the antiplatelet group and 0.96% (95% CI, 0.43%- .60%) in the control group. Bleeding was significantly associated with antiplatelet therapy in multivariate analysis (OR = 4.13; 95% CI = 1.01–17.03; P = .044).[70] Frequent thoracentesis can also be a significant burden and limit quality of life. Although this has never been studied directly, Greener and colleagues,[71] studied factors leading to palliative care consultation among inpatients with advanced heart failure (HF) and found that thoracentesis was the most significant factor (OR = 4.125, 95% CI = 2.023–8.411) on multivariable analysis.

Indwelling pleural catheters

The use of IPCs for CHF-induced PE was first reported in 2009[72] in a small case series (n = 5). Majid and colleagues[73] compared thoracoscopic talc pleurodesis plus IPC versus IPC alone in CHF-induced PE. All patients experienced symptomatic palliation. Spontaneous pleurodesis occurred in 29% of the IPC group over a median of 66 days as compared with 11.5 days in the talc poudrage group, and all patients reported significant symptomatic improvement. Catheter-related infection was reported among 2 participants and was treated with antibiotics alone without catheter removal. In a propensity-matched study by Freeman and colleagues, IPC was compared with thoracoscopic pleurodesis. Patients with IPC had a shorter hospital stay (2 ± 2 days, =<0.001), lower operative morbidity of 2.5% compared with 20% in the thoracoscopic poudrage group, lower readmission rate, and lower mortality (0 vs 5%).

In a recent systematic review and meta-analysis on management of IPCs for non-MPEs, 325 patients from 13 studies were included. CHF-induced PE was the most common cause (50%) of non-MPEs requiring IPC placement. Spontaneous pleurodesis

Table 2
Indwelling pleural catheters in CHF-induced refractory effusion

Study/CHF Ones	Study Design	Sample Size	Symptom Palliation/Patient-Centric Outcomes	Complications (%)	Pleurodesis (%) and Time to Pleurodesis
Herlihy et al,[72] 2009	Single-center retrospective case series	5	NYHA class improved from IV to II	• Empyema: 40% • Death due to empyema (20%)	Not recorded/not recorded
Chalhoub et al,[46] 2011	Single-center retrospective	13	3.8 + 0.4/4 procedure satisfaction score	None	Not recorded/ 113 + 36 d
Srour et al,[76] 2013	Single-center prospective	43	Dyspnea index (BDI, 2.24; 95% CI, 1.53–2.94 vs TDI, 6.19; 95% CI, 5.56–6.82)	• Moderate to large pneumothorax (possibly ex vacuo) (11.6%)	29%/66 d (IQR, 34–242 d)
Freeman et al,[75] 2014	Single-center retrospective propensity matched (IPC vs talc pleurodesis)	40 in the IPC group	Symptom palliation in all patients	None	35%/mean of 150 d
Bhatnagar et al,[47] 2014	Multicenter retrospective	9	Not reported	• Acute renal failure (11%)	44%/median of 38 d
Majid et al,[77] 2016, group 1	Single-center retrospective (Talc pleurodesis + IPC)	15	Immediate postprocedure symptom relief in all patients	• Cellulitis (13%) • Periprocedural hypotension (6%)	80%/median of 11.5 d (range, 2–22 d)
Majid et al,[77] 2016, group 2	Single-center retrospective (IPC alone)	28	Immediate post-procedure symptom relief in all patients	• 3.5% Empyema • 3.5% CPPE • 3.5% Cellulitis	25%/median of 66 d (range, 31–205 d)
Frost et al,[51] 2020	Single-center retrospective	30	No additional intervention needed in 93% of total population	• 16.7% complication (cellulitis, IPC malfunction)	24%/etiology-specific time not available

Abbreviations: BDI, baseline dyspnea index; CHF, congestive heart failure; CPPE, complex parapneumonic effusion; d, day; TDI, traditional dyspnae index.

was achieved in 42.1% (95% CI = 20.1%-64.1%) of CHF-induced PEs. The median time to pleurodesis ranged from 66 to 150 days.[74]

Although most reported studies to date are single center, retrospective with potential selection bias, these results suggest that IPC use in refractory CHF-induced PEs may lead to reduced length of hospital stay and provide symptomatic palliation to patients who would otherwise undergo frequent thoracenteses (Table 2).[46,47,51,72,75–77]

Pleurodesis

Literature on chemical pleurodesis in CHF-induced PE is scant and often includes single-center retrospective studies with heterogeneous population of nonmalignant etiology. In a study comparing IPC drainage (n = 28) with thoracoscopic talc poudrage plus IPC (n = 15) in patients with CHF-induced PEs,[73] the talc poudrage group achieved 80% pleurodesis compared with 25% in the IPC-only group. The median time to IPC removal was 11.5 days (2–22 days). The potential safety and efficacy of IPCs in this study is also confirmed in a propensity-matched comparison of IPC and thoracoscopic pleurodesis by Freeman and colleagues.[75] Patients were divided in 2 groups of 40, with New York heart Association (NYHA) class III or IV HF with no significant difference in age, sex, and functional class. At 6-month follow-up, there was no significant difference in palliation. The patient who underwent pleurodesis had a longer hospital stay of 6 ± 4 days, 23% readmission rate, and 5% mortality. An overall morbidity of 20% was reported in the pleurodesis group as compared with 2.5% in the IPC group with complications including but not limited to respiratory insufficiency, pulmonary embolism, and atrial fibrillation. Results of this study favored use of IPC for palliation compared with thoracoscopic pleurodesis. Prospective randomized trials with focus on patient-centric outcomes comparing chemical pleurodesis versus IPC in patients with refractory CHF-induced PEs are required to further assess their utility.

Prognosis

The presence of PEs in the setting of CHF does not portend a poor outcome. Instead, a refractory PE carries a poor prognosis because it indicates inadequate response to therapy in patients with decompensated heart failure. In one study, PEs found incidentally on routine transthoracic echocardiography (TTE) had 1- and 5 year survival rates of 81% and 70%, respectively.[78] In a study examining the association between PE and 6-month mortality, there was no association with mortality or hospital readmission, with relative risk of 1.393 (95% CI =

0.644–3.014).[79] The effusions mentioned in these studies however were small and did not require thoracentesis.

In a prospective single-center study of patients with non-MPEs by Walker and colleagues,[61] 1-year mortality was as high as 50% [HR = 0.61 (0.44–0.84); P = .02] in patients with CHF-induced effusion (n = 86), which is comparable with 1-year mortality rate (46%) of patients with acute decompensated heart failure admitted to intensive coronary care units.[80] Patients with HH (n = 12) had 1-year mortality of 25% [Hazard Ratio (HR) = 0.23 (0.07–0.71); P = .011];[72] however, mortality is reported to be as high as 48% in studies with larger population of HH.[31]

SUMMARY

Although HF-induced PE and HH are transudative non-MPEs, they are markers of disease severity, associated with significant morbidity and mortality and carry a high symptomatic burden. A systemic and multidisciplinary approach is often required when these effusions become refractory to medical therapy. Treatment decisions depend on goals of treatment and palliation and often need to be highly personalized, particularly in patients with ESLD who maybe future transplant candidates.

DISCLOSURE

The authors have nothing to disclose.

REFERENCES

1. Mercer RM, Corcoran JP, Porcel JM, et al. Interpreting pleural fluid results. Clin Med 2019;19(3):213–7.
2. Research and statistics. GOV.UK. Available at: https://www.gov.uk/search/research-and-statistics. Accessed March 30, 2021.
3. Porcel JM. Management of refractory hepatic hydrothorax. Curr Opin Pulm Med 2014;20(4):352–7.
4. Yoon JH, Kim HJ, Jun CH, et al. Various treatment modalities in hepatic hydrothorax: what is safe and effective? Yonsei Med J 2019;60(10):944–51.
5. Emerson PA, Davies JH. Hydrothorax complicating ascites. Lancet Lond Engl 1955;268(6862):487–8.
6. Johnston RF, Loo RV. Hepatic hydrothorax; studies to determine the source of the fluid and report of thirteen cases. Ann Intern Med 1964;61:385–401.
7. Dumont AE, Mulholland JH. Flow rate and composition of thoracic-duct lymph in patients with cirrhosis. N Engl J Med 1960;263:471–4.
8. Huang P-M, Chang Y-L, Yang C-Y, et al. The morphology of diaphragmatic defects in hepatic hydrothorax: thoracoscopic finding. J Thorac Cardiovasc Surg 2005;130(1):141–5.

9. Huang P-M, Kuo S-W, Chen J-S, et al. Thoraco-scopic mesh repair of diaphragmatic defects in he-patic hydrothorax: a 10-year experience. Ann Thorac Surg 2016;101(5):1921–7.

10. Runyon BA. Paracentesis of ascitic fluid. A safe procedure. Arch Intern Med 1986;146(11): 2259–61.

11. Xiol X, Castellote J, Cortes-Beut R, et al. Usefulness and complications of thoracentesis in cirrhotic pa-tients. Am J Med 2001;111(1):67–9.

12. Meisel S, Shamiss A, Thaler M, et al. Pleural fluid to serum bilirubin concentration ratio for the separation of transudates from exudates. Chest 1990;98(1): 141–4.

13. Bielsa S, Porcel JM, Castellote J, et al. Solving the Light's criteria misclassification rate of cardiac and hepatic transudates. Respirology 2012;17(4): 721–6.

14. Dumont AE, Mulholland JH. Alterations in thoracic duct lymph flow in hepatic cirrhosis: significance in portal hypertension. Ann Surg 1962;156(4): 668–75.

15. Bhattacharya A, Mittal BR, Biswas T, et al. Radioiso-tope scintigraphy in the diagnosis of hepatic hydro-thorax. J Gastroenterol Hepatol 2001;16(3):317–21.

16. Ajmi S, Sfar R, Nouira M, et al. Role of the peritoneo-pleural pressure gradient in the genesis of hepatic hydrothorax. An isotopic study. Gastroentérologie Clin Biol 2008;32(8):729–33.

17. Schuster DM, Mukundan SJ, Small W, et al. The use of the diagnostic radionuclide ascites scan to facili-tate treatment decisions for hepatic hydrothorax. Clin Nucl Med 1998;23(1):16–8.

18. Garcia–Tsao G. Current management of the compli-cations of cirrhosis and portal hypertension: variceal hemorrhage, ascites, and spontaneous bacterial peritonitis. Gastroenterology 2001;120(3):726–48.

19. Garbuzenko DV, Arefyev NO. Hepatic hydrothorax: an update and review of the literature. World J Hep-atol 2017;9(31):1197–204.

20. Morando F, Rosi S, Gola E, et al. Adherence to a moderate sodium restriction diet in outpatients with cirrhosis and ascites: a real-life cross-sectional study. Liver Int 2015;35(5):1508–15.

21. Kumar S, Sarin SK. Paradigms in the management of hepatic hydrothorax: past, present, and future. Hepatol Int 2013;7(1):80–7.

22. Siqueira F, Kelly T, Saab S. Refractory ascites. Gas-troenterol Hepatol 2009;5(9):647–56.

23. Kalambokis G, Fotopoulos A, Economou M, et al. Beneficial haemodynamic and renal sodium handling effects of combined midodrine and octreo-tide treatment in a cirrhotic patient with large hepatic hydrothorax and mild ascites. Nephrol Dial Transpl 2005;20(11):2583.

24. Sourianarayanane A, Barnes DS, McCullough AJ. Beneficial effect of midodrine in hypotensive

cirrhotic patients with refractory ascites. Gastroen-terol Hepatol 2011;7(2):132–4.

25. Rössle M, Siegerstetter V, Huber M, et al. The first decade of the transjugular intrahepatic portosyste-mic shunt (TIPS): state of the art. Liver 1998;18(2): 73–89.

26. Berzigotti A, Seijo S, Reverter E, et al. Assessing portal hypertension in liver diseases. Expert Rev Gastroenterol Hepatol 2013;7(2):141–55.

27. Casado M, Bosch J, García-Pagán JC, et al. Clinical events after transjugular intrahepatic portosystemic shunt: correlation with hemodynamic findings. Gastroenterology 1998;114(6):1296–303.

28. Kok B, Abraldes JG. Patient selection in Transjugular Intrahepatic Portosystemic Shunt (TIPS) for refrac-tory ascites and associated conditions. Curr Hepatol Rep 2019;18(2):197–205.

29. Hung ML, Lee EW. Role of transjugular intrahepatic portosystemic shunt in the management of portal hy-pertension: review and update of the literature. Clin Liver Dis 2019;23(4):737–54.

30. Young S, Bermudez J, Zhang L, et al. Transjugular intrahepatic portosystemic shunt (TIPS) placement: a comparison of outcomes between patients with hepatic hydrothorax and patients with refractory as-cites. Diagn Interv Imaging 2019;100(5):303–8.

31. Singh A, Bajwa A, Shujaat A. Evidence-based re-view of the management of hepatic hydrothorax. Respiration 2013;86(2):155–73.

32. Bercu ZL, Fischman AM, Kim E, et al. TIPS for refrac-tory ascites: a 6-year single-center experience with expanded polytetrafluoroethylene–covered stent-grafts. Am J Roentgenol 2015;204(3):654–61.

33. Perarnau JM, Le Gouge A, Nicolas C, et al. Covered vs. uncovered stents for transjugular intrahepatic portosystemic shunt: a randomized controlled trial. J Hepatol 2014;60(5):962–8.

34. Spencer EB, Cohen DT, Darcy MD. Safety and effi-cacy of transjugular intrahepatic portosystemic shunt creation for the treatment of hepatic hydrotho-rax. J Vasc Interv Radiol 2002;13(4):385–90.

35. Ault MJ, Rosen BT, Scher J, et al. Thoracentesis out-comes: a 12-year experience. Thorax 2015;70(2): 127–32.

36. McVay PA, Toy PT. Lack of increased bleeding after paracentesis and thoracentesis in patients with mild coagulation abnormalities. Transfusion 1991;31(2): 164–71.

37. Shojaee S, Khalid M, Kallingal G, et al. Repeat thor-acentesis in hepatic hydrothorax and non-hepatic hydrothorax effusions: a case-control study. Respir Int Rev Thorac Dis 2018;96(4):330–7.

38. Casoni GL, Gurioli C, Corso R, et al. Hemothorax by intercostal varicose veins in alcoholic liver cirrhosis. Respir Int Rev Thorac Dis 2010;80(1):71–2.

39. Banini BA, Alwatari Y, Stovall M, et al. Multidisci-plinary management of hepatic hydrothorax in

2020: an evidence-based review and guidance. Hepatology 2020;72(5):1851–63.

40. Runyon BA. Introduction to the revised American Association for the Study of Liver Diseases Practice Guideline management of adult patients with ascites due to cirrhosis 2012. Hepatology 2013;57(4): 1651–3.

41. Orman ES, Lok ASF. Outcomes of patients with chest tube insertion for hepatic hydrothorax. Hepatol Int 2009;3(4):582–6.

42. Runyon BA, Greenblatt M, Ming RH. Hepatic hydrothorax is a relative contraindication to chest tube insertion. Am J Gastroenterol 1986;81(7):566–7.

43. Liu LU, Haddadin HA, Bodian CA, et al. Outcome analysis of cirrhotic patients undergoing chest tube placement. Chest 2004;126(1):142–8.

44. Ridha A, Al-Abboodi Y, Fasullo M. The outcome of thoracentesis versus chest tube placement for hepatic hydrothorax in patients with cirrhosis: a nationwide analysis of the national inpatient sample. Gastroenterol Res Pract 2017;2017. https://doi.org/10.1155/2017/5872068.

45. Food and Drug Administration. PleurX pleural catheter and drainage kits. 2001. Rockville, MD. Available at: https://www.accessdata.fda.gov/cdrh_docs/pdf14/K141965.pdf.

46. Chalhoub M, Harris K, Castellano M, et al. The use of the PleurX catheter in the management of non-malignant pleural effusions. Chron Respir Dis 2011;8(3):185–91.

47. Bhatnagar R, Reid ED, Corcoran JP, et al. Indwelling pleural catheters for non-malignant effusions: a multicentre review of practice. Thorax 2014;69(10): 959–61.

48. Chen A, Massoni J, Jung D, et al. Indwelling tunneled pleural catheters for the management of hepatic hydrothorax. a pilot study. Ann Am Thorac Soc 2016;13(6):862–6.

49. Kniese C, Diab K, Ghabril M, et al. Indwelling pleural catheters in hepatic hydrothorax: a single-center series of outcomes and complications. Chest 2019; 155(2):307–14.

50. Shojaee S, Rahman N, Haas K, et al. Indwelling tunneled pleural catheters for refractory hepatic hydrothorax in patients with cirrhosis: a multicenter study. Chest 2019;155(3):546–53.

51. Frost N, Ruwwe-Glösenkamp C, Raspe M, et al. Indwelling pleural catheters for non- malignant pleural effusions: report on a single centre's 10 years of experience. BMJ Open Respir Res 2020;7(1). https://doi.org/10.1136/bmjresp-2019-000501.

52. Li P, Hosseini S, Zhang T, et al. Clinical predictors of successful and earlier removal of indwelling pleural catheters in benign pleural effusions. Respir Int Rev Thorac Dis 2019;98(3):239–45.

53. Mirrakhimov AE, Ayach T, Gray A. Indwelling tunneled pleural catheters for the management of hepatic hydrothorax: a word of caution. Ann Am Thorac Soc 2016;13(8):1432.

54. Hou F, Qi X, Guo X. Effectiveness and safety of pleurodesis for hepatic hydrothorax: a systematic review and meta-analysis. Dig Dis Sci 2016;61(11): 3321–34.

55. Jung Y. Surgical treatment of hepatic hydrothorax: a "four-step approach. Ann Thorac Surg 2016;101(3): 1195–7.

56. Jung Y, Song SY, Na KJ, et al. Minimally invasive surgical strategy for refractory hepatic hydrothorax. Eur J Cardiothorac Surg 2020;57(5):881–7.

57. Cerfolio RJ, Bryant AS. Efficacy of video-assisted thoracoscopic surgery with talc pleurodesis for porous diaphragm syndrome in patients with refractory hepatic hydrothorax. Ann Thorac Surg 2006; 82(2):457–9.

58. Xiol X, Tremosa G, Castellote J, et al. Liver transplantation in patients with hepatic hydrothorax. Transpl Int 2005;18(6):672–5.

59. Walker S, Shojaee S. Nonmalignant pleural effusions: are they as benign as we think?. In: Maskell NA, Laursen CB, Lee YCG, et al, editors. Pleural disease. European Respiratory Society; 2020. p. 218–31. https://doi.org/10.1183/2312508X.10024119.

60. Kataoka H. Pericardial and pleural effusions in decompensated chronic heart failure. Am Heart J 2000;139(5):918–23.

61. Walker SP, Morley AJ, Stadon L, et al. Nonmalignant pleural effusions: a prospective study of 356 consecutive unselected patients. Chest 2017; 151(5):1099–105.

62. Porcel JM, Vives M. Distribution of pleural effusion in congestive heart failure. South Med J 2006;99(1):98–9.

63. Kinasewitz GT, Jones KR. Effusions from cardiac diseases. In: Effusions from cardiac diseases. 2nd edition. CRC Press; 2008. p. 315–21.

64. Han Z-J, Wu X-D, Cheng J-J, et al. Diagnostic accuracy of natriuretic peptides for heart failure in patients with pleural effusion: a systematic review and updated meta-analysis. PLoS One 2015;10(8). https://doi.org/10.1371/journal.pone.0134376.

65. Marinho FCA, Vargas FS, Fabri J, et al. Clinical usefulness of B-type natriuretic peptide in the diagnosis of pleural effusions due to heart failure. Respirol Carlton Vic 2011;16(3):495–9.

66. Porcel JM. Pleural fluid biomarkers: beyond the Light criteria. Clin Chest Med 2013;34(1):27–37.

67. Collins TR, Sahn SA. Thoracocentesis. Clinical value, complications, technical problems, and patient experience. Chest 1987;91(6):817–22.

68. Kataoka H. Ultrasound pleural effusion sign as a useful marker for identifying heart failure worsening in established heart failure patients during follow-up. Congest Heart Fail Greenwich Conn 2012; 18(5):272–7.

69. Faris RF, Flather M, Purcell H, et al. Diuretics for heart failure. Cochrane Database Syst Rev 2012;(2):CD003838.

70. Dangers L, Giovannelli J, Mangiapan G, et al. Antiplatelet drugs and risk of bleeding after bedside pleural procedures: a national multicenter cohort study. Chest 2020. https://doi.org/10.1016/j.chest.2020.10.092.

71. Greener DT, Quill T, Amir O, et al. Palliative care referral among patients hospitalized with advanced heart failure. J Palliat Med 2014;17(10):1115–20.

72. Herlihy JP, Loyalka P, Gnananandh J, et al. PleurX catheter for the management of refractory pleural effusions in congestive heart failure. Tex Heart Inst J 2009;36(1):38–43.

73. Majid A, Kheir F, Fashjian M, et al. Tunneled pleural catheter placement with and without talc poudrage for treatment of pleural effusions due to congestive heart failure. Ann Am Thorac Soc 2015. https://doi.org/10.1513/AnnalsATS.201507-471BC.

74. Patil M, Dhillon SS, Attwood K, et al. Management of benign pleural effusions using indwelling pleural catheters: a systematic review and meta- analysis. Chest 2017;151(3):626–35.

75. Freeman RK, Ascioti AJ, Dake M, et al. A propensity-matched comparison of pleurodesis or tunneled pleural catheter for heart failure patients with recurrent pleural effusion. Ann Thorac Surg 2014;97(6):1872–7.

76. Srour N, Potechin R, Amjadi K. Use of indwelling pleural catheters for cardiogenic pleural effusions. Chest 2013;144(5):1603–8.

77. Majid A, Kheir F, Fashjian M, et al. Tunneled pleural catheter placement with and without talc poudrage for treatment of pleural effusions due to congestive heart failure. Ann Am Thorac Soc 2016;13(2):212–6.

78. Ercan S, Davutoglu V, Altunbas G, et al. Prognostic role of incidental pleural effusion diagnosed during echocardiographic evaluation. Clin Cardiol 2014;37(2):115–8.

79. Davutoglu V, Yildirim C, Kucukaslan H, et al. Prognostic value of pleural effusion, CA-125 and NT-proBNP in patients with acute decompensated heart failure. Kardiol Pol 2010;68(7):771–8.

80. Zannad F, Mebazaa A, Juillière Y, et al. Clinical profile, contemporary management and one-year mortality in patients with severe acute heart failure syndromes: the EFICA study☆. Eur J Heart Fail 2006;8(7):697–705.

Parapneumonic Effusion and Empyema

Dinesh N. Addala, BA, BMBCH, MRCP[a,b,*], Eihab O. Bedawi, MBBS, MRCP[a,b],
Najib M. Rahman, MD, DPhil[a,c]

KEYWORDS

- Pleural infection • Empyema • Parapneumonic effusion

KEY POINTS

- Pleural infection is a spectrum of conditions. Simple parapneumonic effusion refers to pneumonia associated with pleural effusion, whereas complicated parapneumonic effusion and empyema refer to infection of the pleural space.
- The incidence of parapneumonic effusion and empyema is increasing and forms a significant health care burden in terms of mortality and costs.
- The diagnosis of pleural infection must be made using clinical parameters and markers of infection along with sampling of pleural fluid, with pleural fluid pH < 7.2 being the most accurate rapid biomarker.
- Effective treatment of simple parapneumonic effusion can be achieved with antibiotics alone; however, complicated parapneumonic effusion and empyema require early drainage and broad-spectrum antibiotic treatment
- For those that fail drainage and antibiotic treatment, the use of intrapleural tissue plasminogen activator and deoxyribonuclease is safe and effective, and may prevent the need for surgical intervention.

INTRODUCTION

Pleural infection represents a common and often life-threatening condition with an annual incidence of 80,000 across the United Kingdom and United States,[1] reported 30-day mortality of up to 10.5%,[2] and 1-year mortality of more than 19%.[3,4] More than half of the patients with pneumonia develop an associated pleural effusion, with higher morbidity in all groups, including those with "simple" parapneumonic effusions and those with proven infection of the pleural space (empyema or complicated parapneumonic effusion [CPPE]).[5] The clinical burden of parapneumonic effusion and empyema cannot be quantified in terms of mortality alone, with a recent systematic review finding the mean

hospital stay associated with these conditions totaling 19 days, while arising in a frequently co-morbid patient cohort.[5] The costs associated with admission are high, with annual estimates from the United States totaling $500 million,[1] a figure that reflects the high levels of pharmacologic and procedural care required to treat these conditions, including pleural drainage, the increasing use of intrapleural enzyme therapy (IET) with combination tissue plasminogen activator and deoxyribonuclease, as well as surgery.

Although the understanding of microbiology in pleural infection is growing, the cornerstone of treatment remains prompt drainage and initiation of antibiotic therapy, often empirically. Surgery remains predominantly a rescue therapy, used when fluid control and clinical response have not been

Disclosure: The authors have nothing to disclose.
[a] Oxford University Hospitals NHS Foundation Trust; [b] Department of Respiratory Medicine, Churchill Hospital, Old Road, Headington, Oxford OX3 7LE, UK; [c] Oxford NIHR Biomedical Research Centre, John Radcliffe Hospital, Headington OX3 9DU, UK
* Corresponding author.
E-mail address: dnaddala@gmail.com

Clin Chest Med 42 (2021) 637–647
https://doi.org/10.1016/j.ccm.2021.08.001
0272-5231/21/© 2021 Elsevier Inc. All rights reserved.

achieved by these methods; however, the debate regarding early surgery versus medical treatment has not been definitively answered, with ongoing clinical trials looking to provide clarity.[6] The current strategies can often lead to the aforementioned lengthy hospital stays and prolonged courses of antibiotic treatment.[7] Further evidence is required to optimize diagnostics and management of parapneumonic effusion and empyema.

There has been notable progress in several areas over recent years. The characterization of the unique microbiology in pleural infection facilitates clearer guidance in empirical antimicrobial treatment.[8] The routine use of bedside ultrasound in pleural diagnostics has improved the safety of procedures[9] and the specific computed tomography (CT) imaging features of pleural infection are increasingly recognized, which may further improve early diagnosis and treatment.[10] The use of IET provides a valuable added treatment strategy to the decades-old paradigm. This article reviews the current evidence and recent progress in the diagnosis, management, and outcome data in parapneumonic effusion and empyema.

DEFINITIONS AND PATHOPHYSIOLOGY

This article refers frequently to simple parapneumonic effusion, CPPE and empyema. Although this suggests distinct entities, in many patients, there will be a continuous progression through these phases. "Pleural infection" is a term used to encompass CPPE and empyema, referring to the likely presence of bacteria in the pleural space.

Simple parapneumonic effusion is characterized by pleural effusion associated with parenchymal consolidation. Typically, pleural fluid will be free-flowing on ultrasound, not accompanied by pleural enhancement on CT and on aspiration will display a pH>7.2 with negative microbiological culture.[11] It is often the result of undertreated pneumonia, increased pleural membrane permeability secondary to inflammation, and fluid leak into the pleural space. This is known as phase I (exudative).[12]

CPPE is associated with ongoing inflammation of the pleura. The term "complicated" refers to the need for drainage to achieve resolution, and is often associated with bacterial invasion and phagocytes within the pleural space, and the development of fibrin stranding within the pleural fluid. In clinical practice, the pleural fluid pH is likely to be less than 7.2, LDH greater than 1000, and may be culture positive, while ultrasound may demonstrate septation or loculation. This is referred to as phase II (fibrinopurulent), with reduction in fibrinolysis within the pleural space and release of proinflammatory cytokines such as TNF-α.[13]

Empyema is defined by frank pus in the pleural space. It may be associated with either phase II or phase III (organizing phase). The organizing phase is associated with the possible presence of discrete locules on imaging and enhancing visceral pleura on CT. This corresponds with the formation of visceral pleural fibrosis, and fibroblast proliferation within the pleural space. Of note, pleural thickening in this phase may be associated with reduced drainage success and higher likelihood of surgical intervention being required.[14]

DIAGNOSIS
Clinical Presentation

The classical description of nonresolving pneumonic symptoms such as cough, sputum production, and fever, in conjunction with chest pain and the examination findings of a pleural effusion are among the more straightforward pointers to pleural infection. The acuity and severity of these symptoms will often direct a clinician to undertake with urgency the necessary steps of initiating antimicrobial cover and undertaking prompt drainage of pleural fluid. Pleural infection in the cohort of patients with baseline frailty such as the elderly and those with undiagnosed chronic aspiration can be more challenging to establish. This cohort may present with nonspecific constitutional symptoms such as anorexia and malaise with a more insidious presentation.[15] Clinicians must maintain a high index of suspicion to diagnose pleural infection in this subset of patients, in whom delay in diagnosis is common and can lead to higher mortality and requirement of surgical intervention.[16] The overlap in symptoms can cause significant uncertainty between infective and malignant pathology, another potential cause of delayed treatment.

To this end, scoring systems to facilitate risk stratification and prognosis have been of interest. Of these, the RAPID score is the most robustly studied, using age, urea, hospital-acquired infection, and nonpurulence of pleural fluid to predict poor outcome at presentation.[17] RAPID was derived and validated using the MIST-1 and MIST-2 trial cohorts, respectively. The results of the prospective PILOT study (n = 542) stratified patients into low, medium, and high risk using these parameters, with mortality at 3 months of 2.3%, 9.2%, and 29.3%, respectively.[3] The validation of this risk score provides clinicians with an important tool for early identification of patients likely to experience poor outcomes. Targeting pleural infection treatment based on RAPID category is the next logical area for research.

Imaging

The mainstays of imaging in pleural infection remain plain chest radiography, ultrasound, and contrast-enhanced CT. Findings from each are described in **Fig. 1**. Plain chest radiographs are readily available in emergency departments and provide timely information on presence and volume of pleural fluid (see **Fig. 1**A), consolidation, and occasionally the presence of lung abscess. The presence of a pleural effusion should prompt evaluation with ultrasound imaging, which facilitates more detailed assessment with respect to etiology of effusion, and the potential requirement for drainage.[18] Ultrasound findings in transudates or simple parapneumonic effusion will often display anechoic fluid, with little or no septations and freely floating lung.[19] Echogenic fluid appearances point to an inflammatory exudate, or frank pus (see **Fig. 1**B). Septations indicate the presence of fibrin within the effusion and loculations represent discrete collections of fluid that do not communicate. The significance of septations in prognosticating patients with CPPE or empyema is unclear, with data from the PILOT study suggesting that the presence and number of septations did not impact upon 3-month mortality, but did reduce the performance of the RAPID clinical risk score.[20] Loculations can predict drainage failure and individual locules can display different biochemical features when sampled.[21] In cases of loculated pleural effusions, clinicians are advised to make drainage decisions using all clinical information rather than simply relying on the pleural fluid pH or biochemistry from a single locule.

There is a role for CT imaging in pleural infection although timing and indication remain points of discussion. The high sensitivity of contrast CT for complicating pathologies, such as abscess, aberrant drain positioning, and bronchopleural fistula, provides a clear role before IET, surgery, or in patients with worsening clinical parameters 48 hours after drain placement. The high prevalence (in more than 90% of patients with pleural infection)[22]

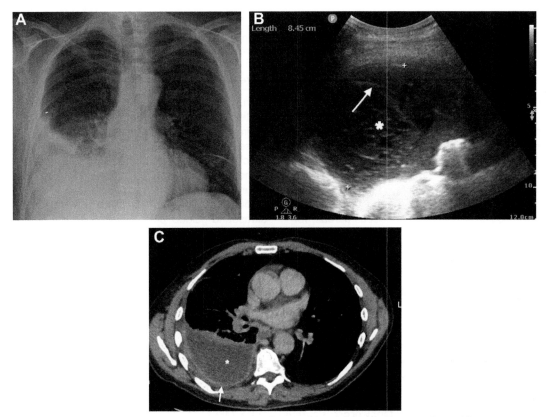

Fig. 1. Imaging modalities demonstrating empyema. All images (*A–C*) from the same patient with proven empyema. (*A*) Chest radiograph demonstrating right lower/mid zone consolidation and pleural effusion. (*B*) Pleural ultrasound image demonstrating echogenic effusion (*white star*) and septation (*white arrow*). (*C*) CT image demonstrating right-sided empyema (*white star*) and parietal pleural enhancement with thickening (*white arrow*).

of parietal pleural enhancement and thickening in pleural infection (see **Fig. 1**C) is well described as the correlate of the inflammatory response of the pleura to pleural infection and the presence of a fibrin capsule.[23] A role for CT scanning earlier may therefore exist as a "rule out" test in patients with suspected pleural sepsis in whom invasive sampling may be contraindicated, such as those on therapeutic anticoagulation. CT imaging with contrast in the pleural venous phase (images captured 20–60s postcontrast injection) provides the optimal means for assessment.

Pleural Fluid Diagnostics

Although the history and basic imaging can alert the clinician to the possibility of pleural infection, the most reliable definitive step for differentiating simple parapneumonic effusion and pleural infection is pleural fluid sampling for biochemistry and microbiological culture.

Microbiology

Microbiological culture is paramount in establishing a causative organism and determining antibiotic choice in the treatment of pleural infection. **Table 1** illustrates the most common organisms identified by setting. The organisms implicated in pneumonia and pleural infection differ, reflecting the divergent host environment of the lung parenchyma versus the relatively hypoxic pleural space.[24] When considering empirical antibiotic choice, it is important to note the variation in microbiology by demographics, including country, age, and community or health care setting.[25,26] A recent systematic review encompassing 10,241 patients is the largest to date on the bacteriology of pleural infection. Overall, the most common organism isolated was *Staphylococcus aureus*, followed by Viridans streptoccocus group, with

Klebsiella and Pseudomonas following these. Of concern to clinicians should be that within *S aureus* isolates, only 67% of community-acquired and 42% of hospital-acquired infections were methicillin sensitive. These findings reenforce the role of oropharyngeal flora harboring organisms causative of pleural infection, with pneumococci and viridans being common isolates, although the mechanisms by which these gain access to the pleura are not entirely clear. Postulated mechanisms include hematogenous spread in the context of poor dental hygiene and recurrent aspiration.[8]

When considering community-acquired versus hospital-acquired infection, the relative risk factors of inpatients must be considered, with higher rates of aspiration and hospital-acquired pneumonia. Accordingly, the rates of gram-negative gut bacteria are higher as is the proportion of methicillin-resistant *S aureus* (MRSA).[27]

Further challenges arise when considering that multiple bacterial isolates occur from almost 13% of cases, despite the relatively poor yield of pleural fluid culture. This almost doubles in metagenomic studies using bacterial DNA sequencing,[28] emphasizing the need for broad antimicrobial cover in pleural infection, even when culture results are positive.

Increasing the Pickup Rate-Technical Factors

With microbiological yield from pleural fluid being limited, consideration has been given to methods to improve culture sensitivity. The simplest of these is to use blood culture bottles for sampling, which increases yield by 20% compared with standard methods.[29] Postulating the nature of pleural fluid to be somewhat abrasive to bacterial proliferation, the AUDIO study illustrated that ultrasound-guided pleural biopsy at the time of chest drain insertion was safe and effective in

Table 1
Frequency of bacterial organisms isolated on pleural fluid culture[8]

	Community-Acquired	Hospital-Acquired
Gram positive	65.1%	51.5%
Gram negative	17.1%	37.5%
Anaerobe	17.8%	11%
Most common specific organism (descending order)	Viridans streptococci (*S milleri* most common) *Streptococcus pneumoniae* *Staphylococcus aureus* (MSSA > MRSA) Enterobacteria Klebsiella Pseudomonas	*Staphylococcus aureus* (MRSA > MSSA) Enterobacteria Enterococci Viridans streptococci Pseudomonas Klebsiella

increasing culture positivity by 25% compared with pleural fluid analysis alone.[30] If borne out in larger studies, the minimal extra equipment and resources required to facilitate this means pleural biopsy as a standard of care may be achievable in many centers. Finally, the use of polymerase chain reaction, targeting 16s ribosomal RNA and subsequent sequencing, has been shown in prospective analysis to increase sensitivity by 50% compared with standard pleural fluid culture.[31] Although impressive, barriers to widespread use include high costs, and amplification of bacterial isolates that are nonpathogenic, thus confounding the clinical picture. As the availability grows, this is an area to be explored further.

Biochemistry

Although positive microbiology is the gold standard in diagnosing CPPE or empyema and guiding antimicrobial choice, pleural fluid culture often requires days to establish and is negative in up to 40% of patients with pleural infection.[26] Hence, the use of pleural fluid biochemistry is valuable, with point of care or rapid turnaround laboratory testing available in most institutions. The presence of frank pus is diagnostic for empyema and further biochemical tests are not required. The primary parameters used are that of pH less than 7.2, glucose less than 2.2 mmol/L, and LDH greater than 1000IU/L to determine inflammatory pleural effusions, that direct treatment for pleural infection. Pleural fluid pH has proven to be the most specific, despite being first described by Light and colleagues in 1973.[32] Data from our own institution has shown that a significant proportion of patients with glucose less than 2.2 and LDH greater than 1000 do so secondary to noninfective diagnoses, the most common being malignancy and connective tissue disease.[33]

The Future of Biomarkers in Pleural Infection

The integration into standard care of biomarkers in both serum and pleural fluid has been relatively unchanged over decades.[7,32] With the growing use of procalcitonin, the performance of this in diagnosing pleural infection was assessed in a prospective clinical trial but disappointingly was found to be equivalent to serum C-reactive protein (CRP) and white cell count. One retrospective study has suggested that pleural fluid CRP greater than 100 can guide chest tube drainage[34]; however, prospective analysis is required. A recent observational study suggests that pleural fluid soluble urokinase plasminogen activator receptor has a high predictive value for IET and surgery requirement, another area that requires further studies.[35]

CLINICS CARE POINTS DIAGNOSTICS

- A high index of suspicion is required to promptly diagnose pleural infection
- Chest radiograph demonstrating a unilateral pleural effusion in the context of infective or constitutional symptoms should always follow on to ultrasound assessment and diagnostic sampling.
- Pleural fluid samples should be sent for culture and sensitivity along with biochemical analysis.
- Pleural fluid pH less than 7.2 remains to date the most accurate indication for drainage.
- The presence of locules on imaging of the pleural space should lower the threshold for chest tube insertion as different locules can display varying characteristics, and render normal biochemical parameters (eg, pH) less meaningful.

TREATMENT STRATEGIES
Antibiotics

Prompt initiation of antibiotics is essential in the management of pleural infection. In culture-positive pleural infection (blood or pleural fluid), targeted antibiotics are advised. In culture pending or negative cases, empirical broad-spectrum antimicrobial cover is indicated, according to local prevalence and resistance profiles.[8] In contrast to the treatment of pneumonia, cover for legionella and mycoplasma is not routinely required with atypical organisms rarely causing pleural infection.[26] Anaerobic cover can be achieved with metronidazole or clindamycin.[36] Gram-positive and gram-negative organisms should be treated, and penicillin-based antibiotics with a β-lactamase inhibitor or a third-generation cephalosporin are recommended.[7,37] Treatment of MRSA has been typically reserved for hospital-acquired infection;[38] however, with the increase in incidence of MRSA within community-associated cases, the addition of vancomycin should be considered in those not improving with standard antimicrobial therapy.

Most antibiotics achieve adequate penetration into the pleural space, with the notable exception of aminoglycosides, which should be avoided in pleural infection.[39] An area lacking in good quality evidence is the duration of antibiotic treatment required, and current practice is based on treatment paradigms in other deep-seated infections such as lung abscess[40] and small retrospective studies. The authors would thus recommend a minimum duration of 4 weeks of antimicrobial therapy (including intravenous and oral routes). There is emerging data that indicate shorter durations may be appropriate, with a small, underpowered randomized trial of 55 patients indicating that 2 weeks of amoxicillin-clavulanate was noninferior to 3 weeks in terms of symptom improvement and preventing recurrence of infection.[41] With the need for antimicrobial stewardship ever-growing, larger studies allowing modification of the current dogma would be welcome.

Chest Drain Insertion and Management

Simple parapneumonic effusions often resolve with antibiotics alone,[7,42] and do not routinely require drainage. Worsening clinical parameters of sepsis, enlarging effusion or the development of septations should prompt resampling of the effusion to assess for progression to CPPE or empyema. Early chest tube insertion is well established as one of the cornerstones in effectively treating CPPE and empyema with delayed insertion leading to increased mortality.[7,43] The seemingly logical premise that a larger diameter tube more readily allows drainage of viscous fluid has not been supported by retrospective analysis of a large randomized controlled trial (RCT) cohort (MIST-1; n = 405). Smaller bore tubes (<14 Fr) do not appear to worsen outcomes in this patient group, and importantly result in reduced pain and improved comfort.[44] The evidence for this is corroborated by other retrospective case series and the MIST-2 trial subanalysis showing no difference in treatment outcomes between small and large bore chest tubes.[10,45,46] Data do exist to suggest that small bore tubes may block more readily; however, this can be overcome by regular saline flush.[47,48] Ultimately, a prospective study, specifically designed to answer the question of drain size, is required.

Intrapleural Enzyme Therapy

Over the last decade, the role of IET has been rife with interest, presenting a viable option to improve drainage and outcomes in pleural infection. The failure of drainage in CPPE and empyema can be attributed to 2 predominating factors: the presence of fibrin septations and increased viscosity due to dead leukocytes and bacterial biofilms. It is perhaps not surprising therefore that the use of intrapleural fibrinolytic monotherapy has not been a success, despite its use dating back over 70 years.[49] In what is to date the largest prospective RCT in pleural infection, the MIST-1 trial reported that intrapleural streptokinase alone did not improve mortality or rates of surgery in pleural infection,[50] the theory prevailing that streptokinase targeted only the fibrin septations, without

addressing viscosity. Thus, the addition of deoxyribonuclease (DNAse) came into focus. DNAse reduces viscosity by breaking down extracellular uncoiled DNA from dead bacteria and leukocytes.[51]

The MIST-2 trial included 210 patients, with the arm that administered alteplase (tPA) in combination with DNAse, resulting in a significant improvement in chest radiograph opacity (the primary endpoint), duration of hospital stay, and need for surgery versus control. In addition, this was associated with a favorable safety profile, specifically a low bleeding risk (3.8%), which has been borne out in larger case series.[10,52] Monotherapy with either agent did not improve outcomes. Despite the encouraging findings, the use of these agents as part of routine care could not be recommended immediately, with two-thirds of pleural infection cases resolving with chest tube drainage and antibiotics alone[50] and small numbers of patients included in the tPA/DNAse arm (n = 52). Additional studies corroborated the findings, with IET finding a niche for the treatment of nondraining CPPE and empyema and for those whom surgery is deemed high risk.[52,53]

The issues of timing and dosage of IET still remain a subject of debate, with international guidelines not specifically addressing these questions.[7,37] To this end, Chadda and colleagues have formed a consensus statement appraising the current evidence to date. This statement notes that most of the patients receiving appropriate antimicrobial cover, clinical and radiological parameters should improve within 24 hours of chest tube insertion. Following the confirmation of loculated pleural collection or lack of drainage, the authors recommend either the use of IET or surgical referral, depending on local expertise and accessibility of minimally invasive surgical techniques. They concluded that IET could be used either initially (at the time of drain insertion) or as subsequent therapy (>24 postdrain insertion).[54] The recommended dosing regime is 10 mg alteplase sequentially with 5 mg DNAse twice per day, with insufficient evidence to recommend alternative dosing. Work in this area has been explored in small numbers, of particular interest a 5 mg alteplase regime showing promising safety and efficacy.[55] In an increasingly elderly, comorbid population,[5] reduced dose fibrinolytics are an appealing prospect for use in patients requiring therapeutic anticoagulation, but safety in this specific subgroup warrants further evaluation.[56]

The issue of costs associated with IET must be addressed, rendering it inaccessible in some health care settings and limiting use in others.

The cost of a 3-day regime of tPA and DNAse is estimated to be £738 (medication costs only)[57,58] in the United Kingdom and $7000 in the United States.[54] Once recent US-based study estimated IET and surgical decortication to be almost equivalent in terms of cost,[59] and the consensus statement notes that cost should not be a deciding factor in IET versus surgery. The balance between IET and surgery is likely to vary immensely between countries.

Surgery

The role of surgery in patients with empyema is well established, providing a valuable treatment modality to remove infected material from the pleural space, and decortication of visceral "rind" to facilitate re-expansion of the lung. This can be done via a video-assisted thoracoscopy (VATS) or a more invasive open thoracotomy. Although the safety profile of VATS and duration of admission (5 vs 8 days) is favorable,[60] mortality rates remain up to 6%, with conversion to open surgery in stage 3 empyema up to 59%.[61] The technical challenges of VATS in this cohort are in establishing adequate access to the pleural space through dense adhesions and achieving adequate decortication.

The question of timing of thoracic surgery is far from straightforward, with delays in surgical intervention consistently predicting conversion to open thoracotomy.[61,62] Although this would appear to add credence to the concept of early surgery, the few clinical trials in this area have been low in numbers, seen higher tube failure rates than medical studies, and included lower median age demographics than comparative medical studies.[63,64] A recent Cochrane review, while finding comparable mortality in surgical and nonsurgical groups, does not sufficiently answer the question, including 6 (of 8 total) pediatric trials. These studies do not also account for the latest developments in IET. As such we are left with current guidelines advocating for a surgical approach in those with failure of chest tube drainage, antibiotics, and IET, and patients not suitable for single lung ventilation or general anesthetic.[7,54] There is the prospect of promising further work in this area, with the currently recruiting MIST-3 RCT assessing the feasibility of pitting standard care versus early IET versus early surgical referral in empyema against one another (ISRCTN18192121).[6] Ultimately, a more nuanced approach may form the "middle ground" in the medical versus surgical debate in empyema, with use of risk scores such as RAPID stratifying those who should be considered for early surgery.

Fig. 2 illustrates a suggested algorithm for the management of parapneumonic effusion and empyema.

CLINICS CARE POINTS

- Prompt drainage and antibiotics should be initiated in all patients with CPPE or empyema
- Empirical antibiotics are often needed and broad-spectrum cover is required
- IET is safe and effective and can be used to improve drainage, for now as a "surgery sparing" option pending further evidence
- Approximately 2 in 3 patients will respond to "standard care" with chest tube drainage and antibiotics
- There is insufficient evidence to support surgery at the point of diagnosis in pleural infection

Alternative Treatments and Future Strategies

Treatment modalities have been explored outside of those discussed earlier. The use of pleural irrigation was demonstrated in the randomized Pleural Irrigation Trial, assessing outcomes with standard medical care versus standard care plus saline irrigation with 250 mL saline 3 times per day (n = 35). The number of patients referred for surgery was significantly lower in the irrigation arm, with improvement in pleural fluid volume compared with controls.[65] Despite small numbers, and a lack of blinding, this is a promising result because of the low-risk nature of saline irrigation, and warrants further assessment in a large multicenter cohort.

Local anesthetic thoracoscopy (LAT) is an intervention with limited data in pleural infection. Although providing obvious utility in clearing septations, it is less well equipped to deal with visceral or pleural thickening where decortication is required. One recent trial has suggested early LAT to be safe and potentially effective, albeit with small numbers (n = 32) and a primary outcome of hospital stay postintervention.[66] In the earlier stage empyema, drainage and IET provide less invasive options, leaving the timing and utility of LAT in the clinical pathway requiring larger-scale trials to define. We would thus conclude that there is currently insufficient data to justify first-line use of medical thoracoscopy for pleural infection treatment outside very selected patients.

Intrapleural antibiotics have been raised as a potential mechanism of "direct delivery" to the pleural space. Although retrospective literature does exist to suggest benefit in postpneumonectomy

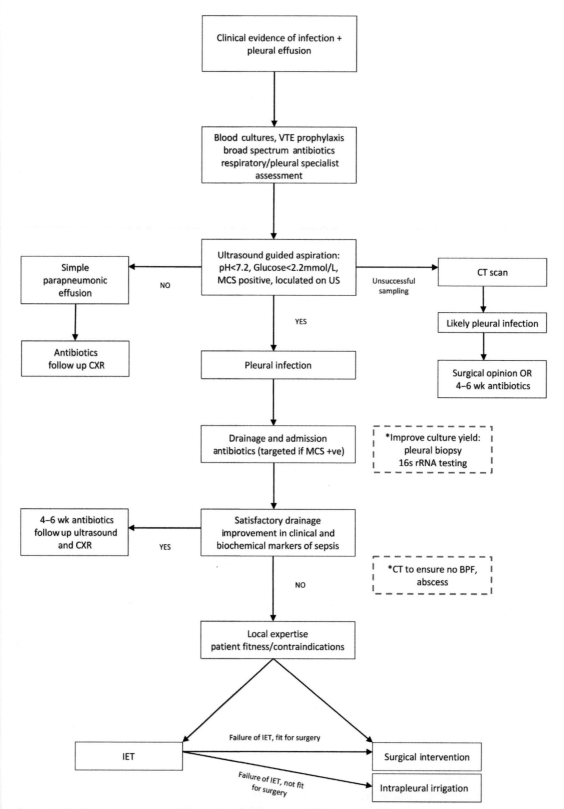

Fig. 2. Suggested treatment algorithm for the management of pleural infection. BPF, bronchopleural fistula; CT, computed tomography; CXR, chest radiograph; IET, intrapleural enzyme therapy; MCS, microscopy, culture, and sensitivity; VTE, venous thromboembolism; US, ultrasound; * denotes optional investigations to improve diagnostics.

empyema,[67] the potential for treatment of nonoperative pleural infection is limited to animal studies and case reports.

SUMMARY

Parapneumonic effusion and empyema are increasingly common entities, associated with high health care costs and morbidity. The outcomes for pleural infection remain poor and treatment currently remains based around modalities that have been in use for many years. The focus areas for progress must involve early diagnosis and tailoring treatment in a "personalized" way to each patient. With this in mind, there are promising signs on the horizon, with molecular techniques to aid identification of causative organisms and an expanding search for improved biomarkers. The more widespread availability of pleural specialist services, allowing early intervention, clarity emerging on IET and trials to establish answers to often posed questions regarding the timing of surgery and IET will guide the management of pleural infection in the years to come.

REFERENCES

1. Grijalva CG, Zhu Y, Nuorti JP, et al. The emergence of parapneumonic empyema in the United States. Thorax 2011;66(8):663–8.
2. Søgaard M, Nielsen RB, Nørgaard M, et al. Incidence, length of stay, and prognosis of hospitalized patients with pleural empyema: a 15-year Danish nationwide cohort study. Chest 2014; 145(1):189–92.
3. Corcoran JP, Psallidas I, Gerry S, et al. Prospective validation of the RAPID clinical risk prediction score in adult patients with pleural infection: the PILOT study. Eur Respir J 2020;56(5):2000130.
4. Brims F, Popowicz N, Rosenstengel A, et al. Bacteriology and clinical outcomes of patients with culture-positive pleural infection in Western Australia: a 6-year analysis. Respirol Carlton Vic 2019;24(2):171–8.
5. Cargill TN, Hassan M, Corcoran JP, et al. A systematic review of comorbidities and outcomes of adult patients with pleural infection. Eur Respir J 2019;54(3):1900541.
6. ISRCTN - ISRCTN18192121: A randomised controlled trial of the feasibility of early administration of clot-busting medication through a chest tube versus early surgery in pleural infection. doi: 10.1186/ISRCTN18192121.
7. Davies HE, Davies RJO, Davies CWH, BTS Pleural Disease Guideline Group. Management of pleural infection in adults: British thoracic society pleural disease guideline 2010. Thorax 2010;65(Suppl 2): ii41–53.
8. Hassan M, Cargill T, Harriss E, et al. The microbiology of pleural infection in adults: a systematic review. Eur Respir J 2019;54(3):1900542.
9. Hassan M, Mercer RM, Rahman NM. Thoracic ultrasound in the modern management of pleural disease. Eur Respir Rev 2020;29:190136.
10. Rahman NM, Maskell NA, West A, et al. Intrapleural use of tissue plasminogen activator and DNase in pleural infection. N Engl J Med 2011;365(6): 518–26.
11. Sundaralingam A, Banka R, Rahman NM. Management of pleural infection. Pulm Ther 2020;7:59–74.
12. Sahn SA. Diagnosis and management of parapneumonic effusions and empyema. Clin Infect Dis 2007; 45(11):1480–6.
13. Alemán C, Alegre J, Monasterio J, et al. Association between inflammatory mediators and the fibrinolysis system in infectious pleural effusions. Clin Sci (Lond) 2003;105(5):601–7.
14. Reichert M, Pösentrup B, Hecker A, et al. Lung decortication in phase III pleural empyema by video-assisted thoracoscopic surgery (VATS)-results of a learning curve study. J Thorac Dis 2018;10(7): 4311–20.
15. El Solh AA, Alhajjhasan A, Ramadan FH, et al. A comparative study of community- and nursing home-acquired empyema thoracis. J Am Geriatr Soc 2007;55(11):1847–52.
16. Ashbaugh DG. Empyema thoracis. Factors influencing morbidity and mortality. Chest 1991;99(5): 1162–5.
17. Rahman NM, Kahan BC, Miller RF, et al. A clinical score (RAPID) to identify those at risk for poor outcome at presentation in patients with pleural infection. Chest 2014;145(4):848–55.
18. Marchetti G, Arondi S, Baglivo F, et al. New insights in the use of pleural ultrasonography for diagnosis and treatment of pleural disease. Clin Respir J 2018;12(6):1993–2005.
19. Svigals PZ, Chopra A, Ravenel JG, et al. The accuracy of pleural ultrasonography in diagnosing complicated parapneumonic pleural effusions. Thorax 2017;72(1):94–5.
20. Corcoran J, Psallidas I, Gerry S, et al. Does the sonographic presence and severity of pleural fluid septation have an impact on clinical outcomes in pleural infection? - data from the Pleural Infection Longitudinal Outcome Study (PILOT). Eur Respir J 2018;52(suppl 62):OA3266.
21. Maskell NA, Gleeson FV, Darby M, et al. Diagnostically significant variations in pleural fluid pH in loculated parapneumonic effusions. Chest 2004;126(6): 2022–4.
22. Kearney SE, Davies CW, Davies RJ, et al. Computed tomography and ultrasound in parapneumonic effusions and empyema. Clin Radiol 2000;55(7):542–7.

23. Stark DD, Federle MP, Goodman PC, et al. Differentiating lung abscess and empyema: radiography and computed tomography. AJR Am J Roentgenol 1983;141(1):163–7.

24. Wrightson JM, Wray JA, Street TL, et al. Absence of atypical pathogens in pleural infection. Chest 2015; 148(3):e102–3.

25. Lin Y-C, Chen H-J, Liu Y-H, et al. A 30-month experience of thoracic empyema in a tertiary hospital: emphasis on differing bacteriology and outcome between the medical intensive care unit (MICU) and medical ward. South Med J 2008;101(5): 484–9.

26. Maskell NA, Batt S, Hedley EL, et al. The bacteriology of pleural infection by genetic and standard methods and its mortality significance. Am J Respir Crit Care Med 2006;174(7):817–23.

27. Corcoran JP, Wrightson JM, Belcher E, et al. Pleural infection: past, present, and future directions. Lancet Respir Med 2015;3(7):563–77.

28. Dyrhovden R, Nygaard RM, Patel R, et al. The bacterial aetiology of pleural empyema. A descriptive and comparative metagenomic study. Clin Microbiol Infect 2019;25(8):981–6.

29. Menzies SM, Rahman NM, Wrightson JM, et al. Blood culture bottle culture of pleural fluid in pleural infection. Thorax 2011;66(8):658–62.

30. Psallidas I, Kanellakis NI, Bhatnagar R, et al. A pilot feasibility study in establishing the role of ultrasound-guided pleural Biopsies in pleural infection (the AUDIO study). Chest 2018;154(4): 766–72.

31. Insa R, Marín M, Martín A, et al. Systematic use of universal 16S rRNA gene polymerase chain reaction (PCR) and sequencing for processing pleural effusions improves conventional culture techniques. Medicine (Baltimore) 2012;91(2):103–10.

32. Light RW, MacGregor MI, Ball WC, et al. Diagnostic significance of pleural fluid pH and PCO2. Chest 1973;64(5):591–6.

33. Addala D, Mercer RM, Lu Q, et al. P101 Inflammatory pleural effusions: differentiating the diagnosis. Thorax 2019;74(Suppl 2):A145–6.

34. Porcel JM, Valencia H, Bielsa S. Factors influencing pleural drainage in parapneumonic effusions. Rev Clin Esp 2016;216(7):361–6.

35. Arnold DT, Hamilton FW, Elvers KT, et al. Pleural fluid suPAR levels predict the need for invasive management in parapneumonic effusions. Am J Respir Crit Care Med 2020;201(12):1545–53.

36. Brook I, Wexler HM, Goldstein EJC. Antianaerobic antimicrobials: spectrum and susceptibility testing. Clin Microbiol Rev 2013;26(3):526–46.

37. Shen KR, Bribriesco A, Crabtree T, et al. The American Association for Thoracic Surgery consensus guidelines for the management of empyema. J Thorac Cardiovasc Surg 2017;153(6):e129–46.

38. Bedawi EO, Hassan M, McCracken D, et al. Pleural infection: a closer look at the etiopathogenesis, microbiology and role of antibiotics. Expert Rev Respir Med 2019;13(4):337–47.

39. Teixeira LR, Sasse SA, Villarino MA, et al. Antibiotic levels in empyemic pleural fluid. Chest 2000; 117(6):1734–9.

40. Kuhajda I, Zarogoulidis K, Tsirgogianni K, et al. Lung abscess-etiology, diagnostic and treatment options. Ann Transl Med 2015;3(13):183.

41. Porcel JM, Ferreiro L, Rumi L, et al. Two vs. three weeks of treatment with amoxicillin-clavulanate for stabilized community-acquired complicated parapneumonic effusions. A preliminary non-inferiority, double-blind, randomized, controlled trial. Pleura Peritoneum 2020;5(1):20190027.

42. Colice GL, Curtis A, Deslauriers J, et al. Medical and surgical treatment of parapneumonic effusions : an evidence-based guideline. Chest 2000;118(4): 1158–71.

43. Meyer CN, Armbruster K, Kemp M, et al. Pleural infection: a retrospective study of clinical outcome and the correlation to known etiology, co-morbidity and treatment factors. BMC Pulm Med 2018;18(1): 160.

44. Rahman NM, Maskell NA, Davies CWH, et al. The relationship between chest tube size and clinical outcome in pleural infection. Chest 2010;137(3): 536–43.

45. Ulmer JL, Choplin RH, Reed JC. Image-guided catheter drainage of the infected pleural space. J Thorac Imaging 1991;6(4):65–73.

46. Crouch JD, Keagy BA, Delany DJ. "Pigtail" catheter drainage in thoracic surgery. Am Rev Respir Dis 1987;136(1):174–5.

47. Horsley A, Jones L, White J, et al. Efficacy and complications of small-bore, wire-guided chest drains. Chest 2006;130(6):1857–63.

48. Davies HE, Merchant S, McGown A. A study of the complications of small bore "Seldinger" intercostal chest drains. Respirol Carlton Vic 2008;13(4):603–7.

49. Tillett WS, Sherry S. The effect in patients of streptococcal fibrinolysin (streptokinase) and streptococcal desoxyribonuclease on fibrinous, purulent, and sanguinous pleural exudations 1. J Clin Invest 1949; 28(1):173–90.

50. U.K. Controlled trial of intrapleural streptokinase for pleural infection | NEJM. Available at: https://www.nejm.org/doi/full/10.1056/nejmoa042473. Accessed February 14, 2021.

51. Hall-Stoodley L, Nistico L, Sambanthamoorthy K, et al. Characterization of biofilm matrix, degradation by DNase treatment and evidence of capsule downregulation in Streptococcus pneumoniae clinical isolates. BMC Microbiol 2008;8(1):173.

52. Piccolo F, Pitman N, Bhatnagar R, et al. Intrapleural tissue plasminogen activator and

deoxyribonuclease for pleural infection. An effective and safe alternative to surgery. Ann Am Thorac Soc 2014;11(9):1419–25.

53. Mehta HJ, Biswas A, Penley AM, et al. Management of intrapleural sepsis with once daily use of tissue plasminogen activator and deoxyribonuclease. Respir Int Rev Thorac Dis 2016;91(2):101–6.

54. Use of fibrinolytics and deoxyribonuclease in adult patients with pleural empyema: a consensus statement - the Lancet Respiratory Medicine. Available at: https://www.thelancet.com/journals/lanres/article/PIIS2213-2600(20)30533-6/fulltext?rss=yes. Accessed February 14, 2021.

55. Popowicz N, Bintcliffe O, De Fonseka D, et al. Dose de-escalation of intrapleural tissue plasminogen activator therapy for pleural infection. The alteplase dose assessment for pleural infection therapy project. Ann Am Thorac Soc 2017;14(6):929–36.

56. Altmann ES, Crossingham I, Wilson S, et al. Intrapleural fibrinolytic therapy versus placebo, or a different fibrinolytic agent, in the treatment of adult parapneumonic effusions and empyema. Cochrane Database Syst Rev 2019;2019(10):CD002312.

57. 2 the technology | Alteplase for treating acute ischaemic stroke | Guidance | NICE. Available at: https://www.nice.org.uk/guidance/ta264/chapter/2-The-technology. Accessed February 14, 2021.

58. Excellence N-TNI for H and C. BNF: British National Formulary - NICE. Available at: https://bnf.nice.org.uk/medicinal-forms/dornase-alfa.html. Accessed February 14, 2021.

59. Shipe ME, Maiga AW, Deppen SA, et al. Cost-effectiveness analysis of fibrinolysis versus thoracoscopic decortication for early empyema. Ann Thorac Surg 2020. https://doi.org/10.1016/j.athoracsur.2020.11.005.

60. Reichert M, Pösentrup B, Hecker A, et al. Thoracotomy versus video-assisted thoracoscopic surgery (VATS) in stage III empyema-an analysis of 217 consecutive patients. Surg Endosc 2018;32(6):2664–75.

61. Stefani A, Aramini B, Casa G, et al. Preoperative predictors of successful surgical treatment in the management of parapneumonic empyema. Ann Thorac Surg 2013;96(5):1812–9.

62. Chung JH, Lee SH, Kim KT, et al. Optimal timing of thoracoscopic drainage and decortication for empyema. Ann Thorac Surg 2014;97(1):224–9.

63. Wait MA, Sharma S, Hohn J, et al. A randomized trial of empyema therapy. Chest 1997;111(6):1548–51.

64. Bilgin M, Akcali Y, Oguzkaya F. Benefits of early aggressive management of empyema thoracis. ANZ J Surg 2006;76(3):120–2.

65. Hooper CE, Edey AJ, Wallis A, et al. Pleural irrigation trial (PIT): a randomised controlled trial of pleural irrigation with normal saline versus standard care in patients with pleural infection. Eur Respir J 2015;46(2):456–63.

66. Kheir F, Thakore S, Mehta H, et al. Intrapleural fibrinolytic therapy versus early medical thoracoscopy for treatment of pleural infection. Randomized controlled clinical trial. Ann Am Thorac Soc 2020;17(8):958–64.

67. Ng T, Ryder BA, Maziak DE, et al. Treatment of postpneumonectomy empyema with debridement followed by continuous antibiotic irrigation. J Am Coll Surg 2008;206(6):1178–83.

Pleural Tuberculosis

Jane A. Shaw, MBChB, MMed (Int), MPhil (Pulm), FCP (SA), Cert Pulm (SA)[a],*,
Coenraad F.N. Koegelenberg, MBChB, MMed (Int), FCP (SA), FRCP (UK), Cert Pulm (SA), PhD[b]

KEYWORDS

• Tuberculosis • Pleural effusion • Pleuritis • Empyema • Biomarkers

KEY POINTS

• Tuberculosis (TB) is a common cause of pleural effusions throughout the world. The incidence in any geographic region is related to the background TB incidence, and the proportion of people living with human immunodeficiency virus.

• TB pleural effusions arise because of an effusive T-helper cell type 1 inflammatory response to *Mycobacterium tuberculosis* antigen in the pleural space, which upsets the balance of Starling forces that determine pleural fluid formation/resorption.

• TB effusions are paucibacillary, so usual tests for mycobacteriologic confirmation have low yields. The best yield is obtained through culture of tissue obtained at thoracoscopy, which is not universally available. Histopathological yield is high on pleural biopsy by all methods.

• Polymerase chain reaction-based tests are highly specific to TB but have relatively poor sensitivity in pleural fluid and pleural tissue. The main benefits of using these tests include their rapidity, and the opportunity to confirm drug sensitivity.

• Surrogate biomarkers of TB infection perform well in the diagnosis of pleural TB, most notably adenosine deaminase and interferon-γ.

• All TB effusions should be treated. The current recommended regimen is 6 months of isoniazid and rifampicin with 2 months of ethambutol and pyrazinamide. Routine administration of corticosteroids is not recommended.

• Loculated effusions should be drained. The addition of intrapleural fibrinolytics may be helpful.

• Surgery is often indicated for the management of TB empyema and its long-term consequences.

INTRODUCTION

Tuberculosis (TB) is the leading cause of death from a single infectious agent worldwide.[1] Despite TB being both preventable and curable, an estimated 10 million people fell ill with TB in 2019, and approximately 1.4 million people died of this disease.[2] TB is a disease of poverty and vulnerability, disproportionately affecting low- and middle-income countries. Although pulmonary TB is the commonest manifestation, up to 25% of patients initially present with the extrapulmonary forms, of which lymphadenitis and pleural TB are the commonest, and this proportion is likely to be even higher in regions where human immunodeficiency virus (HIV) coinfection is prevalent.[3,4] Pleural TB is usually self-limiting, often difficult to diagnose, but should not be neglected. Two-thirds of people with simple TB pleuritis will progress to pulmonary TB within 2 years if left untreated.[5,6] A small proportion of people will develop severe complications, such as TB empyema, bronchopleural fistulas, and long-term functional impairment. The optimal

[a] DST-NRF Centre of Excellence for Biomedical Tuberculosis Research, South African Medical Research Council Centre for Tuberculosis Research, Division of Molecular Biology and Human Genetics, Faculty of Medicine and Health Sciences, Stellenbosch University, PO Box 241, Cape Town 8000, South Africa; [b] Division of Pulmonology, Department of Medicine, Faculty of Medicine and Health Sciences, Stellenbosch University and Tygerberg Academic Hospital, PO Box 241, Cape Town 8000, South Africa
* Corresponding author.
E-mail address: janeshaw@sun.ac.za
Twitter: @OnlyFreshAir (J.A.S.)

Clin Chest Med 42 (2021) 649–666
https://doi.org/10.1016/j.ccm.2021.08.002

regimen for the treatment of pleural TB is still uncertain, as are the indications for surgical intervention. This article reviews the current state of practice in the evolving field of pleural TB.

EPIDEMIOLOGY
The Global Burden of Pleural Tuberculosis

The true burden of pleural TB is difficult to quantify, as often the diagnosis is made on grounds other than definitive bacteriologic confirmation, and notification systems may not differentiate between sites of extrapulmonary TB infection.[4,7] Of the 7.1 million incident cases of TB that were notified worldwide in 2019, 16% were extrapulmonary, with the highest rate of 24% reported in the World Health Organization (WHO) Eastern Mediterranean Region.[2] Africa, which has the highest rate of HIV coinfection, reported a rate of 15% extrapulmonary TB.[2] In the United States, between 3% and 5% of all TB cases are pleural TB.[7,8] Reports from South Africa indicate a higher rate of between 7% and 10% for pleural TB.[9,10] Spain has previously reported that 10% of TB cases are pleural TB.[3] In an older report from a high TB incidence area of Spain, 25% of all pleural effusions were due to TB.[11]

Human Immunodeficiency Virus Coinfection

People living with HIV (PLHIV) are a distinct subpopulation with a higher risk of developing TB disease, of developing extrapulmonary forms of TB, and of dying of TB.[2] Between 40% and 50% of all TB cases in PLHIV are extrapulmonary, and in regions with particularly high background TB prevalence, the rate of extrapulmonary TB may be as high as 70%.[12] In South Africa, pleural TB makes up between 30% and 56% of all cases of extrapulmonary TB in PLHIV, and is, unsurprisingly, the most common cause of an exudative pleural effusion in the area.[13–15]

Drug-Resistant Tuberculosis

Drug-resistant TB (DR-TB) continues to present a major public health threat in many regions of the world. However, reliable data on the rate of DR-TB pleural effusions are sparse. Until recently, drug sensitivity of a TB pleural effusion was inferred from response to treatment, an approach that does not take into account that the natural history of TB effusions is spontaneous resolution.[16] In addition, because of the inherently paucibacillary nature of the disease, most cases of pleural TB do not receive bacteriologic confirmation and therefore drug-sensitivity testing. Existing data suggest that rates of DR-TB pleural effusions are

similar pulmonary DR-TB. In the United States, approximately 6% of all patients with pleural TB between 1993 and 2003 had isolates resistant to Isoniazid (H), and 9.9% were resistant to at least 1 first-line drug, compared with 7.8% and 11.9% for pulmonary TB, respectively.[7] Only 1% was multidrug resistant (MDR).[7] In 1 center in Taiwan between 2001 and 2008, 10% of isolates was resistant to any anti-TB drug, and 2% was MDR.[17] In Greece between 2003 and 2011, 11% of isolates was resistant to any drug, and 3% was MDR.[18] In 1 center in South Korea between 2008 and 2012, 10% was resistant to any anti-TB drug and 2.7% was resistant to any MDR. In Lahore, Pakistan, between April 2016 and August 2017, 9.4% of new pleural TB cases was resistant to H, and 3.2% was resistant to MDR.[19] In Beijing, 2.4% demonstrated Rifampicin (R) resistance.[20]

PATHOPHYSIOLOGY
Pleural Immune Response to Mycobacterium tuberculosis

M tuberculosis (Mtb) gains entry to the pleural space by the rupture of a subpleural caseous focus through the visceral pleura.[21] The parenchymal focus may be small and rapidly cleared by the pulmonary immune response, leaving only the pleural sequelae, or a larger focus of active pulmonary TB, as is often the case with reactivation disease.[22] Pleural mesothelial cells likely modulate the initial inflammatory response to Mtb antigen, secreting chemokines, cytokines, and other proinflammatory mediators, which result in an influx of inflammatory cells.[23] From animal studies with intrapleural instillation of bacillus Calmette-Guerin, it is thought that within the first 24 hours after infection, the predominant cell type in pleural fluid is neutrophils, followed by a large influx of macrophages.[24] A prolonged lymphocytic phase follows, characterized by high levels of T-helper cell type 1 (Th1) cytokines, including interferon gamma (IFN-γ), IFN-γ-inducible protein of 1 kDa, transforming growth factor-β, and tumor necrosis factor (TNF).[25–27] This response is highly compartmentalized and likely very effective at the containment and eradication of Mtb from the pleural space.[28,29]

Development of an Effusion

Biopsy studies have suggested that the pleura proceeds through several phases after infection with Mtb: serofibrinous pleuritis; patchy granulation tissue with predominantly nonnecrotizing granulomas; and finally, confluent granulation tissue with necrotizing granulomas.[30] Healing and clearance of the infection may occur at any stage or progress to empyema. In the serofibrinous pleuritis phase, the integrity of the capillary endothelial cell barrier is compromised by the inflammatory process, and pleural fluid formation accelerates because of loss of resistance.[31] The delicate balance of Starling forces, which usually maintain pleural fluid formation and resorption, is further deranged by the presence of inflammatory proteins in the pleural fluid, increasing the fluid oncotic pressure, and drawing fluid into the space.[32] As a result, the rate of formation exceeds resorption. When granulation tissue begins to form on the pleural surface, the lymphatic stomata, which are responsible for draining pleural fluid into the lymphatics, become occluded, and the effusion accumulates further.[4,32]

Delayed Hypersensitivity, True Pleural Infection, or Both?

How much of a TB effusion is attributable to true pleural infection with Mtb, and how much is because of a perpetuation of the immune response to its antigens is debatable. Leibowitz and colleagues[33] observed that the instillation of Mtb antigen into the pleural space of guinea pigs sensitized to purified protein derivative caused an effusion to develop, but that this response was suppressed by antilymphocyte serum. This, along with the historically poor yield of tests to identify Mtb in the pleural fluid, the Th-1 lymphocyte predominance (with accompanying cytokines) in the pleural fluid, and the spontaneous recovery of most cases of TB effusion, would argue for a Th1-mediated hypersensitivity reaction over ongoing infection. However, new technologies that allow us to culture Mtb in up to 70% of effusions, challenge this dogma. Nonetheless, it is clear that TB effusions have very few organisms, even in the presence of ongoing pleural infection.

CLINICAL FEATURES
Presentation

Pleural TB should be considered in the differential diagnosis of any unilateral pleural effusion.[22,32] It can affect people of any age, both as a manifestation of primary infection and as reactivation of latent TB.[4] It is typically an acute to subacute illness characterized by fever, ipsilateral pleuritic chest pain, and nonproductive cough.[34,35] The patient may have other symptoms, such as dyspnea, night sweats, or weight loss, and occasionally, patients are completely asymptomatic.[7] PLHIV who have a low CD4 count may be older than the average pleural TB patient and have a longer-duration illness.[36] PLHIV are more likely to have

additional evidence of disseminated TB on presentation.[37]

Imaging

On chest radiograph (**Fig. 1**), TB pleural effusions are most commonly unilateral and moderate in size (occupying one-third to two-thirds of the hemithorax).[38,39] However, bilateral effusions and effusions that occupy more than two-thirds of the hemithorax do occur.[38,40] Approximately 20% to 50% of cases will have associated parenchymal infiltrates visible on chest radiograph (**Fig. 2**), often only appreciable after drainage of the effusion.[34,41] Computed tomography (CT) chest scan reveals associated subpleural, peribronchovascular, and/or centrilobular micronodules, interlobular septal thickening, consolidation, or, more rarely, cavitation, in up to 86% of cases of pleural TB (**Fig. 3**).[42,43] Changes typical of TB, especially those suggesting lymphatic spread of infection, may have value in distinguishing pleural TB from other infections.[44] During active infection, both the visceral and the parietal pleura are uniformly thickened, often involving the mediastinal pleural surface.[45] With chronic or healed disease, the pleura may appear thickened and calcified and may be associated with a contracted hemithorax (**Fig. 4**). Thoracic ultrasound findings in pleural TB, which can range between the typical free flowing anechoic effusion, an echogenic effusion, or a complex septated effusion (**Fig. 5**), are nonspecific but valuable in both guiding interventions and identifying features that might suggest alternate diagnoses, such as malignant pleural deposits.[46]

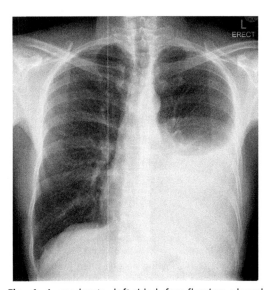

Fig. 1. A moderate left-sided free-flowing pleural effusion from proven pleural TB.

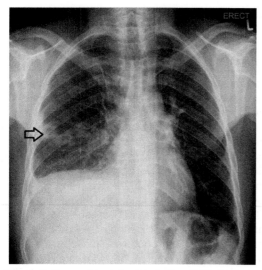

Fig. 2. Patient with right-sided pleural TB had evidence ipsilateral fibrocavitatory parenchymal (*arrow*).

The utility of other imaging modalities, such as ^{18}F-fluorodeoxyglucose (FDG)--PET/CT (**Fig. 6**) and MRI, is still under investigation, and in many settings, the cost of these investigations is prohibitive.

General Pleural Fluid Analysis

The typical TB effusion is a straw-colored exudate with a high lactate dehydrogenase (LDH), high protein content, and lymphocyte proportion of more than 50% with a lymphocyte/neutrophil ratio greater than 0.75.[4] If aspiration is performed early enough in the course of the disease, the predominant cell type is likely to be neutrophils rather than lymphocytes. Similarly, neutrophils are likely to predominate in effusions that complicate, becoming septated or even developing into frank

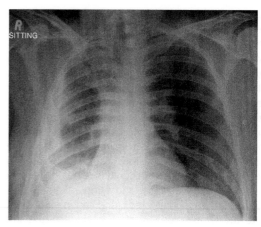

Fig. 4. A chest radiograph of a patient who developed a right-sided fibrothorax with restrictive impairment following apparent uncomplicated pleural TB.

empyema.[47] The pleural fluid glucose is not markedly reduced compared with serum, and the pH is usually greater than 7.3.[4] The combination of low glucose, low pH, and neutrophil predominance suggests chronic active infection, even in the absence of frank pus.[48] A significant proportion of mesothelial cells or eosinophils in the pleural fluid is an unusual finding, but monocytes are often present in high numbers.

DIAGNOSIS
Tests for Mycobacterium tuberculosis

The key difficulty in the diagnosis of TB pleural effusion is the lack of sensitivity of the usual tests to detect Mtb. **Table 1** presents the reported yields for smear microscopy and culture for pleural TB. **Table 2** presents the yields of polymerase chain reaction (PCR)-based techniques for pleural TB.

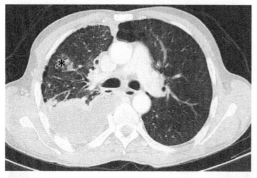

Fig. 3. A CT scan showing a right-sided pleural effusion (confirmed to be secondary to pleural TB) as well as parenchymal involvement (*) with airspace disease.

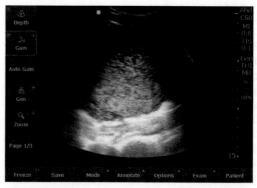

Fig. 5. A low-frequency ultrasound image obtained from a patient with TB empyema who developed a complex nonseptated effusion.

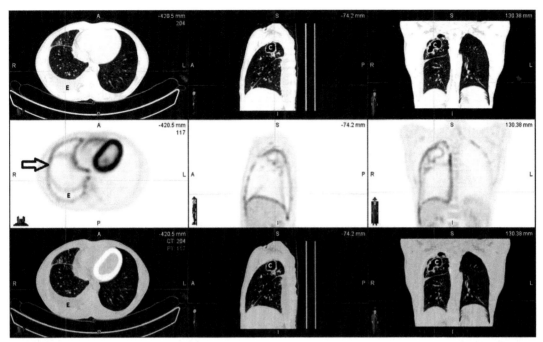

Fig. 6. A PET/CT scan obtained from a patient with active pulmonary and pleural TB. The top row shows the CT images in axial, sagittal, and coronal planes, respectively, with a right-sided pleural effusion (E) associated with apical cavitation (C). The middle row shows the PET images of the same slices in axial, sagittal, and coronal planes, respectively, demonstrating the circumferential uptake of ^{18}F-FDG by the inflamed visceral and parietal (*arrow*) pleura (and pleura lining the interlobar fissure) as well as the rim of the cavity in the parenchyma. The bottom row shows the fused PET/CT images, which combine the anatomic and metabolic features.

Bacteriologic confirmation of infection with Mtb has historically been uncommon in pleural fluid except in complex, purulent effusions (neutrophil predominant),[47,54,57,67] and in PLHIV, who also have a higher yield of sputum culture in pleural TB.[51,56,58] Liquid or broth culture media, such as BACTEC-MGIT semiautomated system (Becton-Dickinson, Franklin Lakes, NJ, USA), have a higher yield than solid culture media, such as Lowenstein-Jensen medium, in most studies where there was direct comparison.[51,54,68] Most TB pleural effusions are paucibacillary and therefore will not meet the threshold ~10,000 organisms per milliliter needed to be visible on smear microscopy, which is still the most readily available test for Mtb in most settings. Culture has a far lower limit of detection but is constrained by the time it takes to get a result, which ranges from 2 to 6 weeks depending on the medium. PCR-based techniques, such as Xpert MTB/RIF (Cepheid, Sunnyvale, CA, USA), are rapid and can detect as few as ~100 organisms per milliliter. Xpert MTB/RIF on pleural fluid has been shown in numerous studies and meta-analyses to be only slightly inferior to liquid culture, but on the whole, disappointing.[61–63,65] The Xpert Ultra cartridge has improved sensitivity over Xpert MTB/RIF in

the diagnosis of pulmonary TB (with a level of detection as low as ~20 organisms per milliliter), but there is no definitive evidence yet that it adds to the diagnosis of pleural TB.[20,69,70] PCR techniques tend to be expensive and are far from universally available, but have the added benefit of detecting R resistance. They should be strongly considered for use on pleural fluid specimens in regions with a high prevalence of DR-TB, despite their low yield. It is worth noting that although the sensitivity is low, the specificity for all tests detecting Mtb directly remains high. The value of sputum testing in pleural TB should not be underestimated, as most patients have concomitant pulmonary parenchymal TB even if not visible on chest radiograph.

Pleural Fluid Biomarkers

There have been many pleural fluid biomarkers assessed for diagnostic utility in TB effusions over the years, but the most well studied are adenosine deaminase (ADA) and IFN-Y. Both these biomarkers have a high diagnostic accuracy in the appropriate setting, and evidence supports using either as a surrogate for Mtb detection in light of the difficulty obtaining definitive

Table 1
The diagnostic yield (% positive) of tests for *Mycobacterium tuberculosis* in pleural tuberculosis

Reference	Pleural Fluid Smear Microscopy	Pleural Fluid Culture			Pleural Tissue Culture	Sputum culture
		Solid Medium	Liquid Medium	Combined or Not Specified		
HIV-negative or not specified						
Chan, 1991[49]	0	23.0				
Maartens, 1991[50]			47.0		71.0	
Seibert, 1991[41]		58.0			66.7	50.0
Valdes, 1998[39]	5.5	36.6			56.4	100.0
Heyderman, 1998[36]	0				33.0	0
Luzze, 2001[51]		12.0	24.0		56.0	15.0
Diacon, 2003[14]		7.0			48.0 (CPB) 76.0 (T)	7.0
Conde, 2003[52]	1.0	10.0			59.0	48.0[a]
Koegelenberg, 2010[53]	0		25.8		63.6	
Ruan, 2012[54]			63.0		39.0	55.0
Von Groote-Bidlingmaier, 2013[55]			60.3			
Marjani, 2016[56]				29.5		38.6
Ko, 2017[57]	0			31.5		33.3
Bielsa, 2019[58]	3.0			18.0		29.0
Wang, 2019[20]	1.4		26.4			
PLHIV						
Heyderman, 1998[36]	18.0				42.0	13.0
Luzze, 2001[51]		43.0	75.0		81.0	27.0
Conde, 2003[52]	8.0	15.0			77.0	77.0[a]
Marjani, 2016[56]				63.0		57.1

Abbreviations: CPB, tissue obtained by closed pleural biopsy; T, tissue obtained by thoracoscopy.
[a] Specifically induced sputum.

mycobacteriologic confirmation. **Table 3** outlines the diagnostic accuracy of the major biomarkers for pleural TB.

Adenosine deaminase

ADA is a purine degrading enzyme with 2 isoforms: ADA1, which is an ubiquitous enzyme found most often in lymphocytes, monocytes, and neutrophils; and ADA2, which is more specific to monocytes and macrophages and is the dominant isoform in TB effusions.[68] It is detected by a low-cost colorimetric test (usually by the Guisti method). ADA will also be elevated in complex parapneumonic effusions, bacterial empyema, lymphoma, rheumatoid arthritis–related effusions, and pleural malignancy, among other conditions, although most of these tend to be ADA1- and neutrophil-predominant. In some regions of the world with a high background of TB prevalence, an elevated ADA (cutoff values vary, but commonly range between 30 and 50 U/

L) in a lymphocyte predominant (or a lymphocyte/neutrophil ratio >0.75), pleural exudate is sufficient evidence to initiate anti-TB treatment, and it is generally not necessary to distinguish between isoenzymes.[91,92] Regions with a low TB prevalence may safely use an ADA less than 30 U/L as a rule-out test for pleural TB in light of its reported negative predictive value (NPV) of 98.9% to 99.7% and sensitivity of 93% to 96.3% in this setting.[93,94] Recently, the utility of the LDH/ADA ratio has been described in both high and low TB prevalence regions, with the benefit of not requiring a cell differential count for interpretation. Blakiston and colleagues[94] showed that in a low TB prevalence region, an LDH/ADA ratio of less than 15 had a sensitivity, specificity, positive predictive value (PPV), and NPV of 89.1%, 84.8%, 17.3%, and 99.5%, respectively. Wang and colleagues[95] found that a ratio of less than 16.2 discriminated between TB effusion and malignancy with a high

Table 2
Meta-analyses of accuracy of polymerase chain reaction–based tests for the diagnosis of pleural tuberculosis

Reference	Studies (n)	Patients (n)	Sample Type	PCR Method	Sensitivity (%, 95%CI)	Specificity (%, 95%CI)
Pai, 2004[59]	14	1513	Pleural fluid	Commercial tests	62.0 (43.0–77.0)	98.0 (96.0–98.0)
	26	1472	Pleural fluid	In-house PCR	71.0 (63.0–78.0)	93.0 (88.0–96.0)
Dinnes, 2007[60]	6	NS	Pleural fluid	Commercial tests	62.0	97.0
	14	NS	Pleural fluid	In-house PCR	76.5	91.0
WHO, 2013[61]	17	1385	Pleural fluid	Xpert MTB/RIF		
				Culture reference standard:	43.7 (24.8–64.7)	98.1 (95.3–99.2)
				Composite reference standard:	17.0 (7.5–34.2)	99.9 (93.7–100)
Denkinger, 2014[62]	14	841	Pleural fluid	Xpert MTB/RIF		
	6	598		Culture reference standard:	46.4 (26.3–67.8)	99.1 (95.2–99.8)
				Composite reference standard:	21.4 (8.8–33.9)	100 (99.4–100)
Penz, 2015[63]	13	1014	Pleural fluid	Xpert MTB/RIF	37.0 (26.0–50.0)	98.0 (95.0–99.0)
Seghal, 2016[64]	21	2167	Pleural fluid	Xpert MTB/RIF		
	10	937		Culture reference standard:	51.4 (43.3–59.7)	98.6 (97.1–99.6)
				Composite reference standard:	22.7 (12.8–36.9)	99.8 (97.2–99.9)
Kohli, 2018[65]	30	4097	Pleural fluid	Xpert MTB/RIF		
	5	405		Culture reference standard:	50.9 (39.7–62.8)	99.2 (98.2–99.5)
				Composite reference standard:	18.4 (9.9–30.7)	98.2 (94.8–99.5)
	4	207	Pleural tissue	Xpert MTB/RIF	30.5 (3.5–77.8)	97.4 (92.1–99.3)
Kohli, 2021[66]	25	3065	Pleural fluid	Xpert MTB/RIF		
	10	1024		Culture reference standard:	49.5 (39.8–59.9)	98.9 (97.6–99.7)
				Composite reference standard:	18.9 (11.5–27.9)	98.9 (97.6–99.7)
	4	207	Pleural tissue	Xpert MTB/RIF		
	1	55		Culture reference standard:	0–85.0[a]	97.0–100[a]
				Composite reference standard:	0[a]	98.0[a]
	4	398	Pleural fluid	Xpert ULTRA		
	2	263		Culture reference standard:	75.0 (58.0–86.4)	87.0 (63.1–97.9)
				Composite reference standard:	61.0 and 38.0[a]	96.0 and 99.0[a]

Xpert MTB/RIF and Xpert ULTRA, both performed on the GeneXpert platform from Cepheid (Sunnyvale).
Abbreviations: 95% CI, 95% confidence interval; NS, not specified.
[a] Meta-analysis not performed.

Table 3
The diagnostic accuracy of selected pleural fluid biomarkers for the diagnosis of pleural tuberculosis

Biomarker	Sensitivity (%)	Specificity (%)	AUC	References[a]
ADA	86.0–93.0	88.0–93.0	0.93–0.97	Goto, 2003[71] Greco, 2003[72] Liang, 2008[73] Morisson, 2008[74] Gui, 2014[75] Aggarwal, 2016[76] Aggarwal, 2019[77] Palma, 2019[78]
IFN-Υ	87.0–89.0	97.0	0.99	Greco, 2003[72] Jiang, 2007[79]
IGRAs	75.0–94.0	79.0–90.0	0.88–0.96	Zhou, 2011[80] Pang, 2015[81] Zhou, 2015[82] Aggarwal, 2015[83] Li, 2015[84]
IL-27	92.0–94.0	90.0–97.0	0.95–0.98	Li, 2017[85] Zeng, 2017[86] Wang, 2018[87] Liu, 2018[88]
TNF-α	85.0	80.0	0.89	Li, 2016[89]
IP-10	84.0	90.0	0.90	Tong, 2017[90]

Abbreviations: AUC, area under the receiver-operating-curve; IP-10, interferon-γ-inducible protein of 10 kDa.
[a] All references are meta-analyses. Note, these meta-analyses are complicated by the different cutoff points, and the different background TB prevalence in the component studies.

degree of accuracy. In the authors' study of 228 patients suspected of having pleural TB, an LDH/ADA ratio less than 12.5 had a sensitivity, specificity, PPV, and NPV of 86%, 88%, 94%, and 72%, respectively.[96] An LDH/ADA ratio less than 10 outperformed an ADA ≥40 U/L alone, but the test with the highest diagnostic accuracy remained the combination of an ADA ≥40 with a lymphocyte-predominant effusion.[96]

Unstimulated interferon-gamma
Pleural fluid IFN-Υ, a cytokine released by activated macrophages and T lymphocytes, has consistently shown high diagnostic accuracy for pleural TB, but its use is limited at present by the lack of a well-defined cutoff value. These IFN-Υ assays are laboratory-based enzyme-linked immunosorbent assays. Recently, Antrum Biotech (South Africa) developed the InterGam Rapid Immuno Suspension Assay (IRISA-TB), which has a reported sensitivity, specificity, PPV, and NPV of 89.8%, 96.5%, 93.6%, and 94.2%, respectively, in pleural fluid, and a rapid turn-around time.[70]

Interferon-gamma release assays
IFN-Υ release assays (IGRAs), such as the QuantiFERON-TB Gold (QIAGEN) and T-SPOT.TB

(Oxford Immunotec), quantify the IFN-Υ released by T lymphocytes in response to stimulation with Mtb antigens. Historically, they have not performed well in pleural TB, although data from a few recent studies suggest that when performed on pleural fluid, they are better than IGRAs on peripheral blood and may have a diagnostic accuracy equal to ADA.[97,98] More data would be needed to confirm this.

Interleukin-27 and other biomarkers
Similar to IFN-Υ and ADA, the Th1 cytokine interleukin-27 (IL-27) has been subject to meta-analysis and shows promising diagnostic utility. The number acquired by multiplying the IL-27 and ADA values (the IL-27 and ADA product) has been shown to have a sensitivity of up to 100% in 2 studies, independent of the background TB prevalence.[99,100] Measuring the pleural fluid/serum IL-27 gradient had a sensitivity and specificity of 97% and 99%, respectively, in 1 report.[101] IL-27 is a member of the IL-12 family and appears to be overexpressed by all cells in the pleural cavity in a TB effusion.[101] It is measured by an enzyme-linked immunosorbent assay, currently used mainly in a research context. The optimal cutoff remains to be found, as those studies range from 390 ng/L to more than 1000 ng/L.[91]

The list of other biomarkers tested for usefulness in diagnosing pleural TB is long and includes lysozyme (including the pleural fluid/serum lysozyme ratio), IL-2 (and the IFN-Y/IL-2 ratio), IFN-Y-induced protein of 10 kDa, neopterin, malondialdehyde, protein carbonyl, pleural decoy receptor-3, TNF-α, TNF soluble receptor-1, hyaluronic acid, leptin, fibronectin, IL-1β, IL-8, IL-6, soluble IL-6 receptor, IL-33, IL-35, soluble IL-2 receptor, soluble CD-26, D-dimers, superoxide dismutase, caspase-cleaved cytokeratin-18, and complement.[4,91,102] So far, none have outperformed those already in common use, and ADA remains the cheapest of these tests in most countries.[103]

Acquiring Pleural Tissue

The benefit of a diagnostic approach using pleural biopsy is that the finding of caseating granulomas is sufficient for the diagnosis of pleural TB, even in the absence of demonstrating Mtb in the tissue. In fact, if the pretest probability is high enough, even a finding of noncaseating granulomas is sufficient.[32] The overall diagnostic yield of pleural biopsy in TB effusions is high (69%–97%, with higher yields in PLHIV, complex effusions, and TB empyema), although there is variation with the method of biopsy.[36,104] Thoracoscopy is generally acknowledged to have the highest yield. In a seminal paper by Diacon and colleagues,[14] thoracoscopy identified 100% of TB effusions, and 76% of biopsies were culture positive. However, in the same study, the yield for ultrasound-guided closed needle biopsy with an Abram's needle was also high (79%). The combination of ultrasound-guided thoracentesis and closed pleural biopsy has been shown to have a sensitivity of 88.9% for pleural TB, and is less invasive, less expensive, and more easily available than thoracoscopy.[105] The authors' unit prefers the Abram's needle to a cutting needle biopsy, such as the Tru-Cut needle, as the yield is higher (81.8% vs 65.2%), and ultrasound guidance to CT guidance because of ease of access and cost.[53] The authors caution clinicians against performing closed pleural biopsy without any image guidance, as this is unsafe.

MANAGEMENT
Antituberculosis Treatment

Currently, the recommended treatment of pleural TB is the same as for pulmonary TB: a 6-month course consisting of a 2-month intensive phase with 4 drugs (H, R, pyrazinamide, and ethambutol, annotated as 2HRZE), followed by a 4-month maintenance continuation phase with only 2 drugs (4HR).[106,107] Most patients will experience a resolution of their symptoms

after 2 weeks to 2 months of conventional treatment, although the radiographic effusion may take longer to resolve completely.[32] A commonly used alternative regimen omits ethambutol from the intensive phase if the risk of DR-TB is low (6HR2Z).[3] This regimen was recently compared with 6HR alone in 200 HIV-negative patients who were followed up for 8 years. The 2 regimens were found to have similar efficacy, and 6HR was associated with significantly fewer treatment-related adverse effects.[108] Shorter treatment regimens or regimens with fewer drugs have been proposed for simple TB effusions, and good outcomes have been reported in small studies for several regimens, including 1HR followed by twice weekly doses of HR for 5 months, 4HR2Z, and 6HR.[109–111]

In general, patients with complex effusions, patients with frank TB empyema, and PLHIV who are not on antiretroviral treatment (ART) are likely to need extended anti-TB treatment, although the optimal duration and regimen are not known.[32,112] Where the pleura is thickened and diseased, anti-TB drug penetration into the pleural space is variable and may be subtherapeutic.[113–116] Although there is a concern that this may drive the emergence of drug resistance, there is very little direct evidence of this as yet.[116] There may be a role for intrapleural instillation of anti-TB medication, and for therapeutic drug monitoring, but at present the evidence is sparse.[114,115]

The treatment of DR-TB is complex, involving long, tailored regimens with multiple old, new, and repurposed anti-TB drugs, many of which have a high degree of toxicity.[117] This becomes even more complex in PLHIV, as many antiretrovirals have significant interactions with anti-TB drugs, and the timing of ART initiation varies with the duration of TB treatment and the CD4 cell count.[117] The world desperately needs innovations in treatment strategies for both drug-sensitive and DR-TB. Currently, there are at least 22 new and repurposed TB drugs and at least 16 new regimens in clinical trials.[2] However, pleural TB is very often neglected in this rapidly evolving field.

Approximately 25% of patients will experience a "paradoxic response" to treatment shortly after initiation.[42] This is a transient worsening of radiologic features, enlargement of the effusion, and worsening of pulmonary infiltrates, accompanied by worsening of symptoms. It is more common in young, healthy men, and if severe, may require treatment with corticosteroids.[44,118]

Corticosteroids

There is very little evidence for benefit from the use of corticosteroids in pleural TB. In 1988, Lee and colleagues[119] randomized 40 patients with pleural TB to placebo or oral prednisolone and reported a significantly reduced time to resolution of symptoms in the intervention group (2.4 days vs 9.2 days), a significantly faster time to complete reabsorption (54.5 days vs 123.2 days), but no difference in residual pleural thickening (RPT). In 1995, Galarza and colleagues[120] randomized 117 patients with pleural TB to 4 weeks of corticosteroids or placebo and found no statistically significant difference in any outcomes, but there were numerically fewer patients with RPT after treatment in the intervention group. In 1996, Wyser and colleagues[121] randomized 74 patients with pleural TB to placebo or oral prednisone for 4 weeks and found a statistically significant shorter time to resolution of symptoms in the intervention group but no difference in RPT. Bang and colleagues[122] randomized 83 patients with proven pleural TB to corticosteroid treatment or placebo in 1997 and reported a statistically significantly shorter time to resolution of symptoms, and a trend toward a faster time to radiographic resolution and lower incidence of pleural adhesions in the treatment group, which did not reach significance. In 1999, Lee and colleagues[123] randomized 82 patients to steroids or placebo and reported a higher incidence of complete resolution of the radiographic effusion, and a significantly lower incidence of RPT at the end of treatment. Elliott and colleagues[124] specifically looked at PLHIV with pleural TB. They randomized 197 patients to oral prednisolone or placebo. Their primary outcome, mortality rate, was not different between groups, and as expected, they found a statistically significant increase in the incidence of Kaposi sarcoma in the treatment group.

At present, corticosteroids are not recommended for the routine management of pleural TB, but further study of this topic is warranted.[106,125]

Drainage and Intrapleural Fibrinolytics

Small studies have suggested a benefit for early drainage of TB effusions, but the evidence is conflicting.[126,127] However, the evidence favoring the use of intrapleural fibrinolytics is growing, as summarized in **Table 4**. Importantly, these interventions have not been assessed for long-term patient-centered measures of benefit.

COMPLICATIONS
Residual Pleural Thickening

RPT is the commonest complication of pleural TB (see **Fig. 4**). One randomized trial of corticosteroids in pleural TB found evidence of RPT greater than 2 mm in 50% of patients on chest radiograph

and 53% to 60% of patients on CT at 24 weeks after initiation of treatment.[121] In a systematic review of the prevalence and pattern of imaging-defined post-TB lung disease, 4 studies reported RPT greater than 10 mm in 20% to 46% of 223 patients treated for pleural TB.[133] The severest form of RPT is fibrothorax, generally defined as uniform RPT greater than 10 mm with fusion of the visceral and parietal pleura, on all pleural surfaces, leading to encasement and contracture of the hemithorax.[134] Reported frequency of this complication varies, and data are sparse.

RPT has been associated with a mild to moderate restrictive impairment on pulmonary function testing in approximately 10% of patients, which may improve over time, and may be worse with increasing degree of pleural thickening, but is likely independent of specific pleural fluid characteristics and treatment.[49,135–137] When RPT results in a trapped lung (restriction of lung expansion by fibrous visceral pleural peel without fusion of the visceral and parietal layers), the patient may experience marked dyspnea, which requires surgical intervention, provided the underlying lung is viable.[134]

Tuberculosis Empyema

Considered by some to be a distinct disease entity from TB pleuritis, TB empyema is a chronic infection of the pleura by Mtb, which drives an influx of neutrophils, accumulation of neutrophilic debris, and necrosis throughout all layers of the pleura, and a purulent pleural collection.[138,139] This often results in a complex loculated effusion, with thickened, calcified pleura and trapped lung. Theoretically, TB empyema can be a sequela of simple TB pleuritis; can arise from direct local spread from a bronchopleural fistula, ruptured subpleural lung abscess, thoracic lymph node or subdiaphragmatic collection; or may be from hematogenous spread from a distant focus.[22] It may be a complication of TB-related pneumonectomy and in the past was associated with such interventions as Lucite-ball plombage, oleothorax, and therapeutic pneumothorax.[22] Patients may present with minimal symptoms and are rarely systemically ill. The CT chest scan shows thickening of both layers of pleura (with or without calcification depending on the duration) surrounding a viscous fluid collection (**Fig. 7**).[140] There may be associated extrapleural fat proliferation, subpleural abscess, or peripheral bronchopleural fistula present.[44] The yield for bacteriologic tests is higher in TB empyemas than other TB pleural effusions.[4] A minority of patients respond well to anti-TB treatment without drainage; however, concerns have been raised regarding poor drug

Table 4
Intrapleural fibrinolytics for the treatment of tuberculosis pleural effusions

Reference	Design	Population	Intervention	Control	Outcomes
Kwak, 2004[128]	Randomized trial, no blinding	43 patients with loculated TB pleural effusion Intervention: 21 Control: 22	Intrapleural urokinase daily, via pigtail catheter starting when drainage was <100 mL/d, until <50 mL/d Background therapy with anti-TB treatment	Anti-TB treatment only	Less RPT in intervention group than control group (9.5% vs 45.5% with ≥10 mm) ($P = .017$) Improved resolution of radiographic pleural effusion at end of treatment in intervention group (100% of intervention group had >75% improvement compared with 77.3% of control group)
Cases Viedma, 2006[129]	Randomized trial, no blinding	29 patients with loculated TB pleural effusion Intervention: 12 Control: 17	Intrapleural urokinase 12 hourly until drainage was <50 mL/d Background therapy with anti-TB treatment	Simple drainage and suction, with anti-TB treatment	Less RPT in intervention group compared with control at end of treatment (8 mm vs 15 mm) ($P<.05$) Higher drainage volume in intervention group (1487 mL vs 795 mL) ($P<.01$)
Chung, 2008[130]	Double-blinded, randomized, placebo-controlled trial	44 patients with loculated TB pleural effusion Intervention: 22 Control: 22	Intrapleural streptokinase daily via pigtail catheter until drainage was <50 mL/d Background therapy with anti-TB treatment	Intrapleural normal saline daily via pigtail catheter until drainage was <50 mL/d, with anti-TB treatment	Higher rate of CXR improvement at 3 d, complete drainage at 3 d in intervention group ($P<.01$) Faster time to relief of dyspnea (2 d vs 5 d) in intervention group ($P = .018$) Higher volume of pleural fluid drained

(continued on next page)

Table 4
(continued)

Reference	Design	Population	Intervention	Control	Outcomes
					(2.6 L vs 1.3 L) (P = .016) Reduced time from treatment to discharge (7 d vs 10 d) (P = .02)
Cao, 2015[131]	Randomized trial, no blinding	171 patients with free-flowing TB pleural effusion Intervention: 86 Control: 85	Intrapleural urokinase daily for 3 d, starting when drainage was <50 mL/d. Background therapy with anti-TB treatment	Simple drainage and anti-TB treatment	Incrementally higher FVC and TLC in intervention group compared with control at the end of treatment (87.2% vs 83.7% and 95.1% vs 91.7%, respectively) (P<.01) Less RPT >10 mm in intervention group (0% vs 9.0%) (P<.05) Lower incidence of blunting of costophrenic angle (5.1% vs 19.5%) and chest pain on inhalation (9.0% vs 28.6%) (P<.05 and P<.01, respectively)
Barthwal, 2016[132]	Observational, retrospective	59 patients with loculated TB pleural effusion who failed tube drainage	Intrapleural fibrinolysis with either streptokinase or urokinase 8 hourly for 24 h, repeated once if needed	—	37/59 (62.7%) responded to therapy, defined as >500 mL of cumulative drainage and complete or near-complete radiological resolution

Abbreviations: FVC, forced vital capacity; TLC, total lung capacity.

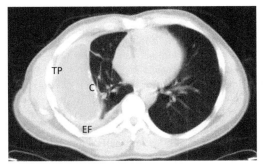

Fig. 7. CT scan obtained from a patient with long-standing, complicated pleural TB (organizing phase) showing a loculated pleural fluid collection with a thickened pleural peel (TP), calcifications (C), and extrapleural fat (EF).

penetration into the pleural space, as well as differential penetration that may lead to the emergence of drug resistance.[113–116] Patients almost invariably require surgery to remove the focus of infection, clear the purulent fluid, and prevent progression to fibrothorax.[4] Decortication through open thoracotomy or video-assisted thoracoscopic surgery has shown reasonable efficacy, although the optimal timing of intervention is unclear.[141–143]

Lipid Effusions

TB is one of the commonest causes of a pseudochylothorax (a cholesterol pleural effusion) worldwide, and it usually arises from a long-standing untreated TB effusion and empyema.[144,145] Invariably, at the time of presentation, the pleura is markedly thickened, and the lung is trapped. The CT chest images are indistinguishable from long-standing complex TB effusions, and the diagnosis should always be entertained in such a situation.[48] A high level of suspicion must also be maintained on pleural fluid analysis, as the pleural fluid only has the typical milky appearance in about half of proven pseudochylothorax cases.[144] The diagnosis is confirmed by a pleural fluid cholesterol level greater than 5.18 mmol/L (>200 mg/dL). Interventions must be guided by the patient's symptoms, level of functional impairment, and evidence (or absence) of ongoing infection. In the authors' environment, pseudochylothorax as a result of previous untreated pleural TB is often an incidental finding, which requires no intervention.

A chylothorax, a pleural effusion containing chylomicrons, triglycerides greater than 1.24 mmol/L (>110 mg/dL), and cholesterol less than 5.18 mmol/L (<200 mg/dL), is a rare manifestation of TB, usually caused by obstruction or erosion of the thoracic duct by TB lymphadenitis rather than pleural infection per se.[146]

SUMMARY

TB is the leading infectious cause of death worldwide, and globally TB remains one of the commonest causes of pleural exudates, particularly in regions with a high TB incidence and in PLHIV. TB pleural effusions are lymphocyte-rich exudates with high ADA, with a low yield on mycobacterial culture. TB pleurisy can also present as loculated neutrophil-predominant effusions, which mimic parapneumonic effusions. Rarely, they can present as frank TB empyema, containing an abundance of mycobacteria. A high proportion of patients have parenchymal involvement on chest imaging. The diagnosis is confirmed by detection of Mtb in sputum, pleural fluid, or pleural tissue, and the recent advent of liquid medium culture techniques has increased the microbiological yield dramatically, but the paucibacillary nature of TB effusions may make mycobacteriologic confirmation challenging. Where the prevalence of TB is high, the presence of a lymphocyte predominant exudate with a high ADA has a high PPV. In low-prevalence areas, a low ADA makes TB very unlikely, and pleural biopsy should be performed to confirm the diagnosis. Pleural biopsy for liquid culture and susceptibility testing must also be considered where the prevalence of DR-TB is high. Treatment regimens are identical to those administered for pulmonary TB. Surgical intervention may be required in loculated effusions and empyemas.

CLINICS CARE POINTS

- Adenosine deaminase should be interpreted with caution in the absence of a differential cell count on the pleural fluid. The pleural fluid lactate dehydrogenase:adenosine deaminase ratio is helpful in this scenario.

- Extremely high pleural fluid adenosine deaminase levels greater than 250 are unlikely to be tuberculosis.

- Closed pleural biopsy has a high yield for pleural tuberculosis but must be performed under image guidance.

- Sputum is often positive for tuberculosis even in the absence of obvious parenchymal disease on chest radiograph.

- In regions with a high prevalence of drug-resistant tuberculosis, diagnosis based only on surrogate biomarkers is discouraged.

- Do not forget to check triglycerides and cholesterol on pleural effusions.

DISCLOSURE STATEMENT

The authors have nothing to disclose.

REFERENCES

1. World Health Organisation. Global health estimates 2016: deaths by cause, age, sex, by country and by region, 2000-2016 2018. Available at: https://www.who.int/healthinfo/global_burden_disease/estimates/en/.
2. World Health Organisation. Global tuberculosis report 2020 2020. Available at: https://www.who.int/teams/global-tuberculosis-programme/tb-reports.
3. Porcel JM. Tuberculous pleural effusion. Lung 2009;187(5):263–70.
4. Shaw JA, Diacon AH, Koegelenberg CFN. Tuberculous pleural effusion. Respirology 2019;24(10):962–71.
5. Patiala J. Initial tuberculous pleuritis in the Finnish armed forces in 1939-1945 with special reference to eventual postpleuritic tuberculosis. Acta Tuberc Scand Suppl 1954;36:1–57.
6. Roper WH, Waring JJ. Primary serofibrinous pleural effusion in military personnel. Am Rev Tuberc 1955;71(5):616–34.
7. Baumann MH, Nolan R, Petrini M, et al. Pleural tuberculosis in the United States: incidence and drug resistance. Chest 2007;131(4):1125–32.
8. Prevention C for DC and. Reported tuberculosis in the United States, 2017. Atlanta, GA: US Department of Health and Human Services, CDC; 2018. p. 2017.
9. Karstaedt AS. Extrapulmonary tuberculosis among adults: experience at Chris Hani Baragwanath Academic hospital, Johannesburg, South Africa. S Afr Med J 2013;104(1):22–4.
10. Edginton ME, Wong ML, Phofa R, et al. Tuberculosis at Chris Hani Baragwanath Hospital : numbers of patients diagnosed and outcomes of referrals to district clinics. Int J Tuberc Lung Dis 2005;9(4):398–402.
11. Valdes L, Alvarez D, Valle JM, et al. The etiology of pleural effusions in an area with high incidence of tuberculosis. Chest 1996;109(1):158–62.
12. Sharma SK, Mohan A. Extrapulmonary tuberculosis. Indian J Med Res 2004;120(4):316–53.
13. Hoogendoorn JC, Ranoto L, Muditambi N, et al. Reduction in extrapulmonary tuberculosis in context of antiretroviral therapy scale-up in rural South Africa. Epidemiol Infect 2017;145(12):2500–9.
14. Diacon AH, Van de Wal BW, Wyser C, et al. Diagnostic tools in tuberculous pleurisy: a direct comparative study. Eur Respir J 2003;22(4):589–91.
15. Friedrich SO, Von Groote-Bidlingmaier F, Diacon AH. Xpert MTB/RIF assay for diagnosis of pleural tuberculosis. J Clin Microbiol 2011;49(12):4341–2.
16. Skouras VS, Kalomenidis I. Drug resistance in patients with tuberculous pleural effusions. Curr Opin Pulm Med 2018;24(4):374–9.
17. Shu C-C, Wang J-T, Wang J-Y, et al. In-hospital outcome of patients with culture-confirmed tuberculous pleurisy: clinical impact of pulmonary involvement. BMC Infect Dis 2011;11:46.
18. Anastasakos V, Skouras V, Moschos C, et al. Patterns of drug resistance among patients with tuberculous pleural effusion in Greece. Int J Tuberc Lung Dis 2017;21(3):309–13.
19. Tahseen S, Ambreen A, Masood F, et al. Primary drug resistance in extra-pulmonary tuberculosis: a hospital-based prospective study from Pakistan. Int J Tuberc Lung Dis 2019;23(8):900–6.
20. Wang G, Wang S, Yang X, et al. Accuracy of Xpert MTB/RIF Ultra for the diagnosis of pleural TB in a Multicenter Cohort study. Chest 2020;157(2):268–75.
21. Stead WW, Eichenholz A, Stauss HK. Operative and pathologic findings in twenty-four patients with syndrome of idiopathic pleurisy with effusion, presumably tuberculous. Am Rev Tuberc 1955;71(4):473–502.
22. Gopi A, Madhavan SM, Sharma SK, et al. Diagnosis and treatment of tuberculous pleural effusion in 2006. Chest 2007;131(3):880–9.
23. Murali R, Park K, Leslie KO. The pleura in health and disease. Semin Respir Crit Care Med 2010;31(6):649–73.
24. Antony VB, Sahn SA, Antony AC, et al. Bacillus Calmette-Guerin-stimulated neutrophils release chemotaxins for monocytes in rabbit pleural spaces and in vitro. J Clin Invest 1985;76(4):1514–21.
25. Antony VB, Repine JE, Harada RN, et al. Inflammatory responses in experimental tuberculosis pleurisy. Acta Cytol 1983;27(3):355–61.
26. da Cunha Lisboa V, Ribeiro-Alves M, da Silva Corrêa R, et al. Predominance of Th1 immune response in pleural effusion of patients with tuberculosis among other Exudative Etiologies. J Clin Microbiol 2019;58(1). https://doi.org/10.1128/JCM.00927-19.
27. Mitra DK, Sharma SK, Dinda AK, et al. Polarized helper T cells in tubercular pleural effusion: phenotypic identity and selective recruitment. Eur J Immunol 2005;35(8):2367–75.
28. Sharma SK, Mitra DK, Balamurugan A, et al. Cytokine polarization in miliary and pleural tuberculosis. J Clin Immunol 2002;22(6):345–52.
29. D'Attilio L, Diaz A, Fernandez RDV, et al. The neuro-endocrine-immune relationship in pulmonary and pleural tuberculosis: a better local profile in pleural fluid. Int J Tuberc Lung Dis 2018;22(3):321–7.
30. ABRAMS WB, SMALL MJ. Current concepts of tuberculous pleurisy with effusion as derived from pleural biopsy studies. Dis Chest 1960;38:60–5.

31. Akulian J, Yarmus L, Feller-Kopman D. The evaluation and clinical Application of pleural physiology. Clin Chest Med 2013;34(1):11–9.

32. Light RW. Update on tuberculous pleural effusion. Respirology 2010;15(3):451–8.

33. Leibowitz S, Kennedy L, Lessof MH. The tuberculin reaction in the pleural cavity and its suppression by antilymphocyte serum. Br J Exp Pathol 1973;54(2):152–62.

34. Berger HW, Mejia E. Tuberculous pleurisy. Chest 1973;63(1):88–92.

35. Levine H, Szanto PB, Cugell DW. Tuberculous pleurisy. An acute illness. Arch Intern Med 1968;122(4):329–32.

36. Heyderman RS, Makunike R, Muza T, et al. Pleural tuberculosis in Harare, Zimbabwe: the relationship between human immunodeficiency virus, CD4 lymphocyte count, granuloma formation and disseminated disease. Trop Med Int Health 1998;3(1):14–20.

37. Richter C, Perenboom R, Mtoni I, et al. Clinical features of HIV-seropositive and HIV-seronegative patients with tuberculous pleural effusion in Dar es Salaam, Tanzania. Chest 1994;106(5):1471–5.

38. Andreu J, Cáceres J, Pallisa E, et al. Radiological manifestations of pulmonary tuberculosis. Eur J Radiol 2004;51(2):139–49.

39. Valdes L, Alvarez D, San Jose E, et al. Tuberculous pleurisy: a study of 254 patients. Arch Intern Med 1998;158(18):2017–21.

40. Porcel JM, Vives M. Etiology and pleural fluid characteristics of large and massive effusions. Chest 2003;124(3):978–83.

41. Seibert AF, Haynes JJ, Middleton R, et al. Tuberculous pleural effusion. Twenty-year experience. Chest 1991;99(4):883–6.

42. Ko JM, Park HJ, Kim CH. Pulmonary changes of pleural TB: up-to-date CT imaging. Chest 2014;146(6):1604–11.

43. Kim HJ, Lee HJ, Kwon S-Y, et al. The prevalence of pulmonary parenchymal tuberculosis in patients with tuberculous pleuritis. Chest 2006;129(5):1253–8.

44. Ko JM, Park HJ, Cho DG, et al. CT differentiation of tuberculous and non-tuberculous pleural infection, with emphasis on pulmonary changes. Int J Tuberc Lung Dis 2015;19(11):1361–8.

45. Skoura E, Bomanji J, Zumla A, et al. Imaging in tuberculosis. Int J Infect Dis 2015;32:87–93.

46. Koegelenberg CFN, Von Groote-Bidlingmaier F, Bolliger CT. Transthoracic ultrasonography for the respiratory physician. Respiration 2012;84(4):337–50.

47. Koh W-J. Progression of tuberculous pleurisy: from a lymphocyte-predominant free-flowing effusion to a neutrophil-predominant loculated effusion. Tuberc Respir Dis (Seoul) 2017;80(1):90–2.

48. Shaw JA, Ahmed L, Koegelenberg CFN. Effusions related to TB. In: Maskell NA, Laursen CB, Lee YG, et al, editors. ERS monograph: pleural disease. European Respiratory Society; 2020. p. 172–92. https://doi.org/10.1183/2312508X.10004420.

49. Chan CHS, Arnold M, Chan CY, et al. Clinical and pathological features of tuberculous pleural effusion and its long-term Consequences. Respiration 1991;58(3–4):171–5.

50. Maartens G, Bateman ED. Tuberculous pleural effusions: increased culture yield with bedside inoculation of pleural fluid and poor diagnostic value of adenosine deaminase. Thorax 1991;46(2):96–9.

51. Luzze H, Elliott AM, Joloba ML, et al. Evaluation of suspected tuberculous pleurisy: clinical and diagnostic findings in HIV-1-positive and HIV-negative adults in Uganda. Int J Tuberc Lung Dis 2001;5(8):746–53.

52. Conde MB, Loivos AC, Rezende VM, et al. Yield of sputum induction in the diagnosis of pleural tuberculosis. Am J Respir Crit Care Med 2003;167(5):723–5.

53. Koegelenberg CFN, Bolliger CT, Theron J, et al. Direct comparison of the diagnostic yield of ultrasound-assisted Abrams and Tru-Cut needle biopsies for pleural tuberculosis. Thorax 2010;65(10):857–62.

54. Ruan S-Y, Chuang Y-C, Wang J-Y, et al. Revisiting tuberculous pleurisy: pleural fluid characteristics and diagnostic yield of mycobacterial culture in an endemic area. Thorax 2012;67(9):822–7.

55. von Groote-Bidlingmaier F, Koegelenberg CF, Bolliger CT, et al. The yield of different pleural fluid volumes for Mycobacterium tuberculosis culture. Thorax 2013;68(3). https://doi.org/10.1136/thoraxjnl-2012-202338.

56. Marjani M, Yousefzadeh A, Tabarsi P, et al. Yield of mycobacteriological study in diagnosis of pleural tuberculosis among Human immune deficiency virus-infected patients. Int J Mycobacteriology 2016;5(Suppl 1):S112–3.

57. Ko Y, Kim C, Chang B, et al. Loculated tuberculous pleural effusion: Easily identifiable and clinically useful predictor of positive mycobacterial culture from pleural fluid. Tuberc Respir Dis (Seoul) 2017;80(1):35–44.

58. Bielsa S, Acosta C, Pardina M, et al. Tuberculous pleural effusion: clinical characteristics of 320 patients. Arch Bronconeumol 2019;55(1):17–22.

59. Pai M, Flores LL, Hubbard A, et al. Nucleic acid amplification tests in the diagnosis of tuberculous pleuritis: a systematic review and meta-analysis. BMC Infect Dis 2004;4:6.

60. Dinnes J, Deeks J, Kunst H, et al. A systematic review of rapid diagnostic tests for the detection of tuberculosis infection. Health Technol Assess 2007;11(3):1–196.

61. World Health Organisation. Automated real-time nucleic acid amplification technology for rapid and simultaneous detection of tuberculosis and rifampicin resistance: xpert MTB/RIF assay for the diagnosis of pulmonary and extrapulmonary TB in adults and children, policy update 2013. Available at: https://apps.who.int/iris/handle/10665/112472.

62. Denkinger CM, Schumacher SG, Boehme CC, et al. Xpert MTB/RIF assay for the diagnosis of extrapulmonary tuberculosis: a systematic review and meta-analysis. Eur Respir J 2014;44(2): 435–46.

63. Penz E, Boffa J, Roberts DJ, et al. Diagnostic accuracy of the Xpert® MTB/RIF assay for extra-pulmonary tuberculosis: a meta-analysis. Int J Tuberc Lung Dis 2015;19(3):278–84. i-iii.

64. Sehgal IS, Dhooria S, Aggarwal AN, et al. Diagnostic performance of Xpert MTB/RIF in tuberculous pleural effusion: systematic review and meta-analysis. J Clin Microbiol 2016;54(4):1133–6.

65. Kohli M, Schiller I, Dendukuri N, et al. Xpert ® MTB/ RIF assay for extrapulmonary tuberculosis and rifampicin resistance. Cochrane Database Syst Rev 2018;8(8):CD012768.

66. Kohli M, Schiller I, Dendukuri N, et al. Xpert MTB/ RIF Ultra and Xpert MTB/RIF assays for extrapulmonary tuberculosis and rifampicin resistance in adults. Cochrane Database Syst Rev 2021;1: CD012768.

67. Zhao T, Chen B, Xu Y, et al. Clinical and pathological differences between polymorphonuclear-rich and lymphocyte-rich tuberculous pleural effusion. Ann Thorac Med 2020;15(2):76–83.

68. Porcel JM. Advances in the diagnosis of tuberculous pleuritis. Ann Transl Med 2016;4(15):282.

69. Perez-Risco D, Rodriguez-Temporal D, Valledor-Sanchez I, et al. Evaluation of the Xpert MTB/RIF Ultra assay for direct detection of Mycobacterium tuberculosis Complex in smear-negative extrapulmonary samples. J Clin Microbiol 2018;56(9). https://doi.org/10.1128/JCM.00659-18.

70. Meldau R, Randall P, Pooran A, et al. Same-day tools, including Xpert Ultra and IRISA-TB, for rapid diagnosis of pleural tuberculosis: a prospective observational study. J Clin Microbiol 2019;57(9). https://doi.org/10.1128/JCM.00614-19.

71. Goto M, Noguchi Y, Koyama H, et al. Diagnostic value of adenosine deaminase in tuberculous pleural effusion: a meta-analysis. Ann Clin Biochem 2003;40(Pt 4):374–81.

72. Greco S, Girardi E, Masciangelo R, et al. Adenosine deaminase and interferon gamma measurements for the diagnosis of tuberculous pleurisy: a meta-analysis. Int J Tuberc Lung Dis 2003;7(8): 777–86.

73. Liang Q-L, Shi H-Z, Wang K, et al. Diagnostic accuracy of adenosine deaminase in tuberculous pleurisy: a meta-analysis. Respir Med 2008; 102(5):744–54.

74. Morisson P, Neves DD. Evaluation of adenosine deaminase in the diagnosis of pleural tuberculosis: a Brazilian meta-analysis. J Bras Pneumol 2008; 34(4):217–24.

75. Gui X, Xiao H. Diagnosis of tuberculosis pleurisy with adenosine deaminase (ADA): a systematic review and meta-analysis. Int J Clin Exp Med 2014; 7(10):3126–35.

76. Aggarwal AN, Agarwal R, Sehgal IS, et al. Meta-analysis of Indian studies evaluating adenosine deaminase for diagnosing tuberculous pleural effusion. Int J Tuberc Lung Dis 2016;20(10):1386–91.

77. Aggarwal AN, Agarwal R, Sehgal IS, et al. Adenosine deaminase for diagnosis of tuberculous pleural effusion: a systematic review and meta-analysis. PLoS One 2019;14(3):e0213728.

78. Palma RM, Bielsa S, Esquerda A, et al. Diagnostic accuracy of pleural fluid adenosine deaminase for diagnosing tuberculosis. Meta-analysis of Spanish studies. Arch Bronconeumol 2019;55(1):23–30.

79. Jiang J, Shi H-Z, Liang Q-L, et al. Diagnostic value of interferon-gamma in tuberculous pleurisy: a metaanalysis. Chest 2007;131(4):1133–41.

80. Zhou Q, Chen Y-Q, Qin S-M, et al. Diagnostic accuracy of T-cell interferon-γ release assays in tuberculous pleurisy: a meta-analysis. Respirology 2011;16(3):473–80.

81. Pang C-S, Shen Y-C, Tian P-W, et al. Accuracy of the interferon-gamma release assay for the diagnosis of tuberculous pleurisy: an updated meta-analysis. PeerJ 2015;3:e951.

82. Zhou X-X, Liu Y-L, Zhai K, et al. Body fluid interferon-γ release assay for diagnosis of extrapulmonary tuberculosis in adults: a systematic review and meta-analysis. Sci Rep 2015;5:15284.

83. Aggarwal AN, Agarwal R, Gupta D, et al. Interferon gamma release assays for diagnosis of pleural tuberculosis: a systematic review and meta-analysis. J Clin Microbiol 2015;53(8):2451–9.

84. Li ZZ, Qin WZ, Li L, et al. Accuracy of enzyme-linked immunospot assay for diagnosis of pleural tuberculosis: a meta-analysis. Genet Mol Res 2015;14(3):11672–80.

85. Li M, Zhu W, Khan RSU, et al. Accuracy of interleukin-27 assay for the diagnosis of tuberculous pleurisy: a PRISMA-compliant meta-analysis. Medicine (Baltimore) 2017;96(50):e9205.

86. Zeng N, Wan C, Qin J, et al. Diagnostic value of interleukins for tuberculous pleural effusion: a systematic review and meta-analysis. BMC Pulm Med 2017;17(1):180.

87. Wang W, Zhou Q, Zhai K, et al. Diagnostic accuracy of interleukin 27 for tuberculous pleural effusion: two prospective studies and one metaanalysis. Thorax 2018;73(3):240–7.

88. Liu Q, Yu Y-X, Wang X-J, et al. Diagnostic accuracy of interleukin-27 between tuberculous pleural effusion and Malignant pleural effusion: a meta-analysis. Respiration 2018;95(6):469–77.

89. Li M, Luo Z, Zhu W, et al. Diagnostic accuracy of tumor necrosis factor-alpha assay for tuberculous pleurisy: a PRISMA-compliant meta-analysis. Medicine (Baltimore) 2016;95(48):e5510.

90. Tong X, Lu H, Yu M, et al. Diagnostic value of interferon-γ-induced protein of 10kDa for tuberculous pleurisy: a meta-analysis. Clin Chim Acta 2017;471:143–9.

91. Skouras VS, Kalomenidis I. Pleural fluid tests to diagnose tuberculous pleuritis. Curr Opin Pulm Med 2016;22(4):367–77.

92. Burgess LJ, Maritz FJ, Le Roux I, et al. Combined use of pleural adenosine deaminase with lymphocyte/neutrophil ratio. Increased specificity for the diagnosis of tuberculous pleuritis. Chest J 1996;109(2):414–9.

93. Sivakumar P, Marples L, Breen R, et al. The diagnostic utility of pleural fluid adenosine deaminase for tuberculosis in a low prevalence area. Int J Tuberc Lung Dis 2017;21(6):697–701.

94. Blakiston M, Chiu W, Wong C, et al. Diagnostic performance of pleural fluid adenosine deaminase for tuberculous pleural effusion in a low-incidence setting. J Clin Microbiol 2018;56(8). https://doi.org/10.1128/JCM.00258-18.

95. Wang J, Liu J, Xie X, et al. The pleural fluid lactate dehydrogenase/adenosine deaminase ratio differentiates between tuberculous and parapneumonic pleural effusions. BMC Pulm Med 2017;17(1):168.

96. Beukes A, Shaw JA, Diacon AH, et al. The utility of pleural fluid lactate dehydrogenase to adenosine deaminase ratio in pleural tuberculosis. Respiration 2020. https://doi.org/10.1159/000509555.

97. Yang X, Zhang J, Liang Q, et al. Use of T-SPOT.TB for the diagnosis of unconventional pleural tuberculosis is superior to ADA in high prevalence areas: a prospective analysis of 601 cases. BMC Infect Dis 2021;21(1):4.

98. Luo Y, Tan Y, Yu J, et al. The performance of pleural fluid T-SPOT.TB assay for diagnosing tuberculous pleurisy in China: a two-Center prospective Cohort study. Front Cell Infect Microbiol 2019;9:10. Available at: https://www.frontiersin.org/article/10.3389/fcimb.2019.00010.

99. Skouras VS, Magkouta SF, Psallidas I, et al. Interleukin-27 improves the ability of adenosine deaminase to rule out tuberculous pleural effusion regardless of pleural tuberculosis prevalence. Infect Dis (London, England) 2015;47(7):477–83.

100. Valdes L, San Jose E, Ferreiro L, et al. Interleukin 27 could be useful in the diagnosis of tuberculous pleural effusions. Respir Care 2014;59(3):399–405.

101. Yang W-B, Liang Q-L, Ye Z-J, et al. Cell origins and diagnostic accuracy of interleukin 27 in pleural effusions. PLoS One 2012;7(7):e40450.

102. Zhang M, Li D, Hu Z-D, et al. The diagnostic utility of pleural markers for tuberculosis pleural effusion. Ann Transl Med 2020;8(9):607.

103. Sharma SK, Banga A. Pleural fluid interferon-gamma and adenosine deaminase levels in tuberculosis pleural effusion: a cost-effectiveness analysis. J Clin Lab Anal 2005;19(2):40–6.

104. Lewinsohn DMDA, Leonard MK, LoBue PA, et al. Official American thoracic society/infectious diseases society of America/Centers for disease Control and prevention clinical practice guidelines: diagnosis of tuberculosis in adults and Children. Clin Infect Dis 2017;64(2):111–5.

105. Koegelenberg CF, Irusen EM, von Groote-Bidlingmaier F, et al. The utility of ultrasound-guided thoracocentesis and pleural biopsy in undiagnosed pleural exudates. Thorax 2015;70(10):995–7.

106. Sharma SK, Ryan H, Khaparde S, et al. Index-TB guidelines: Guidelines on extrapulmonary tuberculosis for India. Indian J Med Res 2017;145(4):448–63.

107. WHO. Guidelines for Treatment of Drug-Susceptible Tuberculosis and Patient Care.; 2017. doi:10.1586/17476348.1.1.85

108. Garcia-Rodriguez JF, Valcarce-Pardeiro N, Alvarez-Diaz H, et al. Long-term efficacy of 6-month therapy with isoniazid and rifampin compared with isoniazid, rifampin, and pyrazinamide treatment for pleural tuberculosis. Eur J Clin Microbiol Infect Dis 2019. https://doi.org/10.1007/s10096-019-03651-7.

109. Bouayad Z, Aichane A, Trombati N, et al. [Treatment of pleural tuberculosis with a short 4-month regimen: preliminary results]. Tuber Lung Dis 1995;76(4):367–9.

110. Dutt AK, Moers D, Stead WW. Tuberculous pleural effusion: 6-month therapy with isoniazid and rifampin. Am Rev Respir Dis 1992;145(6):1429–32.

111. Canete C, Galarza I, Granados A, et al. Tuberculous pleural effusion: experience with six months of treatment with isoniazid and rifampicin. Thorax 1994;49(11):1160–1.

112. Ahmad Khan F, Minion J, Al-Motairi A, et al. An updated systematic review and meta-analysis on the treatment of active tuberculosis in patients with HIV infection. Clin Infect Dis 2012;55(8):1154–63.

113. Elliott AM, Berning SE, Iseman MD, et al. Failure of drug penetration and acquisition of drug resistance in chronic tuberculous empyema. Tuber Lung Dis 1995;76(5):463–7.

114. Long R, Barrie J, Peloquin CA. Therapeutic drug monitoring and the conservative management of chronic tuberculous empyema: case report and review of the literature. BMC Infect Dis 2015;15:327.

115. Long R, Barrie J, Stewart K, et al. Treatment of a tuberculous empyema with simultaneous oral and

intrapleural antituberculosis drugs. Can Respir J 2008;15(5):241–3.

116. Iseman MD, Madsen LA. Chronic tuberculous empyema with bronchopleural fistula resulting in treatment failure and progressive drug resistance. Chest 1991;100(1):124–7.

117. World Health Organization. WHO consolidated Guidelines on drug-resistant tuberculosis treatment 2019. Available at: https//www.who.int/tb/publications/2019/consolidated-guidelines-drug-resistant-TB-treatment/en/.

118. Al-Majed SA. Study of paradoxical response to chemotherapy in tuberculous pleural effusion. Respir Med 1996;90(4):211–4.

119. Lee CH, Wang WJ, Lan RS, et al. Corticosteroids in the treatment of tuberculous pleurisy. A double-blind, placebo-controlled, randomized study. Chest 1988;94(6):1256–9.

120. Galarza I, Cañete C, Granados A, et al. Randomised trial of corticosteroids in the treatment of tuberculous pleurisy. Thorax 1995;50(12):1305–7.

121. Wyser C, Walzl G, Smedema JP, et al. Corticosteroids in the treatment of tuberculous pleurisy. A double-blind, placebo-controlled, randomized study. Chest 1996;110(2):333–8.

122. Bang J, Kim M, Kwak S, et al. Evaluation of steroid therapy in tuberculous pleurisy - a prospective, randomized study. Tuberc Respir Dis 1997;44(1):52–8.

123. Lee B, Jee H, Choi J, et al. Therapeutic effect of prednisolone in tuberculous pleurisy - a prospective study for the prevention of the pleural adhesion. Tuberc Respir Dis 1999;46(4):481–8.

124. Elliott AM, Luzze H, Quigley MA, et al. A randomized, double-blind, placebo-controlled trial of the use of prednisolone as an adjunct to treatment in HIV-1-associated pleural tuberculosis. J Infect Dis 2004;190(5):869–78.

125. Ryan H, Yoo J, Darsini P. Corticosteroids for tuberculous pleurisy. Cochrane Database Syst Rev 2017;3:CD001876.

126. Lai Y-F, Chao T-Y, Wang Y-H, et al. Pigtail drainage in the treatment of tuberculous pleural effusions: a randomised study. Thorax 2003;58(2):149–51.

127. Bhuniya S, Arunabha DC, Choudhury S, et al. Role of therapeutic thoracentesis in tuberculous pleural effusion. Ann Thorac Med 2012;7(4):215–9.

128. Kwak SM, Park CS, Cho JH, et al. The effects of urokinase instillation therapy via percutaneous transthoracic catheter in loculated tuberculous pleural effusion: a randomized prospective study. Yonsei Med J 2004;45(5):822–8.

129. Cases Viedma E, Lorenzo Dus MJ, Gonzalez-Molina A, et al. A study of loculated tuberculous pleural effusions treated with intrapleural urokinase. Respir Med 2006;100(11):2037–42.

130. Chung C-L, Chen C-H, Yeh C-Y, et al. Early effective drainage in the treatment of loculated tuberculous pleurisy. Eur Respir J 2008;31(6):1261–7.

131. Cao G-Q, Li L, Wang Y-B, et al. Treatment of free-flowing tuberculous pleurisy with intrapleural urokinase. Int J Tuberc Lung Dis 2015;19(11):1395–400.

132. Barthwal MS, Marwah V, Chopra M, et al. A Five-year study of intrapleural Fibrinolytic therapy in loculated pleural Collections. Indian J Chest Dis Allied Sci 2016;58(1):17–20.

133. Meghji J, Simpson H, Squire SB, et al. A systematic review of the prevalence and pattern of imaging Defined post-TB lung disease. PLoS One 2016;11(8):e0161176.

134. Jantz MA, Antony VB. Pleural fibrosis. Clin Chest Med 2006;27(2):181–91.

135. Candela A, Andujar J, Hernandez L, et al. Functional sequelae of tuberculous pleurisy in patients correctly treated. Chest 2003;123(6):1996–2000.

136. Barbas CS, Cukier A, de Varvalho CR, et al. The relationship between pleural fluid findings and the development of pleural thickening in patients with pleural tuberculosis. Chest 1991;100(5):1264–7.

137. Bolliger CT, de Kock MA. Influence of a fibrothorax on the flow/volume curve. Respiration 1988;54(3):197–200.

138. Sonmezoglu Y, Turna A, Cevik A, et al. Factors affecting morbidity in chronic tuberculous empyema. Thorac Cardiovasc Surg 2008;56(2):99–102.

139. English JC, Leslie KO. Pathology of the pleura. Clin Chest Med 2006;27(2):157–80.

140. Sahn SA, Iseman MD. Tuberculous empyema. Semin Respir Infect 1999;14(1):82–7.

141. Bagheri R, Haghi SZ, Dalouee MN, et al. Effect of decortication and pleurectomy in chronic empyema patients. Asian Cardiovasc Thorac Ann 2016;24(3):245–9.

142. Chen B, Zhang J, Ye Z, et al. Outcomes of Video-assisted thoracic surgical decortication in 274 patients with tuberculous empyema. Ann Thorac Cardiovasc Surg 2015;21(3):223–8.

143. Kumar A, Asaf BB, Lingaraju VC, et al. Thoracoscopic decortication of stage III tuberculous empyema is effective and safe in selected cases. Ann Thorac Surg 2017;104(5):1688–94.

144. Lama A, Ferreiro L, Toubes ME, et al. Characteristics of patients with pseudochylothorax-a systematic review. J Thorac Dis 2016;8(8):2093–101.

145. Ryu JH, Tomassetti S, Maldonado F. Update on uncommon pleural effusions. Respirology 2011;16(2):238–43.

146. Rajagopala S, Kancherla R, Ramanathan RP. Tuberculosis-Associated Chylothorax: case report and systematic review of the literature. Respiration 2018;95(4):260–8.

Chylothorax and Pseudochylothorax

Cassandra M. Braun, MD, Jay H. Ryu, MD*

KEYWORDS

- Chylothorax • Pseudochylothorax • Yellow nail syndrome • Lymphangioleiomyomatosis

KEY POINTS

- Chylothorax and pseudochylothorax both represent rare forms of pleural effusion and commonly present with a milky white appearance to the pleural fluid.
- The etiology, pathogenesis, management, and clinical implications of a diagnosis of chylothorax and pseudochylothorax are quite different. Pleural fluid analysis is key to differentiate the two.
- Chylothorax is characterized by the presence of chylomicrons, a pleural fluid triglyceride level of greater than 110 mg/dL (1.24 mmol/L), and a cholesterol level of less than 200 mg/dL (5.2 mmol/L).
- Pseudochylothorax is characterized by a neutrophil-predominant exudate and has a cholesterol level ≥200 mg/dL (5.2 mmol/L), whereas the triglyceride level is usually less than 50 mg/dL (0.56 mmol/L).

INTRODUCTION

Most pleural effusions are encountered in the setting of an underlying disorder, with the vast majority of pleural effusions being due to malignancy, heart failure, or infection. Herein, we review uncommon types of pleural effusions encountered in clinical practice that have distinct clinical presentation and pleural fluid characteristics: chylothorax and pseudochylothorax. We also discuss uncommon diseases with well-recognized association with these types of pleural effusions: yellow nail syndrome (YNS) and lymphangioleiomyomatosis (LAM). Recognition of these entities is important because each is associated with distinct pathogenesis and management.

CHYLOTHORAX

Chylothorax, also commonly known as chylous pleural effusion, is defined by the presence of chyle in the pleural cavity. Chyle is a lymphatic fluid rich in lymphocytes, immunoglobulins, electrolytes, vitamins, water, and lipids, and has a characteristically white, milky, and opalescent appearance. The thoracic duct transports chyle and typically originates from the cisterna chyli in the abdomen. It then traverses the aortic diaphragmatic hiatus running posteriorly in the thorax between the azygous vein and the aorta on the right side. At the level of the fifth to seventh thoracic vertebrae, it then crosses to the left chest and enters the venous system at the juncture of the left jugular and subclavian veins. Of note, substantial variation in anatomy (40%–60% of patients) has been observed, and tributaries to the main thoracic duct are not uncommon.[1,2]

A chylous effusion can result from trauma or a benign or malignant disease process leading to occlusion or disruption of the thoracic duct with leakage of lymph into the pleural space (**Table 1**).

Dr C.M. Braun is an Assistant Professor of Medicine at the Mayo Clinic College of Medicine, Rochester MN, USA, and her areas of research interest include pleural diseases, thoracic oncology, interstitial lung diseases, and critical care medicine. Dr J.H. Ryu is David E. and Bette H. Dines Professor of Medicine at the Mayo Clinic College of Medicine, Rochester, MN, USA. His areas of research interest include interstitial lung diseases and pleural diseases. The authors have no commercial or financial conflicts of interest or funding sources to disclose.
Division of Pulmonary and Critical Care Medicine, Mayo Clinic, Gonda 18 South, 200 First Street, Southwest, Rochester, MN 55905, USA
* Corresponding author.
E-mail address: ryu.jay@mayo.edu

Clin Chest Med 42 (2021) 667–675
https://doi.org/10.1016/j.ccm.2021.08.003
0272-5231/21/© 2021 Elsevier Inc. All rights reserved.

Table 1
Etiology of chylothorax

Traumatic	Nontraumatic
Surgical: • Esophageal • Thoracic • Cardiac (coronary artery bypass graft) • Thoracolumbar fusion • Cervical node dissection	Malignancy: most are lymphoma Idiopathic partial or complete obstruction of the thoracic duct Congestive heart failure Nephrotic syndrome Cirrhosis
Penetrating trauma (gunshot or knife wounds)	Mediastinal lymphadenopathy
Hyperextension of the spine	Pulmonary lymphangioleiomyomatosis
Vertebral fracture	Yellow nail syndrome
Blunt trauma to the chest (falls, motor vehicle accident)	Sarcoidosis
Cough	Congenital chylothorax (lymphangiectasias, Down syndrome, Noonan syndrome)
Childbirth	Paragonimiasis and filariasis
Weightlifting	Thrombosis of the superior vena cava or subclavian vein
Central venous catheterization	Constrictive pericarditis
	Thyroid goiter
	Migration of chylous ascites through diaphragm defects
	Prior mediastinal radiotherapy

Most patients with chylothorax will have a unilateral pleural effusion, the side being dependent on the anatomic level at which the chyle leak is located. The degree of injury and patient diet will dictate the rate at which fluid accumulates in the pleural space and as such there may be a variable latency period of 2 days to several weeks before a patient becomes symptomatic.[2] If left untreated, patients with recurrent and large chylothorax may develop resultant hypovolemia, malnutrition, significant electrolyte imbalances and vitamin deficiencies, and immunosuppression.[2]

The diagnosis of chylothorax is made by pleural fluid analysis. Traditional teaching has set diagnostic criteria for chylothorax of a pleural fluid triglyceride level of greater than 110 mg/dL (1.24 mmol/L) and a cholesterol level of less than 200 mg/dL (5.2 mmol/L). In addition, the pleural fluid to serum triglyceride ratio should be >1 and the pleural fluid to serum cholesterol ratio less than 1. Notably, when the triglyceride level in pleural fluid is found to be <50 mg/dL (0.56 mmol/L) the diagnosis of chylothorax is unlikely.[2,3] Most (80%) chylous pleural effusions will be characterized as exudative by the Light criteria.[4] In prior studies when a chylous pleural effusion is found to be transudative in nature, the underlying etiologies included hepatic cirrhosis, nephrotic syndrome, amyloidosis, and obstruction of the superior vena cava.[4,5]

Classically, chylothorax is associated with a milky white appearance of the pleural fluid; however, gross appearance of the fluid can be variable and may be present in fewer than 50% of cases.[4,6] It should be noted that empyema can also result in appearance of a milky white fluid mimicking chylous effusion. To differentiate the two, centrifugation of the pleural fluid sample can be done, which will illustrate a difference in the supernatant between empyema and chylous effusion, as shown in **Fig. 1**. Notably, patients who are fasting or in a postoperative state at the time of pleural fluid sampling may not demonstrate the classic milky appearance but still meet criteria for chylothorax. Similarly, when triglyceride levels fall within the range of 50 to 110 mg/dL, there is diagnostic uncertainty and thus the clinician must remain vigilant in their consideration and workup for this diagnosis. The presence of chylomicrons in the pleural fluid is pathognomonic of chylothorax and can be identified through use of lipoprotein electrophoresis.[3] It should be noted that although lipoprotein electrophoresis remains the gold standard for diagnosis (with reported 83% sensitivity and

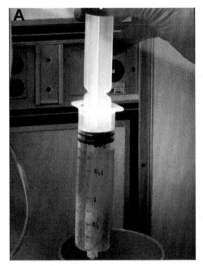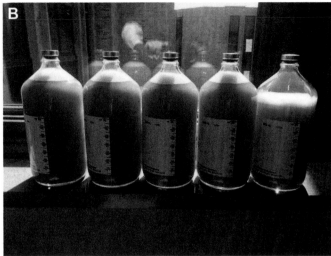

Fig. 1. (*A*) Image of pleural fluid secondary to empyema illustrating settling of the neutrophilic debris and presence of a clear supernatant fluid. (*B*) Image of pleural fluid secondary to a chylous pleural effusion demonstrating persistence of an opaque supernatant. (*Courtesy of* Dante Schiavo, MD and David Midthun, MD Rochester MN.)

100% specificity), it may not be widely available in diagnostic laboratories because of the cost and labor intensity.[3]

Once the diagnosis is established via pleural fluid analysis, the clinician's next step is to ascertain the location and etiology of the chyle leak. Imaging studies, including computed tomography of the chest, MRI of the chest and abdomen, pedal or intranodal lymphangiography, and radionuclide lymphoscintigraphy are most often used.[7] Other means to locate the leak can include the addition of methylene blue to a fat source, such as cream, to help highlight the site of the leak under direct visualization with thoracoscopy.

Treatment of chylous effusions can consist of either conservative (medical) therapy or procedural/surgical intervention, or a combination of the two (**Box 1**, **Fig. 2**). One approach is dietary changes consisting of a high-carbohydrate and high-protein, low-fat diet with focus on ingestion of primarily medium-chain triglycerides that are directly absorbed into the portal circulation.[2] The use of total parenteral nutrition has also been used with complete bowel rest. Administration of octreotide or somatostatin are adjunctive pharmacologic options for management of chylothorax alongside dietary measures. Somatostatin is an endogenous hormone and octreotide is a synthetic long-acting somatostatin analogue that reduce lymph flow and can be administered intravenously or subcutaneously.[8,9] The mechanism by which lymph flow is reduced is thought to be via decreased intestinal absorption of fats, decreased concentration of triglycerides in the thoracic duct, and reduction in splanchnic blood flow, as well as hepatic venous pressures.[10] In most reports, if octreotide or somatostatin is used, the reduction in pleural fluid output is seen within 2 to 3 days, and thus investigators have advocated using a time-limited trial of 1 week.[8]

Box 1
Management options in chylothorax

Observation

Treat underlying condition

Dietary measures: medium-chain triglyceride diet, trial of nil by mouth and total parenteral nutrition

Thoracentesis

Chest tube or indwelling pleural catheter placement

Somatostatin or octreotide

Percutaneous embolization or interruption of the thoracic duct

Pleurodesis via chest tube

Surgical interventions:

- Mechanical or chemical pleurodesis
- Pleurectomy
- Thoracic duct repair or ligation
- Lympho-venous anastomosis
- Pleuro-peritoneal shunting

Adapted from: Ryu JH, Tomassetti S, Maldonado F. Update on uncommon pleural effusions. *Respirology.* 2011;16(2):238-243.

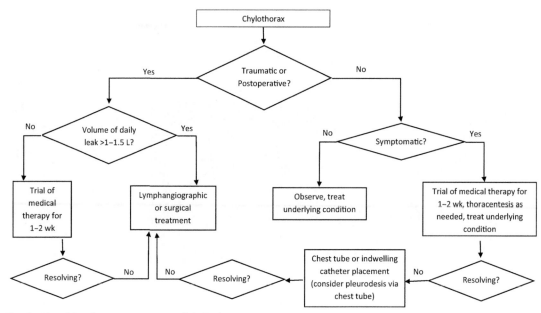

Fig. 2. Algorithm for management of chylothorax.

In cases of postoperative or traumatic chylothorax, the use of the preceding conservative (medical) therapies for up to 2 weeks may result in resolution of the chyle leak for approximately 50% of patients without need for other intervention.[2,11,12] However, in patients who have undergone certain procedures, such as esophagectomy, early procedural or surgical intervention is associated with significantly better mortality outcomes compared with conservative management.[2] Surgical duct ligation or lymphangiography with percutaneous thoracic duct embolization (TDE) is warranted, particularly when the volume of daily chyle leak exceeds 1 to 1.5 L in a day for more than 5 to 7 days. The main limiting factor in successful treatment via lymphangiography with percutaneous TDE is whether the cisterna chyli can be cannulated. In review of several series, the success rate of TDE varied between 38% and 79%, with failure to cannulate the cisterna in these series attributed to body habitus, contrast reaction, or unfavorable anatomy.[13–15] The most used embolic agents include metallic coils, Gelfoam, cyanoacrylate glue, or ethyl vinyl alcohol[15] (**Fig. 3**). In postoperative cases, surgical ligation of the thoracic duct has reported success rates of 85% to 90% in resolution of chylothorax.[15] Other surgical interventions used include placement of a pleuroperitoneal shunt, mass supradiaphragmatic ligation of the thoracic duct, pleural decortication, pleurectomy, and surgical pleurodesis.[11,16] In cases of malignant chylothorax or when the thoracic duct is unidentifiable, talc

pleurodesis has demonstrated good success rates in prevention of recurrent chylothorax.[2]

PSEUDOCHYLOTHORAX (CHOLESTEROL EFFUSION)

Pseudochylothorax is a rare form of pleural effusion, also known as cholesterol pleural effusion, and is less common than chylothorax. Pseudochylothorax is usually unilateral and is due to the accumulation of cholesterol or lecithin-globulin complexes in the pleural space. It is characterized by accumulation of turbid or milky white pleural fluid. Despite the similar gross appearance to chylous pleural effusions, these 2 forms of pleural effusions have different etiology, pathogenesis, and clinical implications. Approximately one-third of patients are asymptomatic at presentation.[16–18] The most common etiologies of pseudochylothorax include tuberculous pleurisy, chronic rheumatoid pleuritis, chronic pneumothorax, trapped lung, and chronic hemothorax.[17–21] Rarely, pseudochylothorax is seen with pleural paragonimiasis, echinococcosis, malignancy, or trauma[17–19,21,22] (**Table 2**).

The diagnosis of pseudochylothorax is established by pleural fluid analysis. Unlike in chylothorax, chylomicrons are not present in pseudochylothorax.[4,17] Cholesterol crystals may be seen on microscopy and have the typical rhomboid shape. Pleural fluid in pseudochylothorax is a neutrophil-predominant exudate and has a cholesterol level ≥ 200 mg/dL (5.2 mmol/L), while

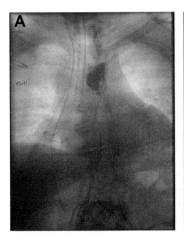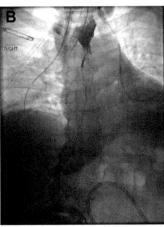

Fig. 3. (*A*) Lymphangiogram demonstrating leaking oil-based contrast (Lipiodol) pooling in the upper mediastinum in a patient after Ivor Lewis Esophagectomy. (*B*) Thoracic duct was embolized using micro coils and cyanoacrylate glue with resolution of the leak.

the triglyceride level is usually less than 50 mg/dL (0.56 mmol/L). Sometimes, triglyceride level may be elevated in pseudochylothorax, but the pleural fluid cholesterol to triglyceride ratio is always greater than 1.[17]

Pseudochylothorax is generally seen in patients with thickened or calcified pleural surfaces and chronic exudative pleural effusions, usually of 5 years' duration or longer.[17,18,23] The exact pathogenesis of pseudochylothorax remains unclear, but the high concentration of cholesterol in the pleural fluid was believed to originate from degraded erythrocytes and neutrophils that are poorly absorbed through a thickened pleural surface. Pseudochylothorax has often been considered a form of lung entrapment in the setting of chronic inflammation.[17] However, the necessity of chronic pleuritis and significant pleural thickening in the development of pseudochylothorax has been called into question. Wrightson and colleagues[19] reported 6 patients with pseudochylothorax that occurred with a short duration of symptoms and in the absence of a thickened pleura. Five of these patients had rheumatoid arthritis and 1 had seronegative inflammatory arthritis. Thus, pseudochylothorax should be included in the differential diagnosis for patients with unexplained pleural effusions, even in the absence of a long history or marked pleural thickening.

In most cases, pseudochylothorax is associated with a benign course and no specific therapy is required. Therapeutic thoracentesis may be needed if the patient has increasing pleural effusion with symptoms. In some patients, aggressive treatment of the underlying disease (tuberculosis or rheumatoid arthritis) may lead to control or resolution of pseudochylothorax.[19,21] Decortication and pleurodesis may be attempted in patients with recurrent symptomatic pseudochylothorax that is not controlled by nonsurgical means.[19,21]

YELLOW NAIL SYNDROME

YNS is a rare disorder characterized by the triad of yellow and thickened nails, lymphedema, and pleural effusion or other respiratory abnormality, including bronchiectasis and chronic sinusitis (**Fig. 4**).[16,24–26] Originally described by Samman and White[27] in 1964 in a case series of 13 patients, there have since been at least 160 cases reported in the literature.[16,24] As some of the findings in YNS may resolve over time, it has been suggested that the presence at any given time of 2 of the triad of manifestations is sufficient to establish the diagnosis of YNS.[28]

Table 2 Etiology of pseudochylothorax	
Common Etiologies	**Rare Etiologies**
Tuberculous pleurisy	Pleural paragonimiasis
Chronic rheumatoid pleuritis	Echinococcosis
Chronic pneumothorax	Malignancy
Chronic hemothorax	Trauma

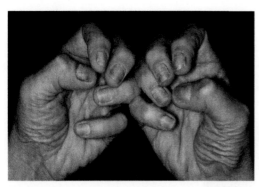

Fig. 4. Typical appearance of nails in YNS characterized by discoloration, thickening, and slow growth. (*Courtesy of* Emily Bendel, MD Rochester MN.)

The pathogenesis of this rare syndrome remains poorly understood. Various anatomic abnormalities of the lymphatic ducts, including lymphatic hypoplasia, dilatations, and extensive collateral lymphatic networks, have been noted on lymphangiography in patients with YNS.[16,27,29] Other investigators have noted functional lymphatic abnormalities based on results of lymphoscintigraphy.[30,31] Histologically, conflicting results have been reported, with some investigators noting dilated lymphatic capillaries in the pleura, whereas others have described relatively normal-appearing lymphatic vessels.[16,25,32] At the present time, functional lymphatic disorder rather than structural disease is favored as the shared pathogenic mechanism for the development of pleural effusions and lymphedema.[16,24,31]

Although a few case reports of familial YNS exist, the evidence to date suggests that the lymphatic dysfunction observed in YNS is an acquired disorder rather than a heritable one.[24] Environmental exposures, including smoking, do not appear to play a role in the pathogenesis of the disease. The recurrent observation that severe respiratory infections often predate the development of lymphedema has led to speculation that infections may serve as a trigger that overwhelms a preexisting dysfunctional lymphatic network, that is, a 2-hit process, and leads to clinical manifestations of YNS.[24,30,31]

YNS has been described in association with a variety of conditions, including malignancy, lymphoproliferative disorders, immunodeficiency states, connective tissue disorders, endocrinopathies, obstructive sleep apnea, Guillain–Barré syndrome, xanthogranulomatous pyelonephritis, and tuberculosis.[24,33] Several cases of antirheumatic drug-induced YNS have been reported in patients with rheumatoid arthritis who were treated with gold, penicillamine, or bucillamine.[33,34]

There is no gender predilection in YNS, which typically presents between the fourth and sixth decades.[24,25] Abnormal nails are the most common manifestation described in patients with YNS, as the diagnosis is hardly ever considered otherwise. Aside from the discoloration, nail abnormalities include slow growth, thickening, transverse ridging, excessive curvature from side to side, uneven pigmentation, diminished lunulae, and onycholysis. The nail findings may vary over time. Several investigators have reported some improvement in the nail abnormalities with better control of the respiratory manifestations or decongestive therapy for lymphedema.[24,25,32,35] The use of topical steroids, azole antifungal agents, or vitamin E has been described, although the evidence supporting their use remains scarce.[24,33]

Lymphedema is present in the vast majority of patients with YNS (80%) and is the presenting symptom in one-third of the cases.[24,25,36] The lower extremities are most affected in a symmetric fashion with nonpitting edema. Lymphedema may also occur in the upper extremities, face, and occasionally in the peritoneal cavity with ascites. Lymphedema tends to persist, although improvements have sometimes been noted with decongestive therapy such as low-pressure compression pumps.[24,37]

Respiratory manifestations are variable.[24,25,36] Bronchiectasis and recurrent lower respiratory tract infections are present in almost half of the patients. Chronic sinusitis is present in 40% of patients.[25] Pleural effusions, usually bilateral, are seen in approximately 40% of cases. Pleural fluid typically shows a lymphocyte-predominant exudate by protein criterion, but in the transudative range by cholesterol and lactate dehydrogenase parameters.[25,36] Chylothorax accounts for 30% of pleural effusions seen in patients with YNS.[25]

Most clinical manifestations of YNS are generally manageable with supportive measures. The management of pleural effusions is tailored to the size of the effusions, associated symptoms, and the clinical context. Therapeutic thoracenteses may suffice in controlling symptomatic pleural effusions, with pleurodesis being considered for managing recurrent symptomatic effusions.[25] Thoracic duct ligation is also an option in the treatment of persistent chylothorax. Respiratory manifestations of bronchiectasis can be controlled with a combination of postural drainage and other bronchopulmonary hygiene measures, along with judicious use of antimicrobial therapy.

Relatively little is known about the natural history of YNS, but the long-term prognosis appears generally favorable.[24,25] The largest case series suggests that life expectancy is only modestly reduced when compared with that of the general population.[25] Progression to respiratory failure rarely occurs.

LYMPHANGIOLEIOMYOMATOSIS

Pulmonary LAM is a disorder characterized by proliferation of abnormal smooth-muscle cells (LAM cells), which is associated with progressive cystic changes in the lung parenchyma.[38,39] LAM may occur sporadically or in association with tuberous sclerosis complex (TSC), an inheritable multiorgan hamartomatosis. Sporadic LAM affects approximately 1 in 400,000 adult women, whereas in TSC-LAM occurs in approximately 30% to 40% of adult women with TSC.[40] Characteristic manifestations of LAM include diffuse pulmonary cysts, progressive exertional dyspnea, hemoptysis, renal angiomyolipoma, recurrent pneumothorax, and increased incidence of meningioma.[40] LAM is now believed to be a low-grade slow-growing neoplasm. This disease is most commonly seen in women, believed to be accelerated by estrogen, and as such typically manifests before menopause around the third to fourth decade of life.

Pleural effusion is seen in 20% to 40% of patients with LAM during the course of the disease and is usually chylous.[38,41,42] The development of chylothorax in LAM likely results from obstruction or disruption of lymphatic vessels or the thoracic duct by proliferating LAM cells.[43–45] Chylothorax in LAM is more often unilateral and does not appear to correlate with the severity of parenchymal lung disease (**Fig. 5**).[41,42] Not all patients with chylothorax in LAM require therapeutic intervention. Management is tailored to the size and clinical effects of the chylous pleural effusion and has included low-fat diet, therapeutic thoracentesis, pleurodesis, pleurectomy, and thoracic duct ligation.[38,41,42] More recently, the discovery of abnormalities in the TSC1/2 genes, which results in activation of the kinase mammalian target of rapamycin (mTOR), has led to trials using mTOR inhibitors like sirolimus.[40] Sirolimus therapy has been shown to be effective in reducing the size of chylous pleural effusions.[46,47]

SUMMARY

Classically both chylothorax and pseudochylothorax present as a pleural effusion with a characteristic milky white appearance to the pleural fluid. Although both are rare causes of pleural effusion, they have distinct etiologies and clinical implications, and as a result require different management strategies. Pleural fluid analysis of cholesterol and triglyceride levels is key to differentiating the 2 syndromes from one another and to then guide the clinician as to what the best next steps are in evaluation and management. YNS and pulmonary LAM are 2 examples of distinct and rare diseases that are associated with the development of chylothorax.

CLINICS CARE POINTS

- Chylothorax and pseudochylothorax both represent rare forms of pleural effusion and classically present with a milky white appearance to the pleural fluid. However, it is key to differentiate between the two with pleural fluid analysis, as they have distinct etiologies and clinical implications for patients.

- YNS is a rare cause of chylothorax and is associated with the classic triad of findings: yellow and thickened nails, lymphedema, and pleural effusion or other respiratory abnormality including bronchiectasis and chronic sinusitis.

- Chylothorax can occur in 20% to 40% of patients with pulmonary LAM, which is a disorder characterized by proliferation of abnormal smooth-muscle cells (LAM cells) and progressive cystic changes in the lung parenchyma.

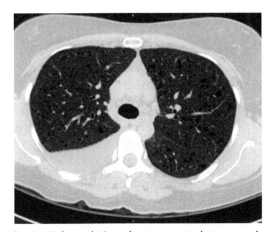

Fig. 5. High-resolution chest computed tomography scan of chylothorax related to LAM. This axial image of a 30-year-old woman with sporadic LAM demonstrates small cystic lesions diffusely throughout both lungs and a moderate-sized right pleural effusion (chylothorax).

REFERENCES

1. Johnson OW, Chick JF, Chauhan NR, et al. The thoracic duct: clinical importance, anatomic variation, imaging, and embolization. Eur Radiol 2016; 26(8):2482–93.

2. Nair SK, Petko M, Hayward MP. Aetiology and management of chylothorax in adults. Eur J Cardio-Thoracic Surg 2007;32(2):362–9.

3. Gibbons SM, Ahmed F. Chylothorax diagnosis: can the clinical chemistry laboratory do more? Ann Clin Biochem 2015;52(Pt 1):173–6.

4. Maldonado F, Hawkins FJ, Daniels CE, et al. Pleural fluid characteristics of chylothorax. Mayo Clinic Proc 2009;84(2):129–33.

5. Diaz-Guzman E, Culver DA, Stoller JK. Transudative chylothorax: report of two cases and review of the literature. Lung 2005;183(3):169–75.

6. Staats BA, Ellefson RD, Budahn LL, et al. The lipoprotein profile of chylous and nonchylous pleural effusions. Mayo Clinic Proc 1980;55(11):700–4.

7. Expert Panel on Vascular I, Interventional R, Majdalany BS, et al. ACR appropriateness criteria((R)) chylothorax treatment planning. J Am Coll Radiol 2017;14(5S):S118–26.

8. Ismail NA, Gordon J, Dunning J. The use of octreotide in the treatment of chylothorax following cardiothoracic surgery. Interactive Cardiovasc Thorac Surg 2015;20(6):848–54.

9. Lopez-Gutierrez JC, Tovar JA. Chylothorax and chylous ascites: management and pitfalls. Semin Pediatr Surg 2014;23(5):298–302.

10. Bello SOZ, Rahamim J. High-dose intravenous octreotide is safe and may be superior to surgery in managing severe postesophagectomy chylothorax in high-risk patients. Ann Thorac Surg 2015;100(1):297–9.

11. Maldonado F, Cartin-Ceba R, Hawkins FJ, et al. Medical and surgical management of chylothorax and associated outcomes. Am J Med Sci 2010; 339(4):314–8.

12. Seriff NS, Cohen ML, Samuel P, et al. Chylothorax: diagnosis by lipoprotein electrophoresis of serum and pleural fluid. Thorax 1977;32(1):98–100.

13. Pamarthi V, Stecker MS, Schenker MP, et al. Thoracic duct embolization and disruption for treatment of chylous effusions: experience with 105 patients. J Vasc Interv Radiol 2014;25(9):1398–404.

14. Itkin M, Kucharczuk JC, Kwak A, et al. Nonoperative thoracic duct embolization for traumatic thoracic duct leak: experience in 109 patients. J Thorac Cardiovasc Surg 2010;139(3):584–9 [discussion 589–90].

15. Reisenauer JS, Puig CA, Reisenauer CJ, et al. Treatment of postsurgical chylothorax. Ann Thorac Surg 2018;105(1):254–62.

16. Ryu JH, Tomassetti S, Maldonado F. Update on uncommon pleural effusions. Respirology 2011;16(2): 238–43.

17. Agrawal V, Sahn SA. Lipid pleural effusions. Am J Med Sci 2008;335(1):16–20.

18. Hillerdal G. Chylothorax and pseudochylothorax. Eur Respir J 1997;10(5):1157–62.

19. Wrightson JM, Stanton AE, Maskell NA, et al. Pseudochylothorax without pleural thickening: time to reconsider pathogenesis? Chest 2009;136(4):1144–7.

20. Garcia-Pachon E, Fernandez LC, Lopez-Azorin F, et al. Pseudochylothorax in pleural effusion due to coronary artery bypass surgery. Eur Respir J 1999; 13(6):1487–8.

21. Garcia-Zamalloa A, Ruiz-Irastorza G, Aguayo FJ, et al. Pseudochylothorax. Report of 2 cases and review of the literature. Medicine 1999;78(3):200–7.

22. Garcia-Zamalloa A. Pseudochylothorax, an unknown disease. Chest 2010;137(4):1004–5. author reply 1005.

23. Sassoon CS, Light RW. Chylothorax and pseudochylothorax. Clin Chest Med 1985;6(1):163–71.

24. Maldonado F, Ryu JH. Yellow nail syndrome. Curr Opin Pulm Med 2009;15(4):371–5.

25. Maldonado F, Tazelaar HD, Wang C-W, et al. Yellow nail syndrome: analysis of 41 consecutive patients. Chest 2008;134(2):375–81.

26. Bramley K, Puchalski JT. Defying gravity: subdiaphragmatic causes of pleural effusions. Clin Chest Med 2013;34(1):39–46.

27. Samman PD, White WF. The "yellow nail" syndrome. Br J Dermatol 1964;76:153–7.

28. Hiller E, Rosenow EC 3rd, Olsen AM. Pulmonary manifestations of the yellow nail syndrome. Chest 1972;61(5):452–8.

29. Nordkild P, Kromann-Andersen H, Struve-Christensen E. Yellow nail syndrome–the triad of yellow nails, lymphedema and pleural effusions. A review of the literature and a case report. Acta Med Scand 1986;219(2):221–7.

30. Bull RH, Fenton DA, Mortimer PS. Lymphatic function in the yellow nail syndrome. Br J Dermatol 1996;134(2):307–12.

31. Cousins E, Cintolesi V, Vass L, et al. A case-control study of the lymphatic phenotype of yellow nail syndrome. Lymphatic Res Biol 2018;16(4):340–6.

32. Solal-Celigny P, Cormier Y, Fournier M. The yellow nail syndrome. Light and electron microscopic aspects of the pleura. Arch Pathol Lab Med 1983; 107(4):183–5.

33. Mishra AK, George AA, George L. Yellow nail syndrome in rheumatoid arthritis: an aetiology beyond thiol drugs. Oxf Med Case Rep 2016;2016(3):37–40.

34. Nakagomi D, Ikeda K, Kawashima H, et al. Bucillamine-induced yellow nail in Japanese patients with rheumatoid arthritis: two case reports and a review of 36 reported cases. Rheumatol Int 2013; 33(3):793–7.

35. Szolnoky G, Lakatos B, Husz S, et al. Improvement in lymphatic function and partial resolution of nails

after complex decongestive physiotherapy in yellow nail syndrome. Int J Dermatol 2005;44(6):501–3.

36. Cordasco EM Jr, Beder S, Coltro A, et al. Clinical features of the yellow nail syndrome. Cleveland Clinic J Med 1990;57(5):472–6.

37. Polat AK, Dang HT, Soran A. Yellow nail syndrome: treatment of lymphedema using low pressure compression. Lymphatic Res Biol 2012;10(1):30–2.

38. Ryu JH, Moss J, Beck GJ, et al. The NHLBI lymphangioleiomyomatosis registry: characteristics of 230 patients at enrollment.[see comment]. Am J Respir Crit Care Med 2006;173(1):105–11.

39. Meraj R, Wikenheiser-Brokamp KA, Young LR, et al. Lymphangioleiomyomatosis: new concepts in pathogenesis, diagnosis, and treatment. Semin Respir Crit Care Med 2012;33(5):486–97.

40. Johnson SR, Cordier JF, Lazor R, et al. European Respiratory Society guidelines for the diagnosis and management of lymphangioleiomyomatosis. Eur Respir J 2010;35(1):14–26.

41. Almoosa KF, McCormack FX, Sahn SA. Pleural disease in lymphangioleiomyomatosis. Clin Chest Med 2006;27(2):355–68.

42. Ryu JH, Doerr CH, Fisher SD, et al. Chylothorax in lymphangioleiomyomatosis. Chest 2003;123(2): 623–7.

43. Glasgow CG, El-Chemaly S, Moss J. Lymphatics in lymphangioleiomyomatosis and idiopathic pulmonary fibrosis. Eur Respir Rev 2012;21(125):196–206.

44. Kumasaka T, Seyama K, Mitani K, et al. Lymphangiogenesis-mediated shedding of LAM cell clusters as a mechanism for dissemination in lymphangioleiomyomatosis. Am J Surg Pathol 2005;29(10): 1356–66.

45. Seyama K, Kumasaka T, Kurihara M, et al. Lymphangioleiomyomatosis: a disease involving the lymphatic system. Lymphatic Res Biol 2010;8(1): 21–31.

46. Taveira-DaSilva AM, Hathaway O, Stylianou M, et al. Changes in lung function and chylous effusions in patients with lymphangioleiomyomatosis treated with sirolimus. Ann Intern Med 2011;154(12): 797–805. W-292-793.

47. Moua T, Olson EJ, Jean HCS, et al. Resolution of chylous pulmonary congestion and respiratory failure in lymphangioleiomyomatosis with sirolimus therapy. Am J Respir Crit Care Med 2012;186(4): 389–90.

Pleural Effusions in the Critically Ill and "At-Bleeding-Risk" Population

Mark Godfrey, MD, Jonathan Puchalski, MD, MEd*

KEYWORDS

• Thoracentesis • Pleural effusion • Bleeding risk • Intensive care

KEY POINTS

• Pleural effusions are common in the intensive care unit (ICU) and in patients with perceived bleeding risks.
• Despite the disease severity in each of these populations, thoracentesis is safe.
• The ICU setting or patient bleeding risks are only parts of a comprehensive and individualized risk-benefit analysis, and they may be superseded by the indications for the pleural procedure or risks of diagnostic or therapeutic delay.

BACKGROUND

Worldwide, pleural effusions contribute to patient suffering from respiratory failure, dyspnea, exercise intolerance, sleep abnormalities, pain, and others. The 2010 British Thoracic Society guidelines indicated that pleural diseases affect 3000 per 1 million people,[1] and estimations include 1.5 million people afflicted in the United States. Malignant pleural effusions account for 125,000 inpatient admissions per year in the United States and a resultant > $5 billion costs.[2] A 2008 analysis reported 127,444 thoracenteses performed in the Medicare population, which accounts for only 15% of the US population, suggesting the number of thoracenteses performed annually in the at-large population is higher than previously suggested.[3]

In the intensive care unit (ICU), pleural effusions may be detected by ultrasound in up to 62% of patients and thoracentesis can change the presumptive diagnosis in up to 45% of patients.[4] In the general population undergoing thoracentesis, up to 42% have been found to have one or more risks for bleeding.[5] Physicians are thus frequently confronted with pleural effusions in patients with comorbidities and risks, and the safety and value of performing thoracentesis in these complicated patients have been questioned.

THORACENTESIS IN THE INTENSIVE CARE UNIT
Prevalence

The reported prevalence of pleural effusion in ICU patients varies greatly depending on the method of patient screening or the ICU population (medical, surgical, trauma, or cardiac ICU patients). Thoracic ultrasound is extremely sensitive for detecting effusions. In a prospective study of ICU patients using chest computed tomography as the comparator, chest radiography (CXR) had a sensitivity, specificity, and diagnostic accuracy for pleural effusion of 65%, 81%, and 69%, respectively, whereas thoracic ultrasound with a single-blinded operator was 100% for all.[6] The effusion prevalence in consecutive medical ICU patients assessed with ultrasound may be as high as 62%.[7] However, given the ability of ultrasound to detect even trivial amounts of fluid, the clinical significance of the effusions in this cohort is questionable: 57 of these effusions (92%) were

Division of Pulmonary, Critical Care and Sleep Medicine, Yale University School of Medicine, 15 York Street, LCI 100, New Haven, CT 06510, USA
* Corresponding author.
E-mail address: jonathan.puchalski@yale.edu

Clin Chest Med 42 (2021) 677–686
https://doi.org/10.1016/j.ccm.2021.08.012
0272-5231/21/© 2021 Elsevier Inc. All rights reserved.

small (ie, only obscuring the costophrenic angle on chest radiograph) and only 11 effusions were successfully sampled.

CXR can overestimate the presence of an effusion in the ICU. In one retrospective cohort, only 35% of "effusions" seen on chest radiographs were confirmed with cross-sectional imaging or ultrasound, and only 10% subsequently underwent a drainage procedure.[8] In another prospective study, up to a quarter of ICU patients had pleural effusion reported on CXR, but when all were subsequently assessed with thoracic ultrasound, only 6.5% had confirmation of a significant effusion (>2 cm depth).[4]

In a large (n = 1351) cohort of ICU patients, 8.4% had effusions that were sizable enough to be detected on radiographs as well as sampled with thoracentesis.[9] A similar prevalence was reported in a retrospective database analysis of over 50,000 ICU admissions, which identified patients with either a diagnosis code for pleural effusion or the presence of pleural fluid laboratory studies in 7.7%.[10] These studies suggest that radiographic methods alone overestimate the prevalence of clinically relevant effusions in the ICU. Uncontrolled retrospective ICU cohorts suggest the prevalence of effusions large enough to be drained is closer to 5% to 10%.

Diagnostic Considerations

The causes of pleural effusion and the biochemical testing to characterize transudates and exudates do not differ in critically ill patients from others.[11] In the ICU setting, volume overload from fluid resuscitation, myocardial depression, hypoalbuminemia, atelectasis, or hepatic hydrothorax are common transudative causes. Exudates may be due to malignant pleural effusion, pancreatitis, pleural infection, or pulmonary embolism, among others. Postoperative effusions in surgical ICU patients may be related to cardiothoracic or major abdominal procedures, traumatic or iatrogenic hemothorax, aortic dissection, or esophageal perforation. In rare circumstances, improper placement or migration of feeding tubes or venous catheters can result in pleural effusions.[12,13] Studies describing the specific etiologies of pleural effusions in ICU patients are often hindered by multiple methodologic limitations, including selection bias for drainage, and as a result tend to have higher proportions of exudative and infectious effusions.[7,10]

Pleural effusion is not a common manifestation of the severe acute respiratory syndrome coronavirus 2 (SARS-CoV-2; "COVID-19"). In a series of 121 patients with symptomatic SARS-CoV-2 infection who were early in the course of illness, pleural effusion was found in only one.[14] In a systematic review of more than 3400 patients where the duration of illness was more heterogenous, pleural effusion was present in only 5.2%, and many of these may be related to hypoalbuminemia or critical illness.[15] It should be noted that SARS-CoV-2 RNA can be isolated in pleural fluid,[16] and all pleural procedures in patients with COVID-19 are potentially aerosol-generating. This has led some physicians to add bleach to the air leak chamber of a chest tube collection device or viral filters to the system.

In the ICU, a presumptive diagnosis for an effusion based on clinical features is often unreliable. Demographic or clinical features have not emerged in patients with effusion and community-acquired pneumonia to reliably indicate empyema, nor do pneumonia-specific or generic sepsis scores predict its development.[17,18] However, there is good quality prospective evidence that thoracentesis augments the clinical decision-making and alters management in the ICU. Fartoukh and colleagues[9] performed a prospective study of all patients admitted to 3 medical ICUs in France. They assessed for the presence of effusion and performed thoracentesis in all who did not have prespecified contraindications (n = 82). They found that the thoracentesis-based diagnosis was different from the presumptive diagnosis in 37 patients (45%), and that management was altered in 31%. There were no prethoracentesis clinical variables that predicted when thoracentesis would be useful. Recently, Fysh and colleagues[4] described a multicenter prospective cohort of ICU patients with pleural effusion, though in this study, the authors left the decision to perform pleural drainage to the discretion of the treating physician. Of 7342 consecutive ICU patients, 226 (3.1%) had clinically significant effusions confirmed on ultrasound and 119 (53%) underwent pleural drainage. Thoracentesis improved the predrainage diagnosis in 91 cases (77%), and in 62 cases (52%), there was a complete change of diagnosis. Although most changes were related to exclusion of pleural infection or malignancy, 22 (19%) revealed previously unsuspected conditions.

Can sonographic features of the effusion reliably suggest an etiology? Unfortunately, though increasingly complex ultrasound characteristics (eg, internal echogenicity or septations) can suggest an effusion will be an exudate, their presence is insensitive and many "simple" appearing fluid collections will be biochemically exudative.[19,20] Taken together, the previous studies demonstrate that there are no clinical or imaging findings that can obviate the need for diagnostic sampling, and that doing so often leads to actionable data.

Therapeutic Considerations

The physiology of pleural effusion drainage is reviewed in more detail in this issue of *Clinics*, and drainage of pleural effusion in mechanically ventilated patients has theoretic benefits in terms of gas exchange, respiratory system mechanics, diaphragmatic function, and hemodynamics.[21] In a systematic review and meta-analysis, Goligher and colleagues[22] described 19 observational studies (n = 1124) assessing the impact of pleural fluid drainage in mechanically ventilated patients. There was a modest but significant improvement in $P_{a}O_{2}$:$F_{i}O_{2}$ ratio of 30.5 (95% confidence interval [CI], 6.4–54.6; P = .013) after drainage, with conflicting results on respiratory mechanics. Subsequent studies have suggested that the presence of a pleural effusion is associated with failure to liberate from mechanical ventilation,[23,24] though the positive impact of drainage on mechanical ventilation duration is unknown.

There are potentially serious negative consequences to expectant management of an effusion in the ICU. In the Fysh and colleagues[4] study described earlier, two-thirds of the 226 identified clinically significant effusions were not drained within 24 hours of identification. In this group of 150 patients managed expectantly, 15 patients (10%) experienced respiratory failure requiring either ICU readmission, medical emergency team activation, noninvasive ventilation, or reintubation together with pleural effusion drainage; 5 of these patients died with irreversible respiratory failure as a contributing cause. An additional 8 patients had missed pleural infections diagnosed on subsequent drainages. The pleural effusion adverse event rate in the expectant management group was 16%, and the 27 patients who were drained required a total of 45 drainage procedures. Compared to the early drainage group (8 pleural effusion-related serious adverse events [PERSAE; 10.5%]), this was not statistically significant for PERSAE. However, there were more overall significant adverse events in the control group (9 [11.8%] vs 35 [23.3%], P < .05).

Technique

Pleural drainage in the ICU is associated with several unique practical challenges. Patient positioning may be hindered by inability to cooperate due to sedation or by intravascular devices (intra-aortic balloon pumps or extracorporeal membrane oxygenation [ECMO] cannulae) that limit position changes, and often an ideal position is not possible. Most ICU patients can achieve a semirecumbent position where the preferred site of drainage is the "triangle of safety" bounded by the pectoralis major, latissimus dorsi, and fifth intercostal space. As summarized by others, the evidence that contemporaneous ultrasound reduces iatrogenic complications in pleural interventions compared to a "blind" approach is so overwhelming that a failure to perform an ultrasound examination is reserved for exceptionally rare, life-threatening emergencies.[25–27] Provision of ultrasound equipment and trained operators should therefore be a priority for any setting where thoracentesis is performed.

Safety

Numerous studies address the safety of pleural procedures in critically ill or mechanically ventilated patients. Early small studies of thoracentesis in ventilated patients (with ultrasound use not described) found a pneumothorax rate of 6% to 10%.[28,29] With the routine use of ultrasound, the rate of pneumothorax is 0% to 7%.[9,30,31] In a surgical ICU cohort of 338 thoracenteses (83 of which occurred in ventilated patients), there were complications in 6 procedures (2%): 2 hemothoraces and 4 pneumothoraces.[32] Among exclusively ventilated patients, there was a 0% to 1.3% rate of pneumothorax following ultrasound-guided thoracentesis.[33,34] In 94 febrile medical ICU patients, 86% of whom were receiving mechanical ventilation, only 2 hemothoraces (2%) were reported after thoracentesis.[35] In other mixed ICU cohorts, with some patients receiving mechanical ventilation and some not, there was a pneumothorax rate of 0% to 4.2%.[36,37] Finally, in a recent prospective cohort of 226 patients receiving pleural drainage in the ICU (the majority receiving small-bore intercostal drains), there were 5 procedure-related adverse events (3 failed insertions, and 1 case each of re-expansion pulmonary edema and parenchymal tube placement).[4]

THORACENTESIS AND THE RISK OF BLEEDING

Thoracentesis is generally considered a low-risk procedure. The use of ultrasound has been shown to decrease the likelihood of hemorrhage by 38.7% in a study of 19,339 thoracenteses in 414 hospitals.[38] Although bleeding complications occur in approximately 1% to 1.5% of patients,[39–41] the bleeding complication rate has been even lower in some studies, with 0.4% of procedures complicated by hemothorax (0.2%) or hematoma in a study including 941 thoracenteses[42] and 0.18% in a study of 9320 thoracenteses.[43]

In and beyond the ICU setting, elevated coagulation parameters, thrombocytopenia, and the use of various medications have traditionally been felt to be associated with higher risks of procedural bleeding, despite a lack of convincing evidence. Although partial thromboplastin time (PTT) and international normalized ratio (INR) "were never intended to, nor have they been shown to assess hemostasis in patients without a history of bleeding,"[44] recent publications still list relative contraindications of the procedures as elevated INR and low platelets.[45] The Turkish Respiratory Society in 2020 recommended ideal conditions including an INR less than 1.5, platelet count greater than 50,000/μL, and a creatinine less than 6 mg/dL when the procedure is nonemergent.[46] The British Thoracic Society Guidelines in 2010 gave a grade C recommendation for having an INR less than 1.5 before thoracentesis[26] Several recent studies offer more information on the safety of thoracentesis in patients with conventionally defined bleeding risks and may help to redefine society guidelines in the future. For example, the Society of Interventional Radiology Consensus Guidelines updated their recommendations in 2019 for patients undergoing percutaneous image-guided interventions. They categorized thoracentesis as a low bleeding risk procedure and did not recommend preprocedural assessment of PT/INR or platelets, but if obtained, correcting INR to ≤ 2.0 to 3.0 and transfusing platelets if less than 20,000/μL. Furthermore, they recommend against withholding unfractionated heparin, low-molecular-weight heparin, clopidogrel and other antiplatelet agents, as well as anticoagulants, before low-risk procedures.[47] This recommendation is a significant change from prior recommendations and the progress is likely based on the following studies.

THORACENTESIS IN PATIENTS WITH THROMBOCYTOPENIA OR AN ELEVATED INR

A summary of studies addressing thoracentesis in patients with abnormal coagulation parameters is summarized in **Table 1**. McVay and Toy[48] (1991) retrospectively found no increased bleeding in patients undergoing thoracentesis or paracentesis with mild to moderate coagulopathy (PT or PTT up to twice midpoint normal range) or mild thrombocytopenia (platelets mostly 50,000–99,000/μL). A PT of 1.5 times midnormal was equivalent to an INR of approximately 2.2 and a PT of 2.0 times midnormal was equivalent to an INR of approximately 3.8. Notably, they performed 57 thoracenteses with an elevated PT, 65 with an elevated PTT, and 24 with thrombocytopenia (7 with platelets

25–48,000/μL) of the 217 pleural procedures. They found that patients with a markedly elevated creatinine (>6 μmol/L) had a higher average hemoglobin drop following the procedure, although only 4 such patients had a thoracentesis.

Bass and White[49] (2005) reviewed 100 thoracenteses in patients with hematologic malignancies. The 2 patients who developed hemothorax had normal platelet and coagulation parameters. Patel and Joshi[50] (2011) reviewed 1076 ultrasound-guided thoracenteses (267 procedures with INR > 1.5 and 58 with platelets <50,000/μL) and found no hemorrhagic complications. Puchalski and colleagues[5] (2013) found that 42% of 312 patients prospectively collected had bleeding risks but no hemothorax during thoracentesis. This study evaluated many bleeding risks including elevated INR, thrombocytopenia, and patients taking medications thought to be associated with a risk of bleeding (clopidogrel, heparin). Renal failure was also included but liberally defined as a creatinine greater than 1.5 μmol/L or those requiring renal replacement therapy and this cohort contained 41 of the 130 "at-risk" patients. Hibbert and colleagues[51] (2013) in the same year demonstrated retrospectively that the bleeding risk was no different in 1009 procedures in those with an INR greater than 1.6 or platelet count less than 50,000/μL compared to those with normal parameters. In 706 procedures without transfusion to correct the abnormal parameters, there were no bleeding events. There were 4 bleeding events in 303 procedures (1.32%) with transfusion, representing 0.4% of the 1009 total procedures. Of these, 1 was a hematoma, 1 was a presumed intercostal artery laceration, and 2 were hemothoraces. Almost all patients had a decrease in hemoglobin within 1 week with a mean decrease of 1.06 (±0.93) g/dL in the group not receiving transfusions before the procedure. This observation was not explained but not attributable to the thoracentesis.

Orlandi and colleagues[52] retrospectively reviewed the use of ultrasound in 436 thoracenteses, with 41 patients having severe thrombocytopenia (<30,000/μL). They found that ultrasound reduced the risk of bleeding and that bleeding was mild in 0.69% of all patients with the complication. The 3 mild bleeding events occurred in the 9 patients with severe thrombocytopenia in whom ultrasound was not used.

Ault and colleagues[43] prospectively analyzed 9320 inpatient thoracenteses (4618 patients; 3796 bilateral thoracenteses). Many patients had more than one procedure. Of the procedures, 359 patients (3.9%) had a platelet count of 20 to 49,000/μL and there were 4 complications, 53

Table 1
Studies evaluating patients with a perceived bleeding risk undergoing thoracentesis

Authors	Bleeding Risk	Number	Results
McVay and Toy[48] 1991, retrospective paracentesis and thoracentesis	Elevated PT/PTT or thrombocytopenia; 217 thoracenteses	Elevated PTT: 65 Elevated PT: 57 Plts<50,000: 7	No increased bleeding risk, although more hemoglobin drop if Cr > 6 mmol/L
Bass et al.[49] 2005, retrospective thoracentesis	Hematologic malignancies (lymphoma, leukemia, post-transplant); 100 thoracenteses	100 patients Plts<50,000: 13 PT/PTT elevation: 14	No bleeding in those at risk; 2/100 patients had hemothorax
Patel and Joshi[50] 2011, retrospective, ultrasound-guided thoracentesis	Elevated INR or thrombocytopenia; 1076 thoracenteses INR available in 822 patients; platelets available in 953	1076 procedures on 605 patients INR>1.5: 267 INR>2: 139 INR>2.5: 59 INR>3: 32 Plts<50,000: 58 (12 of which were <25,000)	No bleeding events
Puchalski et al.[5] 2013, prospective, ultrasound-guided	Various risks factors including INR, thrombocytopenia, renal failure, medications	312 (42% with bleeding risk) INR>1.5: 44 Plts<50,000: 16 Clopidogrel: 14 Heparin: 14	No bleeding events
Hibbert et al.[51] 2013, retrospective, ultrasound-guided	Elevated INR or thrombocytopenia	1009 procedures in 773 patients INR>1.6: 608 procedures without correction Plts<50,000: 113 procedures without correction	No difference but bleeding occurred in the corrected group (1.3 vs 0%)
Ault et al.[43] 2015, prospective	All procedures	9320 procedures Plts 20–49,000: 359 Plts<20,000: 53 INR 1.5–2.99: 2005 INR>3.1: 301	No difference in bleeding in groups comparing INR, PTT, or platelets Hemothorax in 0.05%
Orlandi et al.[52] 2018, retrospective	Thrombocytopenia	41 of 436 patients had plts<30,000	3 (0.69%) patients had topically-controlled bleeding when U/S was not used
Zalt et al.[53] 2012, prospective	Clopidogrel	45 (30 patients)	One superficial hematoma
Mahmood et al.[54] 2014, prospective	Clopidogrel	Thoracentesis: 17 Chest tube: 8	1/25 hemothorax (4%) due to thoracentesis
Patel et al.[55] 2019, retrospective	Clopidogrel, NOAC, and ticagrelor	Clopidogrel: 69 NOAC: 43 Ticagrelor: 3	No bleeding complications
Perl et al.[56] 2020, retrospective	Clopidogrel	Clopidogrel: 88 Control: 169	No difference in bleeding complications
Dangers et al.[57] 2020, multicenter cohort	Antiplatelet drugs	Aspirin: 142 Clopidogrel: 17 Aspirin + Clopidogrel: 22 Aspirin + Prasugrel: 1	Bleeding events: 1.3% Serious bleeding: 0.8% Odds ratio of bleeding using antiplatelets: 3.44 in univariate analysis

(0.57%) had a platelet count of less than 20,000/μL and there were 0 complications, 2005 had an INR 1.5 to 2.99 (21.5%) and there were 20 complications, whereas 301 (3.2%) had an INR greater than 3.1 and there were 5 complications. They found 17 total bleeding episodes (0.18%) of which 5 were hemothoraces (0.05%). The incidence of any complication was higher in patients who were underweight, had an elevated PTT, had greater than 1500 mL of fluid removed, unilateral compared to bilateral procedures, and those with more passes through the skin. There were no associations with bleeding and clinical variables including INR, PTT, or platelets.

THORACENTESIS IN PATIENTS WITH MEDICATION-RELATED BLEEDING "RISKS"

Few studies have evaluated thoracentesis in the presence of medication-induced bleeding risks, such as antiplatelet medications. The Turkish Respiratory Society consensus statement recommends discontinuing antiplatelet medications (Clopidogrel, Prasugrel, Ticagrelor) 5 to 10 days before pleural procedures. They recommend enoxaparin and fondaparinux be held 24 hours, dabigatran and argatroban 48 hours, and direct factor Xa inhibitors (rivaroxaban, apixaban, and edoxaban) at least 24 hours. Notably, there is no recommendation for aspirin.[46] The 2019 recommendations from the Society of Interventional Radiology do not recommend cessation of unfractionated heparin, low-molecular-weight heparin, clopidogrel and other antiplatelet agents, or anticoagulants before thoracentesis.[47]

Zalt and colleagues[53] retrospectively evaluated 45 procedures in 30 patients undergoing thoracentesis while receiving clopidogrel. Patients took clopidogrel within 24 hours and continued use after the procedure. No patient developed hemothorax and 1 patient (2.22%) developed a small hematoma requiring superficial pressure at the puncture site. All patients had a CXR within 72 hours and a complete blood count within 48 hours. One patient had a decrease in hemoglobin by 3 g/dL; this stabilized without intervention and CXR did not show evidence of pleural fluid reaccumulation.

Mahmood and colleagues[54] prospectively examined 25 patients undergoing ultrasound-guided thoracentesis or chest tube placement while receiving clopidogrel and 50 patients as controls. Most (22/25) were concurrently taking aspirin. They assessed for a postprocedural hemoglobin decrease of 2 g/dL or reaccumulation of the pleural effusion within 24 hours. Outpatients were called within 2 weeks to assess for suggestive symptoms. One patient in the clopidogrel group undergoing thoracentesis (1/17 thoracenteses; 5.9%) developed hemothorax requiring chest tube placement and blood transfusion.

Patel and colleagues[55] retrospectively evaluated 115 patients undergoing ultrasound-guided thoracentesis receiving clopidogrel (69), a novel oral anticoagulant (43), or ticagrelor (3) within 24 hours of the procedure. A large proportion of procedures occurred in the presence of multiple bleeding risk factors (45.2%). Postprocedural hemoglobin was obtained within 48 hours in 88 patients (76.5%) and postprocedural radiographs in 58 patients (50.4%). No bleeding complications were identified.

Perl and colleagues[56] retrospectively studied 257 patients (88 on clopidogrel) and found no difference in bleeding events between the groups. Of the patients on clopidogrel, 41 (46%) were also taking aspirin and 2 (2.3%) a dual oral anticoagulant. The single hemothorax occurred in the group not taking clopidogrel, and both groups had 2 patients receive red blood cell transfusion for hemoglobin drops greater than 2 g/dL after the procedure without evidence of hemothorax.

In contrast to the other studies listed, Dangers and Giovannelli[57] conducted a French prospective, multicenter (n = 19) study of patients undergoing thoracentesis, chest tube, and closed pleural biopsies. Of 1124 patients, 182 were on antiplatelet therapy (aspirin: 142; clopidogrel: 17; aspirin plus clopidogrel: 22; aspirin plus prasugrel: 1). Image guidance was used in 77% of the antiplatelet group and 68% of the control group. A total of 377 thoracenteses were included, of whom 74 were on antiplatelet therapy. In over 1000 total pleural procedures, there were 15 bleeding events (6 in the antiplatelet group), 5 of which occurred after thoracentesis (1.3% of total thoracenteses). Two of these were considered serious (0.5% of thoracenteses). The 24-h incidence of bleeding was 1.33% (95% CI, 0.71–2.05) in the whole group, 3.23% (95% CI, 1.08–5.91) in the antiplatelet group, and 0.96% (95% CI, 0.43–1.60) in the control group. All bleeding events were in patients taking aspirin monotherapy, presumptively between 75 and 160 mg. In univariate analysis, the OR for bleeding in the thoracentesis group on antiplatelets was 1.73 (0.28–33.38), $P = .62$. In multivariate analysis, the OR for bleeding was 0.93 (0.10–20.31), $P = .96$. The authors concluded that antiplatelet therapy (meaning aspirin monotherapy in this group) had a significantly increased risk of bleeding in patients undergoing pleural procedures compared with the control group. However, even in a cohort as large as this the absolute bleeding event rate was very low, resulting in wide CIs for their risk estimates. Therefore the authors acknowledged that "pleural procedures may be performed with an acceptable risk when anti-platelet therapy cannot be interrupted."

RISKS ASSOCIATED WITH TRANSFUSION OR MEDICATION WITHDRAWAL

Reversal of INR with fresh frozen plasma or platelet transfusion is not without risk. Transfusion-associated lung injury, volume overload, allergic reaction, viral or bacterial infection, or alloimmunization are all possible complications.[58,59] These risks must be considered when transfusing before thoracentesis given the low risk of bleeding demonstrated in the aforementioned studies.

There are also risks associated with cessation of prescription medications. In patients who undergo coronary stent implantation for ischemic heart disease, stent thrombosis is associated with a mortality rate between 5% and 45%.[60] In a large meta-analysis (30 studies, 221,066 patients, 4276 stent thromboses), after a median of 22 months definite, probable or possible stent thrombosis had occurred in 2.4% of the population. Of this, acute thrombosis occurred in 0.4%, subacute in 1.1%, late in 0.5%, and very late in 0.6%. Definite/probable stent thrombosis was more consistently and commonly associated with stent number/length, extent of coronary disease, and early antiplatelet therapy discontinuation, among others.[61]

Dual-antiplatelet therapy is recommended after stent implantation. However, reasons for stent thrombosis after discontinuation of clopidogrel, for example, are poorly understood. In a small study of patients with drug-eluting coronary stents, long-term (>1 year) clopidogrel use followed by cessation caused rebound platelet hyperreactivity in the subsequent 2 to 6 weeks.[62] Short-term use and cessation may not be associated with major adverse cardiac and cerebrovascular events.[63] Short-term cessation of dabigatran, however, has been shown to cause a paradoxic prothrombotic state associated with platelet aggregability in mice.[64] Additional studies are needed regarding abrupt cessation of antiplatelet or anticoagulant medications and their risks for thrombosis.

INDIVIDUALIZING THERAPY

The decision to perform any procedure, including thoracentesis, is an exercise individualized to each patient. Procedural risks, operator experience, patient characteristics or preference, the risks of transfusions or withdrawal of medications, and the indication and urgency of the procedure must all be integrated. Both diagnostic delay (eg, in the case of pleural infection) or therapeutic delay for a patient who is breathless can have clinical consequences and are poorly captured outcomes in retrospective publications. Bleeding complications related to thoracentesis, with or without additional risk factors, are uncommon and can often be managed conservatively. Therefore, these

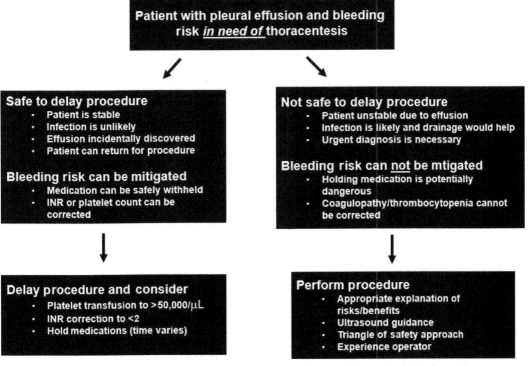

Fig. 1. A proposed approach for performing thoracentesis in patients with perceived bleeding risks.

perceived risks are only one component of a comprehensive risk-benefit analysis, and may be superseded by the indications for the pleural procedure or the antiplatelet agent. An approach to patients with perceived risks for thoracentesis due to these factors is proposed (**Fig. 1**).

SUMMARY

Pleural effusions are a cause of significant morbidity and are frequently encountered in "at-risk" patients, including those in the ICU or patients with presumed risks for bleeding. Thoracentesis in these patients must be considered in the context of diagnostic and therapeutic considerations. In the ICU, an unsuspected diagnosis is not infrequent and respiratory failure may be improved following the procedure. As with all procedures, safety is paramount and use of ultrasound and targeting the approach in the "triangle of safety" may reduce complications. Society guidelines are generally lacking for performing thoracentesis in patients with perceived bleeding risks, but recent and future guidelines may consider growing evidence that the procedure is safe in the setting of coagulation and platelet abnormalities, and in patients on antiplatelet or anticoagulant medications when the procedure is necessary.

CLINICS CARE POINTS

- The use of ultrasound and performing thoracentesis in the "triangle of safety" decreases complications.

- Thoracentesis is clinically useful for diagnostic and therapeutic purposes and is often necessary for ICU patients and those at risk for bleeding.

- When performed in the ICU or in patients with perceived bleeding risks, individualized timing based on the rationale for performing the procedure likely further ensures the generally safe profile of thoracentesis.

DISCLOSURE

The authors have nothing to disclose.

REFERENCES

1. Du Rand I, Maskell N. Introduction and methods: British thoracic society pleural disease guideline 2010. Thorax 2010;65(Suppl 2):ii1–3.
2. Taghizadeh N, Fortin M, Tremblay A. US hospitalizations for malignant pleural effusions: data from the 2012 national inpatient sample. Chest 2017;151(4):845–54.
3. Duszak R Jr, Chatterjee AR, Schneider DA. National fluid shifts: fifteen-year trends in paracentesis and thoracentesis procedures. J Am Coll Radiol 2010;7(11):859–64.
4. Fysh ETH, Smallbone P, Mattock N, et al. Clinically significant pleural effusion in intensive care: a prospective multicenter cohort study. Crit Care Explor 2020;2(1):e0070.
5. Puchalski JT, Argento AC, Murphy TE, et al. The safety of thoracentesis in patients with uncorrected bleeding risk. Ann Am Thorac Soc 2013;10(4):336–41.
6. Xirouchaki N, Magkanas E, Vaporidi K, et al. Lung ultrasound in critically ill patients: comparison with bedside chest radiography. Intensive Care Med 2011;37(9):1488–93.
7. Mattison LE, Coppage L, Alderman DF, et al. Pleural effusions in the medical ICU: prevalence, causes, and clinical implications. Chest 1997;111(4):1018–23.
8. Bates D, Yang N, Bailey M, et al. Prevalence, characteristics, drainage and outcome of radiologically diagnosed pleural effusions in critically ill patients. Crit Care Resusc 2020;22(1):45–52.
9. Fartoukh M, Azoulay E, Galliot R, et al. Clinically documented pleural effusions in medical ICU patients: how useful is routine thoracentesis? Chest 2002;121(1):178–84.
10. Bateman M, Alkhatib A, John T, et al. Pleural effusion outcomes in intensive care: analysis of a large clinical database. J Intensive Care Med 2020;35(1):48–54.
11. Sahn SA. The value of pleural fluid analysis. Am J Med Sci 2008;335(1):7–15.
12. Maisniemi KJ, Koljonen VS. Tension hydrothorax induced by central venous catheter migration in a patient with burns. Br J Anaesth 2006;97(3):423–4.
13. Fonseca VR, Domingos G, Alves P, et al. Placement of nasogastric tube complicated by hydropneumothorax. Intensive Care Med 2015;41(11):1969–70.
14. Bernheim A, Mei X, Huang M, et al. Chest CT findings in coronavirus disease-19 (COVID-19): Relationship to duration of infection. Radiology 2020;295(3):200463.
15. Adams HJA, Kwee TC, Yakar D, et al. Chest CT imaging signature of coronavirus disease 2019 infection: in Pursuit of the Scientific evidence. Chest 2020;158(5):1885–95.
16. Mei F, Bonifazi M, Menzo S, et al. First detection of SARS-CoV-2 by real-time reverse transcriptase-polymerase chain reaction assay in pleural fluid. Chest 2020;158(4):e143–6.
17. Ahmed RA, Marrie TJ, Huang JQ. Thoracic empyema in patients with community-acquired pneumonia. Am J Med 2006;119(10):877–83.

18. Chalmers JD, Singanayagam A, Murray MP, et al. Risk factors for complicated parapneumonic effusion and empyema on presentation to hospital with community-acquired pneumonia. Thorax 2009; 64(7):592–7.

19. Asciak R, Hassan M, Mercer RM, et al. Prospective analysis of the predictive value of sonographic pleural fluid echogenicity for the diagnosis of exudative effusion. Respiration 2019;97(5):451–6.

20. Yang PC, Luh KT, Chang DB, et al. Value of sonography in determining the nature of pleural effusion: analysis of 320 cases. AJR Am J Roentgenol 1992;159(1):29–33.

21. Graf J. Pleural effusion in the mechanically ventilated patient. Curr Opin Crit Care 2009;15(1):10–7.

22. Goligher EC, Leis JA, Fowler RA, et al. Utility and safety of draining pleural effusions in mechanically ventilated patients: a systematic review and meta-analysis. Crit Care 2011;15(1):R46.

23. Dres M, Roux D, Pham T, et al. Prevalence and impact on weaning of pleural effusion at the time of liberation from mechanical ventilation: a multicenter prospective observational study. Anesthesiology 2017;126(6):1107–15.

24. Razazi K, Boissier F, Neuville M, et al. Pleural effusion during weaning from mechanical ventilation: a prospective observational multicenter study. Ann Intensive Care 2018;8(1):103.

25. Evison M, Blyth KG, Bhatnagar R, et al. Providing safe and effective pleural medicine services in the UK: an aspirational statement from UK pleural physicians. BMJ Open Respir Res 2018;5(1):e000307.

26. Havelock T, Teoh R, Laws D, et al. Pleural procedures and thoracic ultrasound: British thoracic society pleural disease guideline 2010. Thorax 2010; 65(Suppl 2):ii61–76.

27. McCracken DJ, Laursen CB, Barker G, et al. Thoracic ultrasound competence for ultrasound-guided pleural procedures. Eur Respir Rev 2019; 28(154):190090.

28. Godwin JE, Sahn SA. Thoracentesis: a safe procedure in mechanically ventilated patients. Ann Intern Med 1990;113(10):800–2.

29. McCartney JP, Adams JW 2nd, Hazard PB. Safety of thoracentesis in mechanically ventilated patients. Chest 1993;103(6):1920–1.

30. Gervais DA, Petersein A, Lee MJ, et al. US-guided thoracentesis: requirement for postprocedure chest radiography in patients who receive mechanical ventilation versus patients who breathe spontaneously. Radiology 1997;204(2):503–6.

31. Lichtenstein D, Hulot JS, Rabiller A, et al. Feasibility and safety of ultrasound-aided thoracentesis in mechanically ventilated patients. Intensive Care Med 1999;25(9):955–8.

32. Petersen S, Freitag M, Albert W, et al. Ultrasound-guided thoracentesis in surgical intensive care patients. Intensive Care Med 1999;25(9):1029.

33. Balik M, Plasil P, Waldauf P, et al. Ultrasound estimation of volume of pleural fluid in mechanically ventilated patients. Intensive Care Med 2006;32(2):318.

34. Mayo PH, Goltz HR, Tafreshi M, et al. Safety of ultrasound-guided thoracentesis in patients receiving mechanical ventilation. Chest 2004; 125(3):1059–62.

35. Tu CY, Hsu WH, Hsia TC, et al. Pleural effusions in febrile medical ICU patients: chest ultrasound study. Chest 2004;126(4):1274–80.

36. Pihlajamaa K, Bode MK, Puumalainen T, et al. Pneumothorax and the value of chest radiography after ultrasound-guided thoracocentesis. Acta Radiol 2004;45(8):828–32.

37. Vignon P, Chastagner C, Berkane V, et al. Quantitative assessment of pleural effusion in critically ill patients by means of ultrasonography. Crit Care Med 2005;33(8):1757–63.

38. Patel PA, Ernst FR, Gunnarsson CL. Ultrasonography guidance reduces complications and costs associated with thoracentesis procedures. J Clin Ultrasound 2012;40(3):135–41.

39. Herman DD, Thomson CC, Brosnhan S, et al. Risk of bleeding in patients undergoing pulmonary procedures on antiplatelet or anticoagulants: a systematic review. Respir Med 2019;153:76–84.

40. Wolfe KS, Kress JP. Risk of procedural hemorrhage. Chest 2016;150(1):237–46.

41. Hooper CE, Welham SA, Maskell NA, British Thoracic S. Pleural procedures and patient safety: a national BTS audit of practice. Thorax 2015;70(2):189–91.

42. Jones PW, Moyers JP, Rogers JT, et al. Ultrasound-guided thoracentesis: is it a safer method? Chest 2003;123(2):418–23.

43. Ault MJ, Rosen BT, Scher J, et al. Thoracentesis outcomes: a 12-year experience. Thorax 2015;70(2): 127–32.

44. Holland L, Sarode R. Should plasma be transfused prophylactically before invasive procedures? Curr Opin Hematol 2006;13(6):447–51.

45. Porcel JM. Chest tube drainage of the pleural space: a concise review for pulmonologists. Tuberc Respir Dis (Seoul) 2018;81(2):106–15.

46. Demirci NY, Deniz K, Bilaceroglu S, et al. Management of bleeding risk before pleural procedures: a consensus statement of Turkish respiratory society – Pleura study group. Eurasian J Pulmonol 2020; 22(2):73–8.

47. Patel IJ, Rahim S, Davidson JC, et al. Society of interventional Radiology consensus guidelines for the periprocedural management of thrombotic and bleeding risk in patients undergoing percutaneous image-guided interventions-Part II: recommendations: endorsed by the canadian association for interventional radiology and the cardiovascular and interventional radiological society of Europe. J Vasc Interv Radiol 2019;30(8):1168–84. e1161.

48. McVay PA, Toy PT. Lack of increased bleeding after paracentesis and thoracentesis in patients with mild coagulation abnormalities. Transfusion 1991;31(2):164–71.

49. Bass J, White DA. Thoracentesis in patients with hematologic malignancy: yield and safety. Chest 2005;127(6):2101–5.

50. Patel MD, Joshi SD. Abnormal preprocedural international normalized ratio and platelet counts are not associated with increased bleeding complications after ultrasound-guided thoracentesis. AJR Am J Roentgenol 2011;197(1):W164–8.

51. Hibbert RM, Atwell TD, Lekah A, et al. Safety of ultrasound-guided thoracentesis in patients with abnormal preprocedural coagulation parameters. Chest 2013;144(2):456–63.

52. Orlandi E, Citterio C, Seghini P, et al. Thoracentesis in advanced cancer patients with severe thrombocytopenia: ultrasound guide improves safety and reduces bleeding risk. Clin Respir J 2018;12(4):1747–52.

53. Zalt MB, Bechara RI, Parks C, et al. Effect of routine clopidogrel use on bleeding complications after ultrasound-guided thoracentesis. J Bronchology Interv Pulmonol 2012;19(4):284–7.

54. Mahmood K, Shofer SL, Moser BK, et al. Hemorrhagic complications of thoracentesis and small-bore chest tube placement in patients taking clopidogrel. Ann Am Thorac Soc 2014;11(1):73–9.

55. Patel PP, Singh S, Atwell TD, et al. The safety of ultrasound-guided thoracentesis in patients on novel oral anticoagulants and clopidogrel: a single-center experience. Mayo Clin Proc 2019;94(8):1535–41.

56. Perl S, Bondarenco M, Natif N, et al. Thoracentesis under clopidogrel is not associated with excessive bleeding events: a cohort study. Respir Res 2020;21(1):281.

57. Dangers L, Giovannelli J, Mangiapan G, et al. Antiplatelet drugs and risk of bleeding after bedside pleural procedures: a national multicenter cohort study. Chest 2021;159(4):1621–9.

58. Kaufman RM, Djulbegovic B, Gernsheimer T, et al. Platelet transfusion: a clinical practice guideline from the AABB. Ann Intern Med 2015;162(3):205–13.

59. Roback JD, Caldwell S, Carson J, et al. Evidence-based practice guidelines for plasma transfusion. Transfusion 2010;50(6):1227–39.

60. Ullrich H, Munzel T, Gori T. Coronary stent thrombosis- predictors and prevention. Dtsch Arztebl Int 2020;117(18):320–6.

61. D'Ascenzo F, Bollati M, Clementi F, et al. Incidence and predictors of coronary stent thrombosis: evidence from an international collaborative meta-analysis including 30 studies, 221,066 patients, and 4276 thromboses. Int J Cardiol 2013;167(2):575–84.

62. Diehl P, Halscheid C, Olivier C, et al. Discontinuation of long term clopidogrel therapy induces platelet rebound hyperaggregability between 2 and 6 weeks post cessation. Clin Res Cardiol 2011;100(9):765–71.

63. Piccolo R, Feres F, Abizaid A, et al. Risk of early adverse events after clopidogrel discontinuation in patients undergoing short-term dual antiplatelet therapy: an individual participant data analysis. JACC Cardiovasc Interv 2017;10(16):1621–30.

64. Kim J, Jang HJ, Schellingerhout D, et al. Short-term cessation of dabigatran causes a paradoxical prothrombotic state. Ann Neurol 2021;89(3):444–58.

Section 3: Pleural Malignancy

Malignant Pleural Effusions

Christopher M. Kapp, MD[a],*, Hans J. Lee, MD[b]

KEYWORDS

- Malignant pleural effusion • Thoracentesis • Indwelling pleural catheter • Talc pleurodesis
- Thoracoscopy

KEY POINTS

- Malignant pleural effusions complicate up to 15% of all patients with a primary malignancy, and an annual incidence of 150,000 cases in the United States alone.
- Diagnosis of malignant pleural effusion is most commonly achieved by thoracentesis (60% on initial thoracentesis), but repeat thoracentesis, computed tomography–guided biopsy, or even thoracoscopy may be required.
- Management centers around improving patient quality of life and can be done with serial thoracentesis, indwelling pleural catheter placement, pleurodesis, or a combination of those.

INTRODUCTION

Malignant pleural effusions (MPEs) are a common complication of cancer, affecting up to 15% of all patients with a primary lung malignancy and an annual incidence in the United States alone of 150,000 cases.[1–3] MPE refers to the accumulation of pleural fluid resultant from an underlying malignancy. An MPE occurs when the lymphatic infrastructure on the parietal pleura is overwhelmed by increased cancer cell production in combination with decreased lymphatic drainage, resulting in accumulation of fluid in the pleural space.[4] The most common underlying cancers at the root of MPE are lung, breast, and lymphoma; however most malignancies have been reported to cause malignant pleural effusions.[5] Diagnosis is attempted with an initial thoracentesis (10%–95% sensitivity based on tumor type) and gradually stepped up to a more invasive thoracoscopy (95% sensitivity) if a definitive diagnosis is eluded.[6–11] The presence of malignant tumor cells in the pleural space upstages a patient's primary cancer to metastatic and is associated with high morbidity and low survivability, with the median survival being 4 to 9 months.[12]

PLEURAL ANATOMY AND PATHOPHYSIOLOGY

The pleural space is defined as the area between the outer surface of the lung and the inner surface of the thorax. Each side of the pleural space (visceral, parietal) is covered with a serous membrane, a smooth and lubricating surface, that combined define the borders of the pleural cavity.[13] The normal pleural cavity is estimated to contain 0.26 mL of fluid per kilogram of bodyweight, primarily produced and absorbed on the parietal surface.[13,14] Fluid production and resorption is dependent on the balance of hydrostatic and oncotic pressure differences between the systemic and pulmonary circulations and the pleural space. The lymphatic vessels in the parietal pleura are capable of resorption of up to a 20-fold increase in pleural liquid formation before being overloaded. In MPE, tumor cells impair drainage of the lymphatic system, leading to fluid accumulation.[4,15,16] Additionally, pleural-based tumor cells have been described to increase fluid production through a cascade of interactions between the host vasculature and immune system. This results in net fluid production related to

a Department of Medicine, Division of Pulmonary, Critical Care, Sleep and Allergy Medicine, University of Illinois at Chicago, 840 South Wood Street, Room 920-N, Chicago, IL 60612, USA; b Section of Interventional Pulmonology, Division of Pulmonary and Critical Care Medicine, Johns Hopkins University, Baltimore, MD, USA
* Corresponding author.
E-mail address: ckapp@uic.edu

Clin Chest Med 42 (2021) 687–696
https://doi.org/10.1016/j.ccm.2021.08.004

plasma extravasation into the pleural space.[4] The combination of decreased resorption and increased production leads to accumulation of MPE. In MPE, postmortem studies suggest that most pleural metastases arise from tumor emboli to the parietal pleura, although other possible mechanisms include direct tumor invasion, hematogenous spread, and lymphatic involvement.[17]

CLINICAL PRESENTATION

Patients can present on a spectrum from completely asymptomatic (15%–25%) to acute respiratory distress, with the most common symptom being dyspnea.[18,19] The physiology behind the presence or lack of breathlessness is not well elucidated, but it is felt it has more to do with displacement of the diaphragm and expansion of the chest wall as opposed to compression of the lung itself.[20] However, the size of the effusion often correlates poorly with the degree of symptoms patients have.[21,22] Frequently co-morbid cardiopulmonary conditions can play a role in the severity of dyspnea.[23] Another less exhibited clinical indicator of an MPE is a dull, pleuritic chest pain or pressure that is, typically more common in mesothelioma.[21] Additional findings on review of systems are consistent with an advanced stage malignancy, including weight loss, malaise, and anorexia.[24] The physical examination is often remarkable for reduced tactile fremitus and dullness to percussion.[21]

IMAGING

Once a pleural effusion is suspected, a confirmatory imaging study is the next best step. Clinicians can choose from a variety of modalities, including bedside ultrasonography (US), chest x-ray (CXR), computed tomography (CT), and fluorodeoxyglucose positron emission tomography (PET-CT) depending on expertise and availability.

Ultrasonography

With the increasingly ubiquitous nature of US, this has become an attractive first imaging test due to its availability, safety, and ability to guide pleural intervention.[24] In addition to its accessibility, US has been shown to be a more sensitive tool for detection of pleural effusion than a CXR, particularly with experienced operators.[25] US is also a useful tool in determining pretest probability for malignant effusions, with pleural thickening >1 cm, pleural nodularity, and diaphragmatic thickening >7 mm highly suggestive of malignant disease (**Fig. 1**).[26] Pleural metastasis usually appears as relatively small hypoechoic

lenticular masses having obtuse margins with the chest wall or large masses with complex echogenicity.[27]

Plain Radiograph

A chest X-ray is often the initial screening test that discovers a pleural effusion (**Fig. 2**). A standard CXR can detect a pleural effusion at roughly 200 mL of volume in PA view, and as little as 50 mL in the lateral view.[28] Pleural plaques, pleural thickening, and rib crowding can all be signs of malignant pleural disease.[27] When patients become symptomatic from a malignant pleural effusion, patients will frequently have moderate to large pleural effusions (80%), and often contralateral shift of the trachea can be seen.[22,29]

Computed Tomography

The British Thoracic Society currently recommends use of a CT scan in all patients with an exudative pleural effusion that do not have a diagnosis after initial thoracentesis.[30] A CT scan can identify features consistent with certain diagnoses and allow for biopsy procedural planning. Nodular pleural thickening, mediastinal pleural thickening, parietal pleural thickening >1 cm, and circumferential pleural thickening have a specificity for pleural malignancy ranging from 78% to 100%.[31–33] Logistic regression was used to retrospectively evaluate CT scan findings most consistent with malignant pleural effusion and these include any pleural lesion >1 cm having the highest probability, but other predictors outside the chest include liver metastasis, abdominal mass, lung mass or nodule, pleural loculation, pericardial effusion, and cardiomegaly.[34]

Positron Emission Tomography-Computed Tomography

PET imaging is commonly used as part of staging evaluation for malignancies; however its value in predicting benign versus malignant disease is limited with a sensitivity of 81% and a specificity of 74%.[35] Where PET is useful, is in helping the proceduralist in determining optimal location for biopsy to obtain adequate tissue (**Fig. 3**).[30,35,36]

DIAGNOSTIC PROCEDURES
Thoracentesis

In persons with a known malignancy or imaging findings suggestive of a malignancy who develop a pleural effusion, the fluid should be sampled to determine etiology.[30,37] Indications for a thoracentesis, or percutaneous drainage of pleural fluid, are limited only by the safety profile of the patient

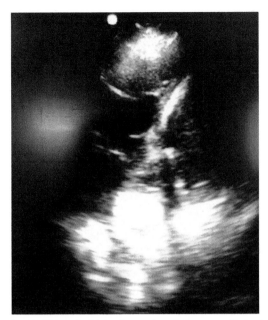

Fig. 1. Pleural thickening related to a malignant pleural effusion as seen on ultrasound.

and the skill of the operator. Ultrasound guidance should be used to improve the safety of the procedure and detection of pleural nodules or pleural thickening can predict the presence of malignancy.[26] Recent studies have shown no increase in risk of bleeding with uncorrected coagulopathy, clopidogrel use, direct oral anticoagulant use, renal disease, and thrombocytopenia.[38–41] In fact, guidelines vary but a platelet count as low as 30,000 has not been associated with increased risk of bleeding.[42] In addition, thoracentesis offers the potential benefit of relief of symptoms and evaluation for an expandable lung.

Fluid characteristics typically show an exudative effusion, but 5% to 10% are transudative by Light's criteria.[43] When suspicion of malignant effusion is high, ensuring an adequate sample for cytologic examination is critical. Optimal volume to be sent for analysis has yet to be determined. Some small studies have described no difference between as little as 25 mL of fluid and as much as 850 mL; however it is suggested that at least 60 mL should be collected, and in cases of large volume thoracentesis some authors recommend providing even more fluid to pathology.[44–47]

Pleural fluid cytology sensitivity for malignancy is 60% but can potentially be increased with a second thoracentesis by 27% with no increased sensitivity thereafter with additional thoracentesis.[30,47] The most likely primary cancers to have a positive cytology from pleural fluid are (in order), ovarian, lung (adeno), breast, and GI all with a sensitivity of greater than 60%.[10] Hematologic, nonadenocarcinoma lung cancer, and mesothelioma carry the lowest sensitivity with mesothelioma as low as single digits in some cases.[10,48–50] Pleural fluid is also being tested for genetic mutations that can help guide therapy, including KRAS and EGFR, with more on the horizon.[51,52]

After at most two successive thoracenteses do not provide a diagnosis, the next step is a pleural biopsy. This can be performed via multiple modalities discussed in the following section.

'Blind' Closed Pleural Biopsy

A blind pleural biopsy is performed using an Abrams or Cope needle and requires less experience, lower cost of equipment, and lower resources than the alternatives discussed in this chapter.[53,54] Blind pleural biopsy increases the diagnostic yield over pleural fluid cytology by 7% to 27% when pleural implants are seen on imaging but up to 50% in mesothelioma.[55,56] Blind pleural biopsies do typically have a lower sensitivity than image-guided pleural biopsy, and this is likely related to being unable to visually inspect the

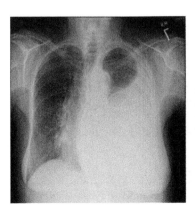

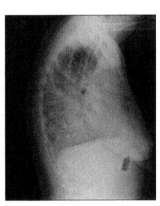

Fig. 2. Chest X-ray showing a large left-sided pleural effusion with contralateral mediastinal shift.

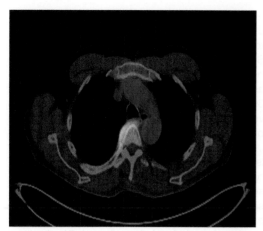

Fig. 3. Pleural thickening on PET/CT with avidity to help plan biopsy.

pleural space and biopsy appropriate tissue.[54,57] Complication rates can be as high as 14.4%, with a 9.4% incidence of pneumothorax.[58]

Image-Guided Biopsy

CT-guided and thoracic ultrasound (TU)–guided biopsy can be performed to obtain pleural tissue for diagnosis, with malignant pleural thickening (see **Fig. 1**) or nodules being targeted. Both modalities show good diagnostic yield, with TU (84%) and CT-guided (76%–100%) accompanied low complication rates.[59,60] In patients with suspected mesothelioma and no pleural effusion, image guidance is preferred over closed pleural biopsy.[61]

Medical Thoracoscopy and Video-Assisted Thoracoscopic Surgery

Medical Thoracoscopy (MT) (also known as pleuroscopy) was popularized by Hans Christian Jacobaeus in 1910.[62] The procedure was originally performed through a cystoscope, and provided a better understanding of pleural disease, serving as the foundation for today's interventions. MT has evolved from its roots into video-assisted thoracoscopic surgery (VATS) and has provided an avenue for multiple diagnostic and therapeutic solutions. MT differs from VATS in that it can be performed in an endoscopy setting (or OR [operating room]), with local anesthesia and/or moderate sedation, single port, and by a pulmonologist or a surgeon. Each of the two methods affords direct visualization and biopsy of pleural nodules, masses, and thickening (**Fig. 4**).

MT has a diagnostic sensitivity for malignant pleural disease of 92.6% when pooling results across 22 case series.[63] Sensitivity remains high

(90.1%) even in patients who first had a nondiagnostic "blind" pleural biopsy.[63] When comparing image-guided biopsy (Abrams Needle) versus MT, the sensitivity for MT was increased but not statistically significantly so.[64] MT with local anesthetic has a low rate of complication and mortality despite the invasive nature of the procedure. Mortality rate related to MT alone is 0.34% and is postulated to be related to use of talc.[63] Significant complications are seen in 1.8% of procedures, and include empyema, hemorrhage, port-site tumor growth (specific to mesothelioma), bronchopleural fistula, and pneumothorax.[65] VATS has similar diagnostic yields and complication rates as MT.

Mesothelioma presents a particular diagnostic challenge, as pleural fluid cytology is diagnostic in under a third of patients.[55,66] In patients whom mesothelioma is suspected, MT or VATS is frequently the tool used to define the disease.[67] Local radiation to the port-site can be considered to prevent seeding, though efficacy of this procedure has not consistently been reproduced and is generally not recommended prophylactically.[67–69]

MANAGEMENT

Once pleural malignancy is confirmed, the crux of management centers around palliation of symptoms and improvement of patient quality of life. The approach to treatment should be individualized based on performance status, tumor type (ie, is there malignant ascites), expected life span, and patient's preferences. While predicted remaining life span is critical in decision making for pleural interventions, it remains challenging for clinicians. Prognostic tools like LENT (based on 4 parameters: LDH level of the pleural fluid, the Eastern Cooperative Oncology Group [ECOG] performance-score, serum neutrophil-to-lymphocyte ratio, tumor histology) and PROMISE (based on clinical and biological parameters to estimate 3-month mortality) can be used to assist in estimating life expectancy.[70,71] Asymptomatic patients with limited life span should be managed much differently than those with symptoms and reasonable survival. Therapeutic thoracentesis should be performed in all symptomatic patients with malignant pleural effusions to determine the effect on breathlessness and to determine the rapidity of recurrence.[5,72] In patients with rapid recurrence, the following strategies can be considered.

Serial Thoracentesis

In select patients, this modality can serve as a destination therapy. Typically, this is

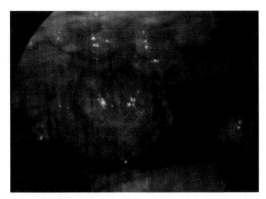

Fig. 4. Thoracoscopic view of tumor implant on the pleural surface of **Fig. 3**.

recommended in patients with far advanced disease and poor performance status. Thoracentesis can be done in the outpatient setting and has a low complication rate, especially with adoption of US to guide needle placement.[73] The amount of fluid that can be removed safely continues to be the focus of debate, with some guidelines recommending only draining 1 to 1.5 L at a time.[17] This is based on concerns for creation of a negative pleural pressure leading to re-expansion pulmonary edema. However, the incidence of re-expansion pulmonary edema is rare (0.10% in one large case series),[74] and the potential symptomatic benefit of fully draining the space likely outweighs the risk. Use of pleural manometry is no longer common practice, but keeping pleural pressure above $-20ccH_2O$ is recommended and can promote safe removal of fluid well past 1.5 L.[75] When clinicians do not have pleural manometry available, patient symptoms of chest pressure can be a surrogate marker and should guide clinicians on the amount of fluid to drain.[76] Method of drainage can be either active aspiration or gravity, and there is no difference in patient symptoms.[77]

Pleurodesis

Pleurodesis is defined as the fusion of the parietal and visceral pleura via creation of extensive adhesions, leading to obliteration of the pleural space and preventing accumulation of a pleural effusion. The exact mechanism of pleurodesis is not fully elucidated, but it is suspected to be related to inflammation and fibrosis via transforming growth factor-β1,[78] interleukin-8, and transforming growth factor-β.[79] Regardless of the mechanism, apposition of the visceral and parietal pleura is required to accomplish successful pleurodesis, unlike in **Fig. 5**. MPE provides a unique challenge for complete apposition, given an often thickened visceral

pleura and incomplete lung re-expansion related to the malignancy itself (ie, nonexpandable lung).[80] When a patient does achieve apposition of the parietal and visceral pleura, it is reasonable to attempt either chemical or mechanical pleurodesis. It remains unclear the relationship on the degree of pleural apposition that predicts pleurodesis success. There are mixed results on using patient symptoms, radiographic imaging, and pleural manometry in predicting success of pleurodesis, but these findings all have a benefit in demonstrating expandable and nonexpandable lung after thoracentesis.[81,82]

Frequently in patients undergoing pleurodesis for a malignancy, a chemical sclerosant is chosen, given the inherent risks of surgery in this ill population. Talc, bleomycin, Corynebacterium parvum, etoposide, povidine-iodine, and doxycycline have all been used as agents to achieve pleurodesis.[83,84] Two large-scale reviews (1168 and 1499 patients) reviewed the efficacy of chemical pleurodesis with complete response occurring in 64% of patients and a relative risk of nonrecurrence at 1.20.[84,85] Talc was found to be the most efficacious of the different sclerosants with no increased mortality, and this appears to be reproducible across multiple studies.[86–91] Talc can be delivered via slurry (suspension form) via chest tube or poudrage (atomized form) via thoracoscopy. Multiple studies have shown no difference in recurrence or complication rates between the two.[65,92] The size of the chest tube may impact success rate of pleurodesis, as one study showed lower failure rates in a 24Fr (24%) versus a 12Fr (30%) chest tube, although pain scores were lower in the 12Fr group.[93]

The most common adverse events associated with pleurodesis are pain (23%) and fever (19%) and likely related to the inflammatory sclerosing process. There have been case reports of acute respiratory failure with talc; however when using graded-size talc, there were no instances of respiratory failure in a series of 558 patients.[94]

Indwelling Pleural Catheter

The use of a tunneled indwelling pleural catheter (IPC) is becoming increasingly common for the management of MPE. A TPC is a silicone tube placed into the pleural cavity, tunneled subcutaneously with a small cuff, and the other end exiting the patient with a one-way valve, allowing for drainage at home or in an ambulatory setting by patients and/or their caregivers.[95] These are excellent mechanisms for palliation of symptoms in the outpatient setting; however patient selection

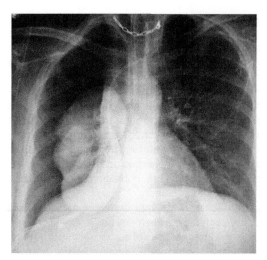

Fig. 5. Malignant pleural effusion leading to trapped lung after evacuation with tube thoracostomy.

is critical for effective use of the catheter and prevention of complications.[96]

There are increasing amounts of data that TPCs are safe and effective in managing patient symptoms and improving quality of life. A large systematic review showed symptomatic improvement in 95.6% of patients and improvement in Borg score immediately after placement.[97,98]

Achievement of pleurodesis is a somewhat hard metric to study, as this is only achievable in patients with significant lung re-expansion; however an IPC is still effective at relieving dyspnea in patients without lung re-expansion. TPC-related pleurodesis has typically been reported to occur at 29 to 59 days after placement.[99–101] Pleurodesis rates vary based on different studies, with overall rates ranging from 45% to 58%.[97,100,102] However, when evaluating patients suitable for pleurodesis (ie, with expandable lung), tha number increases to 70%.[103] It should also be noted, that up to 50% of patients with nonexpendable lung may achieve pleurodesis at 6 months.[104]

IPCs have been compared with various other forms of pleurodesis. In IPC versus doxycycline pleurodesis via tube thoracostomy, there was no significant difference in the degree of symptomatic improvement in dyspnea or quality of life.[105] In IPC versus talc slurry, dyspnea improved in a similar fashion with no difference up to 42 days; however the IPC group did have a significant improvement in dyspnea at 6 months.[98] Additionally, the length of initial hospitalization was shorter in the IPC group (median 0 vs 4 days).[98] Frequency of drainage (daily vs every other day) was evaluated in the ASAP trial, with higher rates of spontaneous pleurodesis in the daily drainage group (47%,

median 54 days) compared with the every other day group (24%, median 90 days).[106]

The incidence of IPC-related infections is low and range from 0% to 12%.[107,108] Fortunately, in patients who have an IPC-related infection, pleurodesis is common and allowed for removal of the catheter in 62% of patients.[108] Having a protocol for prevention of pleural infection, including close follow-up, has been shown to reduce infection rates.[96]

Rapid Pleurodesis

One of the major drawbacks of pleurodesis is that it often necessitates a 5 to 7 day hospitalization,[109] and IPC leads to spontaneous pleurodesis at various rates (45%–70%) and lengths of time (29–90 days).[97,98,106,109,110] The length of time, coupled with an inherent infectious risk, and need for assistance with home drainage does eliminate certain patients' candidacy for an IPC. In these situations, a rapid pleurodesis procedure can be considered. This is a combination of thoracoscopy with talc delivery, as well as IPC insertion simultaneously. This method has been shown to decrease hospital length of stay and duration of IPC use (mean of 8–10 days), while significantly improving quality of life.[111,112] Talc has also been given post-IPC insertion after evidence of good lung re-expansion, with a higher rate of pleurodesis at 35-days than IPC alone.[113]

When considering all of the options for therapy of MPE, IPC does appear to be the most cost-effective option, given the outpatient nature of the procedure and ability to manage fluid removal in the ambulatory setting.[114]

SUMMARY

MPE is a commonly encountered clinical problem with significant associated morbidity. Making a timely diagnosis via thoracentesis or other invasive procedure should be accomplished as quickly as possible. Management centers around patient characteristics and quality of life and should be personalized to fit needs.

CLINICS CARE POINTS

- Malignant pleural effusions occur when cancer is detected in the pleural space, and once diagnosed carry a median survival of 4-9 months.

- Imaging findings suggestive of malignancy include CT or US showing pleural thickening

>1cm, pleural nodularity, diaphragm thickening >7mm, and PET-avidity in the pleural space.

- Initial thoracentesis has a diagnostic sensitivity of 60%. Sensitivity for ovarian, lung (adenocarcinoma), breast, and GI-related malignancies are all >60%; while hematologic malignancy, non-adenocarcinoma lung primary, and mesothelioma all having lower sensitivities.
- Thoracic ultrasound-guided, CT-guided, and medical thoracoscopy-guided biopsies all have good sensitivity for diagnosis at 76% or greater.
- Management of malignant effusions should rely upon patient symptoms, patient desire for procedures (i.e. insertion of indwelling pleural catheter), and life expectancy.

DISCLOSURE

The authors have nothing to disclose.

REFERENCES

1. Clive AO, Jones HE, Bhatnagar R, et al. Interventions for the management of malignant pleural effusions: a network meta-analysis. Cochrane Database Syst Rev 2016;2016(5):CD010529.
2. Bibby AC, Dorn P, Psallidas I, et al. ERS/EACTS statement on the management of malignant pleural effusions. Eur Respir J 2018;52. 1800349.
3. Rodriguez-Panadero F, Borderas Naranjo F, Lopez Mejias J. Pleural metastatic tumours and effusions. Frequency and pathogenic mechanisms in a post-mortem series. Eur Respir J 1989;2:366–9.
4. Stathopoulos GT, Kalomenidis I. Malignant pleural effusion: tumor-host interactions unleashed. Am J Respir Crit Care Med 2012;186:487–92.
5. Antony VB, Loddenkemper R, Astoul P, et al. Management of malignant pleural effusions. Am J Respir Crit Care Med 2000;162:1987–2001.
6. Maturu VN, Dhooria S, Bal A, et al. Role of medical thoracoscopy and closed-blind pleural biopsy in undiagnosed exudative pleural effusions: a single-center experience of 348 patients. J Bronchology Interv Pulmonol 2015;22:121–9.
7. Murthy V, Bessich JL. Medical thoracoscopy and its evolving role in the diagnosis and treatment of pleural disease. J Thorac Dis 2017;9:S1011–21.
8. Boutin C, Cargnino P, Viallat JR. Thoracoscopy in the early diagnosis of malignant pleural effusions. Endoscopy 1980;12:155–60.
9. Dixit R, Agarwal KC, Gokhroo A, et al. Diagnosis and management options in malignant pleural effusions. Lung India 2017;34:160–6.
10. Arnold DT, De Fonseka D, Perry S, et al. Investigating unilateral pleural effusions: the role of cytology. Eur Respir J 2018;52. 1801254.
11. Loveland P, Christie M, Hammerschlag G, et al. Diagnostic yield of pleural fluid cytology in malignant effusions: an Australian tertiary centre experience. Intern Med J 2018;48:1318–24.
12. Meriggi F. Malignant pleural effusion: still a long way to go. Rev Recent Clin Trials 2019;14:24–30.
13. Wang NS. Anatomy of the pleura. Clinchest Med 1998;19:229–40.
14. Miserocchi G. Physiology and pathophysiology of pleural fluid turnover. Eurrespir J 1997;10:219–25.
15. GT S IK. Animal models of malignant pleural effusion. Curr Opin Pulm Med 2009;15:343–52.
16. Psallidas I, Stathopoulos GT, Maniatis NA, et al. Secreted phosphoprotein-1 directly provokes vascular leakage to foster malignant pleural effusion. Oncogene 2013;32:528–35.
17. Antony VB, Loddenkemper R, Astoul P, et al. Management of malignant pleural effusions. Eur Respir J 2001;18:402–19.
18. Estenne M, Yernault JC, De Troyer A. Mechanism of relief of dyspnea after thoracocentesis in patients with large pleural effusions. Amj Med 1983;74:813–9.
19. Cartaxo AM, Vargas FS, Salge JM, et al. Improvements in the 6-min walk test and spirometry following thoracentesis for symptomatic pleural effusions. Chest 2011;139:1424–9.
20. Doelken P, Abreu R, Sahn SA, et al. Effect of thoracentesis on respiratory mechanics and gas exchange in the patient receiving mechanical ventilation. Chest 2006;130:1354–61.
21. Light RW. Clinical practice. Pleural effusion. N Engl J Med 2002;346:1971–7.
22. Chernow B, Sahn SA. Carcinomatous involvement of the pleura: an analysis of 96 patients. Amj Med 1977;63:695–702.
23. Davies HE, Davies RJO, Davies CWH. Management of pleural infection in adults: British Thoracic Society pleural disease guideline 2010. Thorax 2010;65:ii41–53.
24. Feller-Kopman D. Therapeutic thoracentesis: the role of ultrasound and pleural manometry. Curr Opin Pulm Med 2007;13:312–8.
25. Yousefifard M, Baikpour M, Ghelichkhani P, et al. Screening performance characteristic of ultrasonography and Radiography in detection of pleural effusion; a meta-analysis. Emerg (Tehran) 2016;4:1–10.
26. Qureshi NR, Rahman NM, Gleeson FV. Thoracic ultrasound in the diagnosis of malignant pleural effusion. Thorax 2009;64:139–43.
27. Wernecke K. Ultrasound study of the pleura. Eur Radiol 2000;10:1515–23.
28. Blackmore CC, Black WC, Dallas RV, et al. Pleural fluid volume estimation: a chest radiograph prediction rule. Acad Radiol 1996;3:103–9.

29. Maher GG, Berger HW. Massive pleural effusion: malignant and nonmalignant causes in 46 patients. Am Rev Respir Dis 1972;105:458–60.

30. Hooper C, Lee YCG, Maskell N. Investigation of a unilateral pleural effusion in adults: British Thoracic Society pleural disease guideline 2010. Thorax 2010;65:ii4–17.

31. Leung AN, Muller NL, Miller RR. CT in differential diagnosis of diffuse pleural disease. AJR Am J Roentgenol 1990;154:487–92.

32. Hallifax RJ, Haris M, Corcoran JP, et al. Role of CT in assessing pleural malignancy prior to thoracoscopy. Thorax 2015;70:192–3.

33. Traill ZC, Davies RJ, Gleeson FV. Thoracic computed tomography in patients with suspected malignant pleural effusions. Clin Radiol 2001;56: 193–6.

34. Porcel JM, Pardina M, Bielsa S, et al. Derivation and validation of a CT scan scoring system for discriminating malignant from benign pleural effusions. Chest 2015;147:513–9.

35. Porcel JM, Hernandez P, Martinez-Alonso M, et al. Accuracy of fluorodeoxyglucose-PET imaging for differentiating benign from malignant pleural effusions: a meta-analysis. Chest 2015;147:502–12.

36. Wang ZJ, Reddy GP, Gotway MB, et al. Malignant pleural mesothelioma: evaluation with CT, MR imaging, and PET. Radiographics 2004;24:105–19.

37. Feller-Kopman D, Light R. Pleural disease. N Engl J Med 2018;378:740–51.

38. Zalt MB, Bechara RI, Parks C, et al. Effect of routine clopidogrel use on bleeding complications after ultrasound-guided thoracentesis. J Bronchology Interv Pulmonol 2012;19:284–7.

39. Puchalski JT, Argento AC, Murphy TE, et al. The safety of thoracentesis in patients with uncorrected bleeding risk. Ann Am Thorac Soc 2013;10: 336–41.

40. Patel PP, Singh S, Atwell TD, et al. The safety of ultrasound-guided thoracentesis in patients on Novel oral anticoagulants and clopidogrel: a single-center experience. Mayo Clin Proc 2019; 94:1535–41.

41. Puchalski J. Thoracentesis and the risks for bleeding: a new era. Curr Opin Pulm Med 2014; 20:377–84.

42. Orlandi E, Citterio C, Seghini P, et al. Thoracentesis in advanced cancer patients with severe thrombocytopenia: ultrasound guide improves safety and reduces bleeding risk. Clin Respir J 2018;12: 1747–52.

43. Sahn SA. State of the art. The pleura. Am Rev Respir Dis 1988;138:184–234.

44. Swiderek J, Morcos S, Donthireddy V, et al. Prospective study to determine the volume of pleural fluid required to diagnose malignancy. Chest 2010;137:68–73.

45. Abouzgheib W, Bartter T, Dagher H, et al. A prospective study of the volume of pleural fluid required for accurate diagnosis of malignant pleural effusion. Chest 2009;135:999–1001.

46. DeMaio A, Clarke JM, Dash R, et al. Yield of malignant pleural effusion for detection of oncogenic driver mutations in lung adenocarcinoma. J Bronchology Interv Pulmonol 2019;26:96–101.

47. Garcia LW, Ducatman BS, Wang HH. The value of multiple fluid specimens in the cytological diagnosis of malignancy. Mod Pathol 1994;7: 665–8.

48. Ylagan LR, Zhai J. The value of ThinPrep and cytospin preparation in pleural effusion cytological diagnosis of mesothelioma and adenocarcinoma. Diagn Cytopathol 2005;32:137–44.

49. Hsu C. Cytologic detection of malignancy in pleural effusion: a review of 5,255 samples from 3,811 patients. Diagn Cytopathol 1987;3:8–12.

50. Johnston WW. The malignant pleural effusion. A review of cytopathologic diagnoses of 584 specimens from 472 consecutive patients. Cancer 1985;56:905–9.

51. Steinfort DP, Kranz S, Dowers A, et al. Sensitive molecular testing methods can demonstrate NSCLC driver mutations in malignant pleural effusion despite non-malignant cytology. Transl Lung Cancer Res 2019;8:513–8.

52. Wang Y, Liu Z, Yin H, et al. Improved detection of EGFR mutations in the tumor cells enriched from the malignant pleural effusion of non-small cell lung cancer patient. Gene 2018;644:87–92.

53. Walsh LJ, Macfarlane JT, Manhire AR, et al. Audit of pleural biopsies: an argument for a pleural biopsy service. Respir Med 1994;88:503–5.

54. Chakrabarti B, Ryland I, Sheard J, et al. The role of Abrams percutaneous pleural biopsy in the investigation of exudative pleural effusions. Chest 2006; 129:1549–55.

55. Maskell NA, Butland RJA. BTS guidelines for the investigation of a unilateral pleural effusion in adults. Thorax 2003;58:8ii–17.

56. Whitaker D, Shilkin KB. Diagnosis of pleural malignant mesothelioma in life–a practical approach. J Pathol 1984;143:147–75.

57. Baumann MH. Closed pleural biopsy: not dead yet! Chest 2006;129:1398–400.

58. Pereyra MF, San-Jose E, Ferreiro L, et al. Role of blind closed pleural biopsy in the managment of pleural exudates. Can Respir J 2013;20:362–6.

59. Benamore RE, Scott K, Richards CJ, et al. Image-guided pleural biopsy: diagnostic yield and complications. Clin Radiol 2006;61:700–5.

60. Mei F, Bonifazi M, Rota M, et al. Diagnostic yield and safety of image-guided pleural biopsy: a systematic review and meta-analysis. Respiration 2021;100:77–87.

61. Stigt JA, Boers JE, Groen HJ. Analysis of "dry" mesothelioma with ultrasound guided biopsies. Lung Cancer 2012;78:229–33.

62. Shojaee S, Lee HJ. Thoracoscopy: medical versus surgical-in the management of pleural diseases. J Thorac Dis 2015;7:S339–51.

63. Rahman NM, Ali NJ, Brown G, et al. Local anaesthetic thoracoscopy: British Thoracic Society pleural disease guideline 2010. Thorax 2010;65:ii54–60.

64. Metintas M, Ak G, Dundar E, et al. Medical thoracoscopy vs CT scan-guided Abrams pleural needle biopsy for diagnosis of patients with pleural effusions. Chest 2010;137:1362–8.

65. Dresler CM, Olak J, Herndon JE, et al. Phase III intergroup study of talc poudrage vs talc slurry sclerosis for malignant pleural effusion. Chest 2005;127:909–15.

66. Renshaw AA, Dean BR, Antman KH, et al. The role of cytologic evaluation of pleural fluid in the diagnosis of malignant mesothelioma. Chest 1997;111:106–9.

67. Boutin C, Rey F, Viallat JR. Prevention of malignant seeding after invasive diagnostic procedures in patients with pleural mesothelioma. A randomized trial of local radiotherapy. Chest 1995;108:754–8.

68. Clive AO, Taylor H, Dobson L, et al. Prophylactic radiotherapy for the prevention of procedure-tract metastases after surgical and large-bore pleural procedures in malignant pleural mesothelioma (SMART): a multicentre, open-label, phase 3, randomised controlled trial. Lancet Oncol 2016;17:1094–104.

69. O'Rourke N, Garcia JC, Paul J, et al. A randomised controlled trial of intervention site radiotherapy in malignant pleural mesothelioma. Radiother Oncol 2007;84:18–22.

70. Psallidas I, Kanellakis NI, Gerry S, et al. Development and validation of response markers to predict survival and pleurodesis success in patients with malignant pleural effusion (PROMISE): a multicohort analysis. Lancet Oncol 2018;19(7):930–9.

71. Clive AO, Kahan BC, Hooper CE, et al. Predicting survival in malignant pleural effusion: development and validation of the LENT prognostic score. Thorax 2014;69(12):1098–104.

72. Roberts ME, Neville E, Berrisford RG, et al. Management of a malignant pleural effusion: British Thoracic Society pleural disease guideline 2010. Thorax 2010;65:ii32–40.

73. Cavanna L, Mordenti P, Berte R, et al. Ultrasound guidance reduces pneumothorax rate and improves safety of thoracentesis in malignant pleural effusion: report on 445 consecutive patients with advanced cancer. World J Surgoncol 2014;12:139.

74. Ault MJ, Rosen BT, Scher J, et al. Thoracentesis outcomes: a 12-year experience. Thorax 2015;70:127–32.

75. Feller-Kopman D, Berkowitz D, Boiselle P, et al. Large-volume thoracentesis and the risk of reexpansion pulmonary edema. AnnThoracSurg 2007;84:1656–61.

76. Feller-Kopman D, Walkey A, Berkowitz D, et al. The relationship of pleural pressure to symptom development during therapeutic thoracentesis. Chest 2006;129:1556–60.

77. Lentz RJ, Shojaee S, Grosu HB, et al. The impact of gravity vs Suction-driven therapeutic thoracentesis on pressure-related complications: the GRAVITAS multicenter randomized controlled trial. Chest 2020;157:702–11.

78. Shojaee S, Voelkel N, Farkas L, et al. Transforming growth factor-beta1 rise in pleural fluid after tunneled pleural catheter placement: pilot study. J Bronchologyintervpulmonol 2013;20:304–8.

79. Rodriguez-Panadero F, Montes-Worboys A. Mechanisms of pleurodesis. Respiration 2012;83:91–8.

80. Huggins JT, Maldonado F, Chopra A, et al. Unexpandable lung from pleural disease. Respirology 2018;23:160–7.

81. Huggins JT, Sahn SA, Heidecker J, et al. Characteristics of trapped lung: pleural fluid analysis, manometry, and air-contrast chest CT. Chest 2007;131:206–13.

82. Lee HJ, Yarmus L, Kidd D, et al. Comparison of pleural pressure measuring instruments. Chest 2014;146:1007–12.

83. Haddad FJ, Younes RN, Gross JL, et al. Pleurodesis in patients with malignant pleural effusions: talc slurry or bleomycin? Results of a prospective randomized trial. World J Surg 2004;28:749–53.

84. Shaw P, Agarwal R. Pleurodesis for malignant pleural effusions. Cochrane Database Syst Rev 2004;(1):CD002916.

85. Walker-Renard PB, Vaughan LM, Sahn SA. Chemical pleurodesis for malignant pleural effusions. Ann Intern Med 1994;120:56–64.

86. Noppen M, Degreve J, Mignolet M, et al. A prospective, randomised study comparing the efficacy of talc slurry and bleomycin in the treatment of malignant pleural effusions. Acta ClinBelg 1997;52:258–62.

87. Fentiman IS, Rubens RD, Hayward JL. A comparison of intracavitary talc and tetracycline for the control of pleural effusions secondary to breast cancer. EurJ Cancer ClinOncol 1986;22:1079–81.

88. Diacon AH, Wyser C, Bolliger CT, et al. Prospective randomized comparison of thoracoscopic talc poudrage under local anesthesia versus bleomycin

instillation for pleurodesis in malignant pleural effusions. Amj Respircrit Care Med 2000;162:1445–9.

89. Ong KC, Indumathi V, Raghuram J, et al. A comparative study of pleurodesis using talc slurry and bleomycin in the management of malignant pleural effusions. Respirology 2000;5:99–103.

90. Kuzdzal J, Sladek K, Wasowski D, et al. Talc powder vs doxycycline in the control of malignant pleural effusion: a prospective, randomized trial. Med Sci Monit 2003;9:I54–9.

91. Scarci M, Caruana E, Bertolaccini L, et al. Current practices in the management of malignant pleural effusions: a survey among members of the European Society of Thoracic Surgeons. Interact Cardiovasc Thorac Surg 2017;24:414–7.

92. Bhatnagar R, Piotrowska HEG, Laskawiec-Szkonter M, et al. Effect of thoracoscopic talc poudrage vs talc slurry via chest tube on pleurodesis failure rate among patients with malignant pleural effusions: a randomized clinical trial. JAMA 2020;323:60–9.

93. Rahman NM, Pepperell J, Rehal S, et al. Effect of opioids vs NSAIDs and larger vs smaller chest tube size on pain control and pleurodesis efficacy among patients with malignant pleural effusion: the TIME1 randomized clinical trial. JAMA 2015;314:2641–53.

94. Janssen JP, Collier G, Astoul P, et al. Safety of pleurodesis with talc poudrage in malignant pleural effusion: a prospective cohort study. Lancet 2007;369:1535–9.

95. Gillen J, Lau C. Permanent indwelling catheters in the management of pleural effusions. Thorac Surg Clin 2013;23:63–71, vi.

96. Gilbert CR, Lee HJ, Akulian JA, et al. A quality improvement intervention to reduce indwelling tunneled pleural catheter infection rates. Ann Am Thorac Soc 2015;12:847–53.

97. Van Meter ME, McKee KY, Kohlwes RJ. Efficacy and safety of tunneled pleural catheters in adults with malignant pleural effusions: a systematic review. J Gen Intern Med 2011;26:70–6.

98. Davies HE, Mishra EK, Kahan BC, et al. Effect of an indwelling pleural catheter vs chest tube and talc pleurodesis for relieving dyspnea in patients with malignant pleural EffusionThe TIME2 randomized controlled TrialIndwelling pleural catheters vs talc pleurodesis. JAMA 2012;307:2383–9.

99. Tremblay A, Michaud G. Single-Center experience with 250 tunnelled pleural catheter insertions for malignant pleural effusion. Chest 2006;129:362–8.

100. Warren WH, Kalimi R, Khodadadian LM, et al. Management of malignant pleural effusions using the Pleur(x) catheter. Ann Thorac Surg 2008;85:1049–55.

101. Suzuki K, Servais EL, Rizk NP, et al. Palliation and pleurodesis in malignant pleural effusion: the role for tunneled pleural catheters. J Thorac Oncol 2011;6(4):762–7.

102. Warren WH, Kim AW, Liptay MJ. Identification of clinical factors predicting Pleurx catheter removal in patients treated for malignant pleural effusion. Eur J Cardiothorac Surg 2008;33:89–94.

103. Tremblay A, Mason C, Michaud G. Use of tunnelled catheters for malignant pleural effusions in patients fit for pleurodesis. Eur Respir J 2007;30:759–62.

104. Muruganandan S, Azzopardi M, Fitzgerald DB, et al. Aggressive versus symptom-guided drainage of malignant pleural effusion via indwelling pleural catheters (AMPLE-2): an open-label randomised trial. Lancet Respir Med 2018;6:671–80.

105. Putnam JB Jr, Light RW, Rodriguez RM, et al. A randomized comparison of indwelling pleural catheter and doxycycline pleurodesis in the management of malignant pleural effusions. Cancer 1999;86:1992–9.

106. Wahidi MM, Reddy C, Yarmus L, et al. Randomized trial of pleural fluid drainage frequency in patients with malignant pleural effusions. The ASAP trial. Am J Respir Crit Care Med 2017;195:1050–7.

107. Lui MM, Thomas R, Lee YC. Complications of indwelling pleural catheter use and their management. BMJ Open Respir Res 2016;3:e000123.

108. Fysh ET, Tremblay A, Feller-Kopman D, et al. Clinical outcomes of indwelling pleural catheter-related pleural infections: an international multicenter study. Chest 2013;144:1597–602.

109. Putnam JB Jr, Walsh GL, Swisher SG, et al. Outpatient management of malignant pleural effusion by a chronic indwelling pleural catheter. Ann Thorac Surg 2000;69:369–75.

110. Porcel JM, Lui MM, Lerner AD, et al. Comparing approaches to the management of malignant pleural effusions. Expert Rev Respir Med 2017;11:273–84.

111. Reddy C, Ernst A, Lamb C, et al. Rapid pleurodesis for malignant pleural effusions. Chest 2011;139:1419–23.

112. Krochmal R, Reddy C, Yarmus L, et al. Patient evaluation for rapid pleurodesis of malignant pleural effusions. J Thorac Dis 2016;8:2538–43.

113. Bhatnagar R, Keenan EK, Morley AJ, et al. Outpatient talc administration by indwelling pleural catheter for malignant effusion. N Engl J Med 2018;378:1313–22.

114. Shafiq M, Frick KD, Lee H, et al. Management of malignant pleural effusion: a cost-Utility analysis. J Bronchology Interv Pulmonol 2015;22:215–25.

Malignant Pleural Mesothelioma
Updates for Respiratory Physicians

Calvin Sidhu, MBBS, FRACP[a,b,c], Amber Louw, MBBS[b,c,d],
Y.C. Gary Lee, MBChB, PhD, FRACP, FCCP, FRCP[a,b,c,e],*

KEYWORDS

• Pleural • Cancer • Mesothelioma • Effusion • Needle tract • Asbestos

KEY POINTS

- The global incidence of malignant pleural mesothelioma is predicted to continue to rise, especially in developing countries where use of asbestos is less regulated.
- There have been many developments in mesothelioma management, particularly molecular diagnostics and immunotherapy treatment.
- Optimal care of mesothelioma patients requires multidisciplinary involvement of both medical (i.e. pulmonology, medical oncology, radiation oncology, palliative care) and allied health (i.e. dietetics, physiotherapy/exercise physiology) specialties.

INTRODUCTION

Malignant mesothelioma is the result of neoplastic transformation of the mesothelial cells, with more than 80% arising from the pleura. The global incidence of mesothelioma continues to rise. Although the number of cases in developed countries has remained stable, the World Health Organization predicts an exponential increase in mesothelioma cases in developing regions, where underreporting of mesothelioma is also common, due to unregulated use of asbestos.[1–7]

It is important, therefore, that pulmonologists have a solid understanding of malignant pleural mesothelioma (MPM), which has many unique features separating it from other common (eg, lung) cancers. This article aims to update clinicians of key advances of MPM relevant to day-to-day practice in particular new diagnostic tests, management of resultant malignant effusions, and latest advances on treatment. We highlight important unanswered questions that should be the focus of future research.

ETIOLOGY

Asbestos exposure is the most recognized cause of MPM, as asbestos fibers are difficult to degrade once inhaled.[8] The larger the amount of exposure, and the more years after inhalation, the more likely the eventual development of MPM, which typically develops after a lag period of 3 to 4 decades after the initial asbestos exposure.[8] Crocidolite (blue asbestos) has longer and thinner fibers, is more resistant to biodegradation, and is significantly more carcinogenic than chrysotile (white asbestos).[8]

Asbestos is used extensively as insulation material. Workers involved in direct handling of asbestos (eg, mining and transportation) and those using asbestos products (eg, construction workers, electricians, plumbers, carpenters, car manufacturing, and mechanics) are at high risks.[8] There are more men in these occupations, hence a higher incidence of men with MPM. In recent years a "third wave" of MPM has been recognized

[a] Respiratory Medicine, Sir Charles Gairdner Hospital, Perth, Western Australia; [b] Pleural Medicine Unit, Institute for Respiratory Health, Perth, Western Australia; [c] School of Medical & Health Sciences, Edith Cowan University, Perth, Western Australia; [d] National Centre for Asbestos Related Diseases, University of Western Australia; [e] School of Medicine, University of Western Australia, Perth, Western Australia
* Corresponding author. UWA School of Medicine, 533 Harry Perkins Building, QE II Med Ctr, Perth, Western Australia 6009, Australia.
E-mail address: gary.lee@uwa.edu.au

Clin Chest Med 42 (2021) 697–710
https://doi.org/10.1016/j.ccm.2021.08.006
0272-5231/21/© 2021 Elsevier Inc. All rights reserved.

in people who had asbestos exposure from renovations of homes that contained asbestos.

Nevertheless, only a small number of asbestos-exposed subjects develop mesothelioma, raising the possibility of cofactors, especially genetic predisposition. High-risk and low-risk genetic associations have also been described. BRCA-associated protein 1 (BAP-1) syndrome is a recent discovery and a step toward elucidating the genetic predispositions for MPM.[8–10] Patients with this rare autosomal dominant condition have a higher risk for mesothelioma and a range of other uncommon malignancies, such as atypical Spitz tumor, melanomas (uveal/cutaneous), renal cell carcinoma (clear cell), and basal cell carcinomas.[9,10] Familial incidence rates of the syndrome is 6% to 7%, but asbestos exposure is still required for MPM to develop. Patients with BAP-1 syndrome who developed MPM do have a better prognosis than those without the mutations. Mutations to DNA repair gene, such as CDKN2A, PABL-1, and FANCI, also have been found in MPM, and their presence is thought to permit lower asbestos exposure to trigger neoplasia.[8–10] Homologous recombinant repair (HHR) and enhancer of zeste homolog 2 (EZH2) gene mutations also have been reported in patients with MPM.[8–10]

PATHOPHYSIOLOGY

Asbestos fibers trigger many biological changes, including inflammatory cascades, once inhaled into the lung and transverse the pleural space.[11,12] Many downstream reactions have been reported, such as asbestos-driven and macrophage-related phagocytosis causing reactive oxygen species formation, mitotic and chromosomal instability of mesothelial cells, accumulation of carcinogenic asbestos-surface–derived proteins and release of cytokine and growth factors.[11,12] Receptor tyrosine kinases can be activated, causing downstream promotion of Raf-MEK-extracellular signal-related kinases and phosphoinositide-3-kinase-AKT pathways.[11,12] Cyclin-dependent kinase inhibitors can become inactivated causing reduced tumor suppressor activity.[11,12] Neurofibromatosis (NF) type-2 genes can mutate and further reduce availability of tumor-suppressing proteins, such as merlin.[11,12] Aforementioned mutations of BAP-1, an apoptosis regulator, can affect chromosome dynamics, DNA damage responses, and cell-cycle growth regulation to allow MPM to proliferate.[10] It may also alter drug sensitivity. Description of the latest findings of molecular mechanisms underlying MPM are outside the scope of this review and can be found elsewhere.[8,13–15]

HISTOLOGY

MPM mainly consists of 2 histologic subtypes: epithelioid (~70%) and sarcomatoid (~10), including desmoplastic, with a third subtype that contains both histotypes, termed biphasic or mixed (~20).[16] It is increasingly recognized that MPM is a heterogeneous disease, even within the same tumor. The more areas sampled, the more likely it is that a representative of the whole tumor has been obtained. Relevant histologic differential diagnoses considered are subtype dependant; and, include reactive proliferations, metastatic adenocarcinoma, melanoma, and sarcoma.[17]

CLINICAL PRESENTATIONS

Symptoms of MPM are often nonspecific and insidious, hence patients typically present several months from onset of first symptoms. Most (more than 90%) patients present with a pleural effusion, and hence breathlessness (usually on exertion) and/or cough.[18] Chest pain is often related to local soft tissue invasions or neuropathic involvement. Constitutional symptoms, especially weight loss, night sweats, and fatigue, are common but are often underreported and undertreated. Disease progression within the unilateral hemithorax can cause rib invasion, pericardial involvement, lymphangitis, superior vena cava obstruction, esophageal obstruction, recurrent laryngeal nerve palsy, or even transdiaphragmatic spread into the peritoneum (**Fig. 1**). Contralateral disease can also develop with parenchymal lung nodules and pleural involvement. In an autopsy study, distant metastases were common and can involve most extrapulmonary organs, although many are not apparent clinically premortem.[19] Incidental detection from chest imaging performed for other indications can occur.

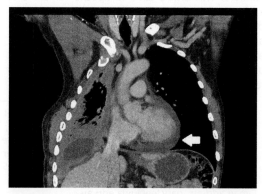

Fig. 1. Right MPM and associated pericardial effusion (*arrow*).

Clinicians therefore should maintain a high level of suspicion of the diagnosis, especially in at-risk individuals with occupational exposure and/or other benign asbestos changes (eg, pleural plaques).

IMAGING

There are no unique pathognomonic features that allow the diagnosis of MPM solely by imaging. Imaging, however, can aid detection of malignant pleural involvement, guide biopsies, and show disease extent and treatment response.

Most patients present with a pleural effusion. Chest radiography may reveal benign asbestos pleuro-pulmonary changes, such as pleural plaques, pleural thickening, and interstitial lung disease, suggestive of asbestosis, blunting of the costophrenic angle from small effusions or pleural thickening, or even reduced hemithorax size (**Fig. 2**). The presence or absence of these features does not define or exclude MPM. In advanced MPM, there may be nodular pleural thickening, pleural masses, pericardial or contralateral pleural effusion, parenchymal tumor infiltrates or lymphangitis, and rib erosion/fractures. Absence of a pleural effusion does not exclude MPM.

Thoracic ultrasonography can help identify pleural effusions and guide drainage and/or biopsies. The presence of parietal pleural thickening >1 cm, pleural nodularity, and diaphragmatic thickening >7 mm were highly suggestive of malignant disease (positive predictive value 100% in a study of 52 patients) but histocytological diagnosis is still needed to differentiate MPM from metastatic cancers.[20]

Computed tomography (CT) is part of the routine workup of patients suspected of MPM. Scanning with a pleural phase enhancement protocol using intravenous contrast can help identify abnormal areas of pleural thickening or nodularity for biopsy, assist with staging, and monitor treatment response. Delayed-phase scanning (230–300 seconds post-contrast injection) was shown in a small prospective study to be better than early phase (30–60 seconds) scanning.[21] Presence of air within the pleural space can serve as a useful contrast to delineate parietal and visceral pleural abnormalities and is the subject of a pilot feasibility (AIR) study.[22]

CT findings of circumferential pleural thickening, pleural thickening >1 cm, pleural nodularity, and mediastinal pleural thickening are proven cardinal features of pleural malignancy (but again not specific for MPM).[23] It can also identify disease invasion into the adjacent soft tissues, hemidiaphragm, vascular structures, or pericardium.

Avidity of pleural tissues on 18-flurodeoxygenase PET is not specific for MPM for diagnostic purposes and previous talc pleurodesis will lead to pleural avidity indefinitely (**Fig. 3**). In selected cases, PET can help target percutaneous biopsy especially in the presence of diffuse pleural thickening[24] (**Fig. 4**). Recent work has shown that PET activity can provide prognostication information in MPM but the data are less convincing for disease monitoring.[25] Its role in selecting patients for salvage treatments is being explored.[26]

Routine use of MRI is not justified, but it remains a focus of research.[21] MRI can help separate

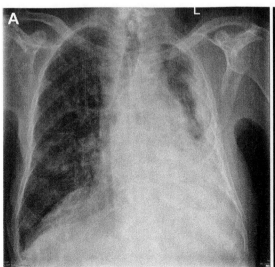
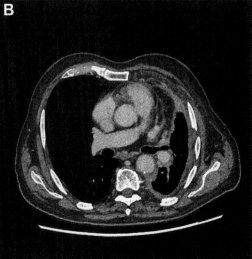

Fig. 2. . Progressive circumferential pleural thickening and hemithorax contraction on chest radiograph (*A*) with corresponding CT (*B*).

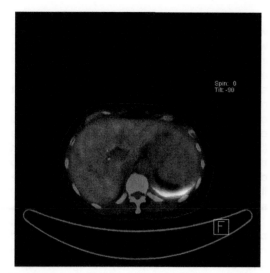

Fig. 3. PET scan showing increased activity in the area of previous talc pleurodesis.

benign from malignant pleural disease but can be limited by availability and costs.[27] Gadolinium contrast-enhanced MRI can assist in clarifying MPM extension into adjacent structures, particularly important when planning surgical resection, and also can be used as an alternative if there are contraindications to the iodine contrast for CTs.[27] Ohno and colleagues[28] compared whole-body MRI with other modalities used for staging MPM. MRI and PET-MRI had a superior diagnostic accuracy of 87% (compared with the 56.5% of other modalities).[28] Whole-body MRI is also

currently being investigated for tumor volume analysis during treatment plus determining survival.[21] Dynamic contrast-enhanced MRI was shown to provide prognostic information in terms of overall survival, such as from contrast-washout graphing, but was not contributory to disease monitoring.[25]

There are ongoing investigations of applying advanced imaging technologies to MPM, such as radiomics with mathematical analysis of tumors and deep learning convolutional neural networks in volumetric segmentational analysis.[29]

DIAGNOSIS

Most patients present with a pleural effusion. Ultrasound-guided sampling of these and cytologic examination can be diagnostic. However, separating malignant mesothelial cells from benign or reactive ones can be challenging, on both cytologic and histologic preparations. The cytologic diagnosis of epithelioid and biphasic MPM have been endorsed by international practice guidelines and is also accepted for medicolegal purposes.[30] The main concern regarding cytologic assessment is the perceived lack of sensitivity; however, this is as high as 70% in some centers.[31] Cytology and histology should be considered complementary.

Recent advances in investigations based on the common molecular alterations seen in the disease have improved the pathologists' ability to distinguish between benign and malignant mesothelial proliferations. Loss of BAP-1 has been found to have a 100% positive predictive value for mesothelioma in the correct clinical setting and can be

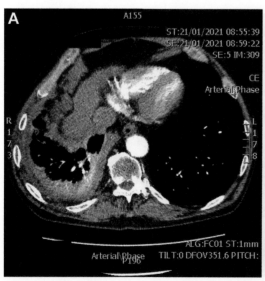

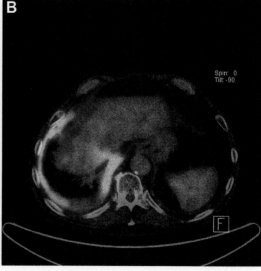

Fig. 4. (*A*) Circumferential pleural thickening on CT chest (*A*) and (*B*) PET scan highlighting areas of tracer avidity and increased activity.

assessed by immunohistochemistry in pleural fluid cells or tissue biopsies.[30] BAP-1 loss is present in most cases of epithelioid MPM and up to two-thirds of biphasic MPM but is less common in the sarcomatoid/desmoplastic variants (**Fig. 5**). Another valuable diagnostic tool is the assessment of homozygous deletion of chromosome 9p21, which encodes *CDKN2A (cyclin-dependent kinase inhibitors 2A)* and *methylthioadenosine phosphorylase (MTAP)*[30,32] (**Fig. 6**). The former is detected using fluorescence in situ hybridization (FISH) and deletion is present in most MPM cases. FISH is a technique requiring specialized equipment and interpretation, which is not available at all pathology centers. The immunohistochemical (IHC) assessment of MTAP has been shown to be a reliable surrogate for the FISH investigation and is quicker to perform.[32,33] These tests can be performed on both cytologic and histologic preparations and can add to the diagnostic

evidence in case assessment. However, lack of identification of an abnormality in any one of these tests does not rule out a mesothelioma diagnosis.

As malignant pleural effusion is more commonly a result of metastatic carcinomas, separating those from MPM is critical. It is recommended that after cytomorphological assessment, initial IHC testing include establishing the mesothelial lineage of abnormal cells with at least 2 mesothelial markers (eg, calretinin, cytokeratin 5/6, Wilms Tumor 1, D2-40).[34] MPM cells are generally expected to show negative staining for adenocarcinoma markers (eg, TTF-1, CEA, Ber-EP4).[34] Other relevant IHC tests that may be performed include epithelial membrane antigen, p53, desmin, glucose-transporter 1, and insulinlike growth factor II messenger RNA-binding protein 3.[35] Detailed discussions of the choice of IHC panel and application of molecular markers have been reviewed elsewhere.[35,36]

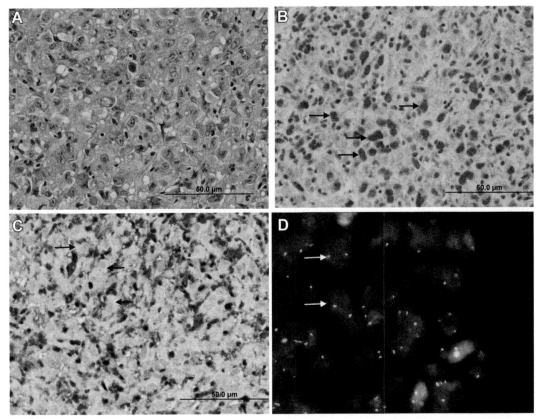

Fig. 5. The tumor is composed of pleomorphic mesothelial cells (*A*) (hematoxylin-eosin, original magnification ×60, scale bar = 50 μm) that demonstrate (*B*) retained nuclear staining for BAP-1 (*arrows* indicate nuclei with retained stain) (BAP-1 immunohistochemistry, original magnification ×60, scale bar = 50 μm). The cells demonstrate loss of cytoplasmic staining for MTAP (indicated by *arrows*) (MTAP immunohistochemistry, original magnification ×60, scale bar = 50 μm) (*C*). Corresponding FISH analysis (*D*) shows homozygous loss of *CDKN2A* (*arrows* indicate such nuclei) (loss of 2 red signals in abnormal nuclei with at least one retained chromosome 9 centromere signal [*green*]). (*Courtesy of* Joanne Peverall and Amber Louw, Diagnostic Genomics, PathWest Laboratory, Nedlands, Australia.)

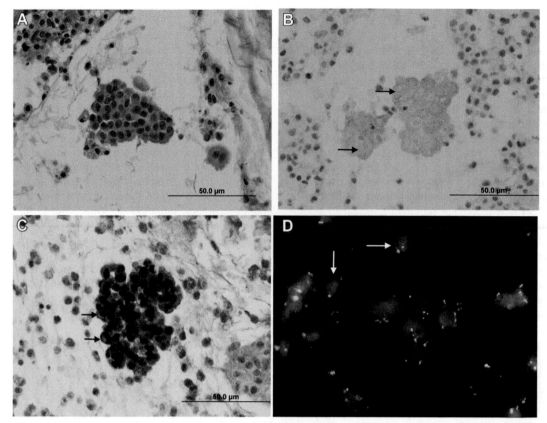

Fig. 6. This cell block demonstrates malignant mesothelioma cells (*A*) (hematoxylin-eosin, original magnification ×60, scale bar = 50 μm) with (*B*) loss of nuclear staining for BAP1 (*arrows*), note the positive inflammatory cells (BAP1 immunohistochemistry, original magnification ×60, scale bar = 50 μm). (*C*) The mesothelioma cells demonstrate retained cytoplasmic staining for MTAP (*arrows*) (MTAP immunohistochemistry, original magnification ×60, scale bar = 50 μm) and the FISH analysis (*D*) shows no loss of *CDKN2A* (*arrows* indicate nuclei) (2 red signals in abnormal nuclei with at least one retained chromosome 9 centromere signal [*green*]). (*Courtesy of* Joanne Peverall and Amber Louw, Diagnostic Genomics, PathWest Laboratory, Nedlands, Australia.)

If the pleural fluid is not diagnostic, pleural tissue sampling will be needed and can be performed via various techniques depending on available resources/expertise, patient fitness, and disease features. Percutaneous biopsy using imaging guidance with ultrasound or CT is the least invasive approach and is appropriate when pleural thickening, especially with nodularity, is detectable (**Fig. 7**). Image guidance is less important in patients with diffuse pleural thickening in which "blind" closed pleural biopsies (eg, with Abram needle) can be considered.

Biopsy under direct vision can be achieved with either medical (pleuroscopy) or surgical (usually video-assisted) thoracoscopy. Pleuroscopy using either rigid or semirigid scopes allow pleural tissue sampling with sedation (instead of general anesthesia) and has a high success rate for malignant pleural diseases. However, the pleura is often diffusely thickened in patients with MPM or benign asbestos thickening. Rigid forceps are needed for biopsy. Cryobiopsy with flexible pleuroscopes is a

new approach that has been shown to be safe and to provide larger and deeper specimens.[37] Caution is required and cryobiopsy usually needs to be combined with initial forceps sampling for best results. Narrow-band imaging and confocal laser electron microscopy are being evaluated but are unlikely to be useful given the large area of the pleura, particularly if there are no significant abnormal areas visualized.[38]

Video-assisted thoracoscopic surgery (VATS) is particularly useful if the patient has a loculated pleural cavity that requires surgical division of adhesions to allow full inspection of the pleura. VATS also permits sampling of the lung, pericardium, and mediastinal pleura, which is not usually safe to perform during pleuroscopy.

BIOMARKERS

Much work has been done to search for MPM biomarkers that could provide potential diagnostic, prognostic, and disease/response monitoring

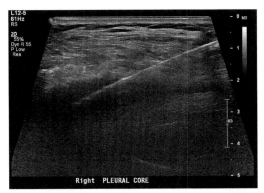

Fig. 7. Ultrasound-guided percutaneous pleural biopsy.

values. However, none of the biomarkers investigated are sensitive or specific enough to be used in isolation.

Soluble mesothelin is a glycoprotein highly expressed in MPM cells and can be detected in serum, pleural fluid, and urine.[39–41] High mesothelin levels in pleural fluid and serum are strongly suggestive of mesothelioma but can also occur in a small percentage of metastatic cancers; normal mesothelin levels do not exclude disease.[40] Data to date do not justify its use as a screening tool for MPM. Mesothelin has been approved for use in treatment monitoring and is best for epithelioid disease and in patients without renal dysfunction (as mesothelin is renally excreted). An elevated (blood or pleural fluid) mesothelin level in a patient with unexplained pleural effusion/thickening demands further investigations even if initial cytology or biopsies are nonmalignant.[39–41]

Many other markers have also been investigated. Osteopontin has a poor sensitivity for MPM, as it can be raised in lung, breast, and colonic malignancies, and not suitable for disease monitoring.[42] Its role in prognostication requires further validation.[42] The initial promising results of fibulin-3 in diagnosis of MPM has failed to be reproduced by other investigators.[42,43] Hyaluronic acid levels are raised in pleural fluid and has shown promising diagnostic value (especially when combined with pleural mesothelin levels to increase overall specificity).[42] Higher levels were correlated with significantly better survival.[42] Serum and pleural fluid vascular endothelial growth factor (VEGF) levels were elevated in MPM, but have not reached sufficient accuracy for clinical use.[42]

STAGING

Different staging systems have been proposed for MPM, such as the tumor-nodal-metastasis (TNM) system from the International Association for Study of Lung Cancer and International Mesothelioma Interest Group.[17,21] Many of the systems were designed to aid planning of surgery (which have not been shown beneficial in randomized trials), and involved invasive or expensive staging investigations (eg, MRI) not otherwise required for clinical care and do not impact clinical management. Future design of staging systems needs to take into consideration the unique nature of MPM, such as its diffuse pleural involvement (rather than a discreet tumor mass such as in lung or breast cancers), difficulty of imaging based on its location, and its multifocal nature (and heterogeneity even within individuals).

PROGNOSIS

MPM is a universally fatal cancer. Reported survival rates vary depending in part on how survival is defined (eg, from date of onset of symptoms, first medical presentation, histologic confirmation, or date of first treatment) and nature of the cohort (those enrolled in clinical, especially surgical trials, are likely to be "fitter" with better expected survival). Overall, a median survival in the range of 8–14 months is often cited, with an estimated 41% 1-year and 12% 3-year survival rate.[18] Treatment has not made dramatic impact on survival (see sections later in this article).

Various predictive factors (often in isolation) have been published. Generally speaking, histologic subtype (epithelioid has significantly better prognosis than sarcomatoid MPM) and performance status are most important.[16,18] The Brim tree can be used to categorize patients' estimated survival into 4 groups depending on performance score (Eastern Cooperative Oncology Group), histologic subtype, weight loss, and reduced hemoglobin and albumin levels.[44] Other comorbidities, presence of chest pain, and high inflammatory markers have also been associated with poorer prognosis.[17] Clinicians must be cautious that significant individual variations exist and any prognostic algorithm can only serve as a rough guide.

Numerous histologic features have been reported to have prognostic significance (eg, BAP-1 loss, homozygous deletion of CDKN2A, high mitotic counts, PDL-1 expression) but have no clinical applications at present.[16] Many of these features are confounded by histologic subtype, and parameters measured may vary within individuals from biopsies to biopsies.

TREATMENT

MPM remains an incurable cancer despite decades of attempts with various therapeutic modalities, singly or in combination. Several features of MPM separate it from other solitary tumors and make it refractory to conventional therapies. MPM arises not as a solitary tumor but numerous foci of disease along the pleura and tumor infiltration of the underlying tissues (and lung) are common. In the absence of curative therapies, treatment should be individualized and take into consideration patients' baseline condition (eg, performance status) and personal wishes.

Surgery has not provided a cure because of the widespread nature of disease involvement of all the pleural surfaces, and often their underlying structures. Radical surgical resections have been attempted, the most common approaches being extrapleural pneumonectomy (EPP) and pleurectomy/decortication (P/D). EPP removes the entire lung, pericardium, diaphragm, parietal pleura, and regional lymph nodes, whereas P/D debulks the pleural tumor with pleurectomy (and often the diaphragm and pericardium) but spares the lung.

Only after many years of practice was EPP subjected to scrutiny of a randomized controlled trial (RCT), the Mesothelioma and Radical Surgery (MARS) trial.[45,46] Patients randomized to undergo EPP suffered from extensive complications and died (median) 5.5 months sooner than those who did not have EPP. Meta-analyses have confirmed that P/D incurs a lower morbidity and mortality when compared with EPP.[45] However, the Meso-VATS multicenter RCT found no survival advantage of P/D over talc pleurodesis in MPM.[47] P/D was associated with prolonged air leak and hospital stay. Current evidence, therefore, does not support the use of radical surgery for MPM, except in the setting of clinical studies.

Important lessons must be learned. Facing an incurable cancer with poor outlook, patients are often desperate to try any new/experimental treatments proposed; however, these treatments must still undergo vigorous scientific examination before they should be offered as a routine practice. Interventions always have risks/complications and, as in the case of EPP, treatment can bring more harm than no treatment.

Radiotherapy has been evaluated in MPM in several settings. Adjuvant hemithoracic radiotherapy has been included in multimodality treatment either as part of neoadjuvant therapy before EPP or used postoperatively. Observational series enrolling highly selected patients with early-stage MPM have provided better overall survival than historical controls, but is likely confounded by selection bias and requires confirmation with randomized trials. Intensity modulated radiotherapy (IMRT) has advantages over conventional radiotherapy and is now incorporated in multimodality studies, such as the IMPRINT study in which IMRT was combined with P/D and induction chemotherapy and showed survival rates of 80% and 59% after 1 and 2 years, respectively.[48] Other studies have investigated the use of IMRT followed by EPP (in the Surgery for Mesothelioma after Radiotherapy trial).[49] Newer radiotherapy technologies, such as proton therapy and Arc therapy, are also being explored.[50,51]

Prophylactic radiotherapy following pleural interventions to prevent procedural tract metastases in MPM was first suggested by a small RCT of 40 patients, and became routine practice in many centers.[52] However, no significant benefits were found in 4 subsequent RCTs of prophylactic radiotherapy, including 2 large multicenter studies that enrolled 578 patients combined.[53,54] Importantly, in the SMART trial, the incidence of symptomatic procedural tract metastases was only 9% in the control (no radiotherapy) group (vs 16%) and adequate symptom control was achieved with radiotherapy when tract metastases developed.[54] Prophylactic radiotherapy is therefore no longer recommended. Instead, patients should be advised to look out for early signs of needle tract metastases, especially if associated with symptoms, when radiotherapy should be considered (**Fig. 8**).

Local radiotherapy for palliation of symptoms (eg, pain from tumor erosion of ribs) should also be used for MPM as for other solitary tumors in suitable circumstances.

Systemic therapy is the only treatment modality that has shown survival (albeit modest) benefits for MPM. Even so, only 4 treatments out of numerous experimental therapies tested have proven to prolong survival in RCTs.

Combination cisplatin-pemetrexed remains the standard-of-care treatment since Vogelzang and

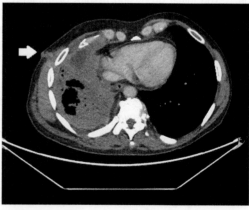

Fig. 8. Malignant mesothelioma catheter tract metastases (*arrow*).

colleagues[55] showed, in 2003, an increased median overall survival of 2.8 months, longer time to progression of 1.8 months, and 25% increased response rate in an RCT (n = 456 patients) when compared with cisplatin alone. Raltitrexed, with cisplatin, showed similar survival benefits in a separate RCT, confirming a class effect of the multifolate agents. It was not until 2016 that further improvement in survival was demonstrated. The MAPS randomized trial (n = 448) showed that addition of bevacizumab (an anti-VEGF agent) to pemetrexed-cisplatin further increased the median survival to ~19 months compared with pemetrexed-cisplatin alone (16 months).[56]

Combination immunotherapy has provided the latest advances in treatment of MPM. In the CheckMate 742 RCT, 605 patients were randomized to combination ipilimumab and nivolumab or pemetrexed-cisplatin chemotherapy.[57] Dual immunotherapy provided greater response rates (32% vs 8%) and improved median survival (18.1 vs 14.1 months; $P = .0020$) over chemotherapy.[57] The benefits were particularly pronounced in non-epithelioid disease, providing for the first time a major improvement for patients with sarcomatoid MPM. Grade 3 to 4 treatment-related adverse events were similar (30% vs 32%) between the groups.

Combining immunotherapy and chemotherapy represents another possible approach. A single-arm phase II (DREAM) trial showed promise combining pemetrexed-cisplatin chemotherapy with durvalumab as front-line treatment.[58] Validation is under way with an RCT.

Use of immunotherapy as second-line therapy has not been as promising. The PROMISE-MESO phase III trial investigated pembrolizumab monotherapy against single-agent chemotherapy in relapsed MPM but did not show significant improved survival.[59] The CTLA-4 antibody, tremelimumab, showed promise in a phase II trial as first-line therapy but use in progressive MPM was shown to be nonsuperior to placebo (DETERMINE study).[60] The MAPS2 phase II trial (n = 125 patients who had progressed on chemotherapy) found nivolumab-ipilimumab produced slightly better disease control (50% vs 44% at 12 weeks) and 1-year survival (58% vs 49%) over nivolumab alone.[61] Nivolumab, a PD-L1 checkpoint inhibitor, as a second-line agent (NivoMes) and third-line agent (MERIT) showed early potential for stabilizing progressive MPM disease.[62] Alternatives such as nintedanib were added to chemotherapy in the LUME-Meso trial but also did not improve survival.[62]

Different treatment targets, such as histone deacetylase, arginosuccinate synthetase-1, and focal adhesion kinase, have been explored in mesothelioma but have not translated into significant disease response.[50,62] Early-phase work manipulating mesothelin has shown promising results, with BAP-1, TP53, and CDKN2A mutations also being investigated.[42,54,63] Vaccines have also been assessed against Wilms tumor-1 (WT-1).[42,54,63] Chimeric antigen receptor T-cell therapy, dendritic cell therapy, and oncolytic viruses against MPM are being explored.[42,54,63]

SYMPTOM PALLIATION

In the absence of curative therapies, the goal of MPM care is primarily symptom control. Palliative care is an important aspect of MPM management.

Psychosocial support is critical to the patient journey, but supportive care standards vary largely among centers and remain a poorly researched area of MPM. An early, open discussion is essential of the incurable nature of the disease, its prognosis, and likely progressive physical deterioration with associated psychosocial and social stresses.

Clinicians need to beware of unique psychological issues that patients with MPM must endure, not seen in other cancers. The long lag time since asbestos exposure means many patients have lived anxiously for decades worrying about disease development. Many may have seen coworkers die of MPM; these encounters often shape their choice of therapies. Anger that they were subjected to occupational risks of asbestos without protection at their workplace is common. Some were even told asbestos was not harmful. Compensation proceedings can be protracted and stressful.

A systematic review of psychosocial assessment of patients with MPM showed that patients and caregivers wanted improvements in the delivery of the diagnosis, emotional support and empathy, patient-centered treatment, honest information their disease progression, and how/when death would occur. Patients generally welcome the input of palliative care teams, and their expertise is important to provide holistic care that covers pharmacologic and nonpharmacological interventions to optimize quality of life (QoL). Interestingly, the recent RESPECT-Meso trial showed routine early referral of all patients with MPM to specialist palliative care was not superior to standard practice (referral when clinically deemed needed).[64] Many possible explanations exist; for example, enrolling centers in the study often had well setup patient support adequate to provide high standard care.

Nutritional support is important in MPM, although seldom investigated. In a recent study of 61 patients with MPM, 44% were pre-sarcopenic and

38% were malnourished.[65] Pre-sarcopenia was associated with poorer activity levels, whereas malnutrition was associated with poorer QoL. In the largest postmortem study of MPM (n = 318), we found that no precise cause of death could be determined in 63 (19.8%) cases even after postmortem.[19] The body mass index was significantly lower in these cases (18.8 ± 4.3), compared with those with identifiable anatomic cause of death (21.0 ± 4.7), raising the possibility of metabolic contribution to the cause of death.

In malignant pleural effusions, breathlessness is the most common symptom at presentation; hence, long-term pleural effusion control to minimize symptoms and preserve QoL is important. There are many myths about breathlessness and pleural effusion that are worth noting. Breathlessness is typically related to the increased work of breathing as a result of the pleural effusion; in particular, the mechanical disadvantages that arise from expansion of the hemithorax to accommodate the fluid and the weight of the effusion.[66] The recently published PLeural Effusion and Symptom Evaluation (PLEASE) study evaluated 150 patients with moderate-to-large pleural effusions before and after pleural fluid drainage (median 1.7 L) and found that removal of the fluid brought symptom relief in approximately three-quarters of the cohort (but not everyone).[67] Improvement in vital signs (including oxygen saturation) were modest compared with the symptom benefits. Hence, clinicians must look for alternative causes (eg, pulmonary emboli) of breathlessness in patients who present with significant hypoxemia or in patients who do not have symptomatic improvement after pleural fluid drainage. Diaphragmatic dysfunction (presumably from the weight of the effusion) was common and improved quickly after drainage. Patients with more severe breathlessness and those with diaphragmatic changes were more likely to enjoy improvement in dyspnea.

In patients with very short expected survival and those with slow fluid recurrence, intermittent therapeutic thoracentesis can be an option. In others, creation of pleurodesis or insertion of an indwelling pleural catheter (IPC) for long-term ambulatory drainage are common options. The recent IPC-Plus study suggested the two can be combined to provide the best benefits.[68]

Pleurodesis can be attempted by instillation of pleurodesing agents (most commonly talc) via a chest tube (or IPC) or by thoracoscopic (medical or surgical) pleurodesis. Three RCTs have shown no advantage of VATS pleurodesis over bedside talc slurry instillation.[18] A recent large (n = 330) RCT also found similar success rates between pleurodesis using talc poudrage during medical thoracoscopy compared with chest tube talc slurry pleurodesis.[18] In a study specifically of malignant effusion in patients with malig pleural effusion (n = 390), surgical pleurodesis showed no advantage over bedside chemical pleurodesis in efficacy (with failure rates of 32% vs 31%, respectively), survival, or total time spent in hospital until death.[18] No clinical, biochemical, or radiographic parameters adequately predict pleurodesis outcome.

IPC is rapidly developing as a treatment option for malignant effusions, including those from MPM. Two RCTs, namely the Therapeutic Intervention of Malignant Effusion (TIME)-2 (n = 106 patients with MPE) and the Australasian Malignant PLeural Effusion (AMPLE) trial (n = 146 patients; 38 with mesothelioma) have shown that IPC offered significant improvement in dyspnea relief and QoL scores from preintervention, and the extent of benefits were similar between IPC and chest tube pleurodesis.[69,70] The AMPLE trial further showed that IPC significantly reduced patients' lifetime hospitalization days by a mean of 3.6 days.[69] Importantly the need for additional ipsilateral pleural procedures was significantly reduced to 4% (vs 22% in those treated with talc slurry pleurodesis). The latest malignant pleural effusion guidelines from the American Thoracic Society (endorsed by the Society of Thoracic Surgeons and Society of Thoracic Radiologists) included IPCs as an alternative to chest tube slurry pleurodesis as front-line definitive therapy.[71]

Recent studies have further optimized the use of IPC. Two RCTs found that daily IPC drainage improves the likelihood of spontaneous pleurodesis compared with symptom-guided (AMPLE-2 trial) or alternate day drainage (ASAP trial).[72,73] In the AMPLE-2 trial (n = 87; 29 had MPM), daily drainage was also associated with better QoL scores measured by EuroQuol-5 Dimension 5 L.[73] The IPC-PLUS trial (n = 154; 23 had MPM) showed that talc slurry can be instilled via the IPC and significantly increased rates of achieving pleurodesis (when compared with placebo) and with better symptom scores and QoL measures.[68]

IPC also remained the recommended choice of treatment for those with nonexpandable lung as well as those who had failed pleurodesis (**Fig. 9**). Complications with IPC use are also important to recognize, including infections and catheter tract metastases, with guidelines having been recently released.[74,75] IPC (with talc pleurodesis) has yet to be compared with surgical (VATS) pleurodesis; this is the subject of the ongoing AMPLE-3 RCT.

Pain syndromes in mesothelioma can have both a somatic and neuropathic component depending on the distribution of disease.[76] This is important to note for determining the optimal analgesia

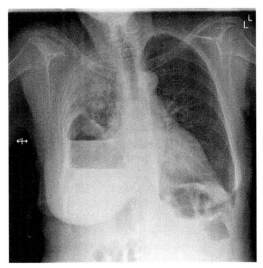

Fig. 9. Nonexpandable lung with hydropneumothorax and IPC.

choice for patients. Somatic pain usually responds to opioid analgesia, which can be initially introduced using immediate-release doses to gauge daily requirements and then converted to more convenient extended-release formulations. Neuropathic pain is managed using antiepileptics such as gabapentin or pregabalin, or antidepressants such as amitriptyline. Newer agents such as tapentadol have also exhibited combination effects and comes in both instant and extended-release forms. Choice of analgesic also can be determined by coexisting symptoms such as night sweats, reduced appetite or anxiety/depression (amitriptyline), uncorrectable or distressing dyspnea (opioids), or need for control of epileptic events (gabapentin/pregabalin). Localized pain can be assisted by corticosteroid if felt to be related to progressive disease and tumoral edema, but radiotherapy also can be considered, as discussed previously.[77] Interventional options including nerve blocks or intrathecal analgesia are considered when pain is refractory to the aforementioned oral or despite escalation to subcutaneous medication infusions. Surgical techniques such as cervical cordotomy have also been shown to provide safe and effective mesothelioma-related pain control but can be limited in its availability.[78]

FUTURE DIRECTIONS

MPM is a cancer of a clear cause; banning of asbestos to prevent future generations of patients is the top priority. Asbestos is a cheap and effective insulation material and its global use continue to grow rather than reduce, according to the World Health Organization data. Clinicians are therefore likely to continue to encounter MPM. However,

the global epidemiology of MPM is changing, and public health and research directions must respond accordingly. In developed countries, the demographics are changing. Because of increasing population longevity, a growing number of elderly patients are diagnosed with MPM from exposure many decades ago. These patients are generally not fit for aggressive therapies (eg, surgery or chemotherapy). The number of younger patients is decreasing rapidly because of prohibition of asbestos use.[3] On the contrary, MPM is rising in many developing countries where clinicians have relatively limited expertise in its diagnosis and management. To have an effective impact on these patients, new treatments need to be affordable and techniques must be available in resource-limited regions.

New experimental therapies for MPM have often been applied to patients without rigorous investigations, and apparent benefits are often confounded by selection bias. Clinicians must be mindful that these unproven therapies can produce more harm (eg, EPP) than benefits. Global collaborations are important to evaluate new diagnostic and therapeutic methods in the fastest way. It is encouraging to see a growing trend of sharing of biobank samples and increasing number of multinational clinical trials.

Until a cure is found, best supportive care remains a key part of MPM management. Control of symptoms, for example, weight loss, fatigue, and reduction in physical activities deserve more investigations. Although all clinicians and patients recognize that psychological support is important, its best delivery requires research and interventions that are clinically evaluated.

CLINICS CARE POINTS

- Detection of loss of BAP-1 protein by immunohistochemistry and deletion of CDKN2A by fluroscence-in-situ-hybridization are new diagnostic tools for malignant pleural mesothelioma, and should be included wherever appropriate to enhance diagnostic yield and accuracy.

- Dual agent immunotherapy (nivolumab and ipilimumab) has been found to significantly improve survival, particularly in sarcomatoid-containing mesothelioma.

- Prognosis remains poor and symptom management, especially breathlessness secondary to malignant pleural effusions, is important to maintain quality-of-life.

DISCLOSURE

The authors have nothing to disclose.

REFERENCES

1. Furuya S, Chimed-Ochir O, Takahashi K, et al. Global asbestos disaster. Int J Environ Res Public Health 2018;15(5):1000.

2. Keshava HB, Tang A, Siddiqui HU, et al. Largely unchanged annual incidence and overall survival of pleural mesothelioma in the USA. World J Surg 2019;43(12):3239–47.

3. Kerger BD. Longevity and pleural mesothelioma: age-period-cohort analysis of incidence data from the Surveillance, Epidemiology, and End Results (SEER) Program, 1973-2013. BMC Res Notes 2018;11(1):337.

4. Le GV, Takahashi K, Park EK, et al. Asbestos use and asbestos-related diseases in Asia: past, present and future. Respirology 2011;16(5):767–75.

5. Diandini R, Takahashi K, Park EK, et al. Potential years of life lost (PYLL) caused by asbestos-related diseases in the world. Am J Ind Med 2013; 56(9):993–1000.

6. Delgermaa V, Takahashi K, Park EK, et al. Global mesothelioma deaths reported to the World Health Organization between 1994 and 2008. Bull World Health Organ 2011;89(10):716–24, 24a–24c.

7. Park EK, Takahashi K, Hoshuyama T, et al. Global magnitude of reported and unreported mesothelioma. Environ Health Perspect 2011;119(4):514–8.

8. Asciak R, George V, Rahman NM. Update on biology and management of mesothelioma. Eur Respir Rev 2021;30(159):200226.

9. Betti M, Aspesi A, Sculco M, et al. Genetic predisposition for malignant mesothelioma: a concise review. Mutat Res 2019;781:1–10.

10. Testa JR, Cheung M, Pei J, et al. Germline BAP1 mutations predispose to malignant mesothelioma. Nat Genet 2011;43(10):1022–5.

11. Sekido Y. Molecular pathogenesis of malignant mesothelioma. Carcinogenesis 2013;34(7):1413–9.

12. Jaurand MC, Fleury-Feith J. Pathogenesis of malignant pleural mesothelioma. Respirology 2005; 10(1):2–8.

13. Yap TA, Aerts JG, Popat S, et al. Novel insights into mesothelioma biology and implications for therapy. Nat Rev Cancer 2017;17(8):475.

14. Wadowski B, De Rienzo A, Bueno R. The molecular basis of malignant pleural mesothelioma. Thorac Surg Clin 2020;30(4):383–93.

15. Blanquart C, Jaurand MC, Jean D. The biology of malignant mesothelioma and the relevance of preclinical models. Front Oncol 2020;10:388.

16. Husain AN, Colby TV, Ordonez NG, et al. Guidelines for pathologic diagnosis of malignant mesothelioma 2017 update of the consensus statement from the international mesothelioma interest group. Arch Pathol Lab Med 2018;142(1):89–108.

17. Geltner C, Errhalt P, Baumgartner B, et al. Management of malignant pleural mesothelioma–part 1: epidemiology, diagnosis, and staging. Wien Klin Wochenschr 2016;128(17):611–7.

18. Bibby AC, Tsim S, Kanellakis N, et al. Malignant pleural mesothelioma: an update on investigation, diagnosis and treatment. Eur Respir Rev 2016; 25(142):472–86.

19. Finn RS, Brims FJH, Gandhi A, et al. Postmortem findings of malignant pleural mesothelioma: a two-center study of 318 patients. Chest 2012;142(5): 1267–73.

20. Qureshi NR, Rahman NM, Gleeson FV. Thoracic ultrasound in the diagnosis of malignant pleural effusion. Thorax 2009;64(2):139–43.

21. Armato SG III, Francis RJ, Katz SI, et al. Imaging in pleural mesothelioma: a review of the 14th international conference of the international mesothelioma interest group. Lung Cancer 2019;130:108–14.

22. Fysh ETH, Thomas R, Tobin C, et al. Air in the pleural cavity enhances detection of pleural abnormalities by CT scan. Chest 2018;153(6):e123–8.

23. Leung AN, Muller NL, Miller RR. CT in differential diagnosis of diffuse pleural disease. AJR Am J Roentgenol 1990;154(3):487–92.

24. de Fonseka D, Underwood W, Stadon L, et al. Randomised controlled trial to compare the diagnostic yield of positron emission tomography CT (PET-CT) TARGETed pleural biopsy versus CT-guided pleural biopsy in suspected pleural malignancy (TARGET trial). BMJ Open Respir Res 2018;5(1):e000270.

25. Hall DO, Hooper CE, Searle J, et al. 18F-Fluorodeoxyglucose PET/CT and dynamic contrast-enhanced MRI as imaging biomarkers in malignant pleural mesothelioma. Nucl Med Commun 2018;39(2):161–70.

26. Incerti E, Broggi S, Fodor A, et al. FDG PET-derived parameters as prognostic tool in progressive malignant pleural mesothelioma treated patients. Eur J Nucl Med Mol Imaging 2018;45(12):2071–8.

27. Wang ZJ, Reddy GP, Gotway MB, et al. Malignant pleural mesothelioma: evaluation with CT, MR imaging, and PET. Radiographics. 2004;24(1):105–19.

28. Ohno Y, Yui M, Aoyagi K, et al. Whole-body MRI: comparison of its capability for TNM staging of malignant pleural mesothelioma with that of coregistered PET/MRI, integrated FDG PET/CT, and conventional imaging. Am J Roentgenol 2019; 212(2):311–9.

29. Pavic M, Bogowicz M, Kraft J, et al. FDG PET versus CT radiomics to predict outcome in malignant pleural mesothelioma patients. EJNMMI Res 2020; 10(1):81.

30. Louw A, Badiei A, Creaney J, et al. Advances in pathological diagnosis of mesothelioma: what

pulmonologists should know. Curr Opin Pulm Med 2019;25(4):354–61.

31. Segal A, Sterrett GF, Frost FA, et al. A diagnosis of malignant pleural mesothelioma can be made by effusion cytology: results of a 20 year audit. Pathology 2013;45(1):44–8.

32. Kinoshita Y, Hida T, Hamasaki M, et al. A combination of MTAP and BAP1 immunohistochemistry in pleural effusion cytology for the diagnosis of mesothelioma. Cancer Cytopathol 2018; 126(1):54–63.

33. Berg KB, Churg AM, Cheung S, et al. Usefulness of methylthioadenosine phosphorylase and BRCA-associated protein 1 immunohistochemistry in the diagnosis of malignant mesothelioma in effusion cytology specimens. Cancer Cytopathol 2020; 128(2):126–32.

34. Woolhouse I, Bishop L, Darlison L, et al. BTS guideline for the investigation and management of malignant pleural mesothelioma. BMJ Open Respir Res 2018;5(1):e000266.

35. Eccher A, Girolami I, Lucenteforte E, et al. Diagnostic mesothelioma biomarkers in effusion cytology. Cancer Cytopathol 2021;129(7):506–16.

36. Sheaff M. Guidelines for the cytopathologic diagnosis of epithelioid and mixed-type malignant mesothelioma: complementary statement from the international mesothelioma interest group, also endorsed by the international academy of cytology and the papanicolaou society of cytopathology. A proposal to be applauded and promoted but which requires updating. Diagn Cytopathol 2020;48(10): 877–9.

37. Thomas R, Karunarathne S, Jennings B, et al. Pleuroscopic cryoprobe biopsies of the pleura: a feasibility and safety study. Respirology 2015;20(2):327–32.

38. Wijmans L, Baas P, Sieburgh TE, et al. Confocal laser endomicroscopy as a guidance tool for pleural biopsies in malignant pleural mesothelioma. Chest 2019;156(4):754–63.

39. Creaney J, Segal A, Olsen N, et al. Pleural fluid mesothelin as an adjunct to the diagnosis of pleural malignant mesothelioma. Dis Markers 2014;2014: 413946.

40. Creaney J, Yeoman D, Naumoff LK, et al. Soluble mesothelin in effusions: a useful tool for the diagnosis of malignant mesothelioma. Thorax 2007; 62(7):569–76.

41. Scherpereel A, Grigoriu B, Conti M, et al. Soluble mesothelin-related peptides in the diagnosis of malignant pleural mesothelioma. Am J Respir Crit Care Med 2006;173(10):1155–60.

42. Arnold DT, Maskell NA. Biomarkers in mesothelioma. Ann Clin Biochem 2018;55(1):49–58.

43. Creaney J, Dick IM, Meniawy TM, et al. Comparison of fibulin-3 and mesothelin as markers in malignant mesothelioma. Thorax 2014;69(10):895–902.

44. Brims FJ, Meniawy TM, Duffus I, et al. A novel clinical prediction model for prognosis in malignant pleural mesothelioma using decision tree analysis. J Thorac Oncol 2016;11(4):573–82.

45. Bueno R, Opitz I, Taskforce IM. Surgery in malignant pleural mesothelioma. J Thorac Oncol 2018;13(11): 1638–54.

46. Treasure T, Lang-Lazdunski L, Waller D, et al. Extra-pleural pneumonectomy versus no extra-pleural pneumonectomy for patients with malignant pleural mesothelioma: clinical outcomes of the Mesothelioma and Radical Surgery (MARS) randomised feasibility study. Lancet Oncol 2011;12(8):763–72.

47. Rintoul RC, Ritchie AJ, Edwards JG, et al. Efficacy and cost of video-assisted thoracoscopic partial pleurectomy versus talc pleurodesis in patients with malignant pleural mesothelioma (MesoVATS): an open-label, randomised, controlled trial. Lancet 2014;384(9948):1118–27.

48. Rimner A, Zauderer MG, Gomez DR, et al. Phase II study of hemithoracic intensity-modulated pleural radiation therapy (IMPRINT) as part of lung-sparing multimodality therapy in patients with malignant pleural mesothelioma. J Clin Oncol 2016; 34(23):2761.

49. Cho BCJ, Donahoe L, Bradbury PA, et al. Surgery for malignant pleural mesothelioma after radiotherapy (SMART): final results from a single-centre, phase 2 trial. Lancet Oncol 2021;22(2):190–7.

50. Scherpereel A, Wallyn F, Albelda SM, et al. Novel therapies for malignant pleural mesothelioma. Lancet Oncol 2018;19(3):e161–72.

51. Sayan M, Mamidanna S, Fuat Eren M, et al. New horizons from novel therapies in malignant pleural mesothelioma. Adv Respir Med 2020;88(4):343–51.

52. Boutin C, Rey F, Viallat JR. Prevention of malignant seeding after invasive diagnostic procedures in patients with pleural mesothelioma. A randomized trial of local radiotherapy. Chest 1995;108(3):754–8.

53. Bayman N, Appel W, Ashcroft L, et al. Prophylactic irradiation of tracts in patients with malignant pleural mesothelioma: an open-label, multicenter, phase III randomized trial. J Clin Oncol 2019;37(14):1200–8.

54. Clive AO, Taylor H, Dobson L, et al. Prophylactic radiotherapy for the prevention of procedure-tract metastases after surgical and large-bore pleural procedures in malignant pleural mesothelioma (SMART): a multicentre, open-label, phase 3, randomised controlled trial. Lancet Oncol 2016;17(8):1094–104.

55. Vogelzang NJ, Rusthoven JJ, Symanowski J, et al. Phase III study of pemetrexed in combination with cisplatin versus cisplatin alone in patients with malignant pleural mesothelioma. J Clin Oncol 2003; 21(14):2636–44.

56. Zalcman G, Mazieres J, Margery J, et al. Bevacizumab for newly diagnosed pleural mesothelioma in the Mesothelioma Avastin Cisplatin Pemetrexed

Study (MAPS): a randomised, controlled, open-label, phase 3 trial. Lancet 2016;387(10026): 1405–14.

57. Baas P, Scherpereel A, Nowak AK, et al. First-line nivolumab plus ipilimumab in unresectable malignant pleural mesothelioma (CheckMate 743): a multicentre, randomised, open-label, phase 3 trial. Lancet 2021;397(10272):375–86.

58. Nowak AK, Lesterhuis WJ, Kok PS, et al. Durvalumab with first-line chemotherapy in previously untreated malignant pleural mesothelioma (DREAM): a multicentre, single-arm, phase 2 trial with a safety run-in. Lancet Oncol 2020;21(9):1213–23.

59. Popat S, Curioni-Fontecedro A, Dafni U, et al. A multicentre randomised phase III trial comparing pembrolizumab versus single-agent chemotherapy for advanced pre-treated malignant pleural mesothelioma: the European Thoracic Oncology Platform (ETOP 9-15) PROMISE-meso trial. Ann Oncol 2020; 31(12):1734–45.

60. Maio M, Scherpereel A, Calabrò L, et al. Tremelimumab as second-line or third-line treatment in relapsed malignant mesothelioma (DETERMINE): a multicentre, international, randomised, double-blind, placebo-controlled phase 2b trial. Lancet Oncol 2017;18(9):1261–73.

61. Scherpereel A, Mazieres J, Greillier L, et al. Nivolumab or nivolumab plus ipilimumab in patients with relapsed malignant pleural mesothelioma (IFCT-1501 MAPS2): a multicentre, open-label, randomised, non-comparative, phase 2 trial. Lancet Oncol 2019;20(2):239–53.

62. Nicolini F, Bocchini M, Bronte G, et al. Malignant pleural mesothelioma: state-of-the-art on current therapies and promises for the future. Front Oncol 2019;9:1519.

63. Yang H, Xu D, Schmid RA, et al. Biomarker-guided targeted and immunotherapies in malignant pleural mesothelioma. Ther Adv Med Oncol 2020;12. 1758835920971421.

64. Hoon SN, Lawrie I, Qi C, et al. Symptom burden and unmet needs in malignant pleural mesothelioma: exploratory analyses from the RESPECT-meso study. J Palliat Care 2021;36(2):113–20.

65. Jeffery E, Lee YCG, Newton RU, et al. Body composition and nutritional status in malignant pleural mesothelioma: implications for activity levels and quality of life. Eur J Clin Nutr 2019;73(10):1412–21.

66. Thomas R, Jenkins S, Eastwood PR, et al. Physiology of breathlessness associated with pleural effusions. Curr Opin Pulm Med 2015;21(4):338–45.

67. Muruganandan S, Azzopardi M, Thomas R, et al. The Pleural Effusion and Symptom Evaluation (PLEASE) study of breathlessness in patients with a symptomatic pleural effusion. Eur Respir J 2020; 55(5):1900980.

68. Bhatnagar R, Keenan EK, Morley AJ, et al. Outpatient talc administration by indwelling pleural catheter for malignant effusion. N Engl J Med 2018; 378(14):1313–22.

69. Thomas R, Fysh ETH, Smith NA, et al. Effect of an indwelling pleural catheter vs talc pleurodesis on hospitalization days in patients with malignant pleural effusion: the AMPLE randomized clinical trial. JAMA 2017;318(19):1903–12.

70. Davies HE, Mishra EK, Kahan BC, et al. Effect of an indwelling pleural catheter vs chest tube and talc pleurodesis for relieving dyspnea in patients with malignant pleural effusion: the TIME2 randomized controlled trial. JAMA 2012;307(22):2383–9.

71. Feller-Kopman DJ, Reddy CB, DeCamp MM, et al. Management of malignant pleural effusions. An Official ATS/STS/STR clinical practice guideline. Am J Respir Crit Care Med 2018;198(7):839–49.

72. Wahidi MM, Reddy C, Yarmus L, et al. Randomized trial of pleural fluid drainage frequency in patients with malignant pleural effusions. The ASAP trial. Am J Respir Crit Care Med 2017;195(8):1050–7.

73. Muruganandan S, Azzopardi M, Fitzgerald DB, et al. Aggressive versus symptom-guided drainage of malignant pleural effusion via indwelling pleural catheters (AMPLE-2): an open-label randomised trial. Lancet Respir Med 2018;6(9):671–80.

74. Gilbert CR, Wahidi MM, Light RW, et al. Management of indwelling tunneled pleural catheters: a modified delphi consensus statement. Chest 2020; 158(5):2221–8.

75. Miller CRJ, Chrissian AA, Lee YCG, et al. Key highlights from the American association for bronchology and interventional pulmonology evidence-Informed guidelines and expert panel report for the management of indwelling pleural catheters. Chest 2021; 159(3):920–3.

76. MacLeod N, Kelly C, Stobo J, et al. Pain in malignant pleural mesothelioma: a prospective characterization study. Pain Med 2016;17(11):2119–26.

77. Macleod N, Price A, O'Rourke N, et al. Radiotherapy for the treatment of pain in malignant pleural mesothelioma: a systematic review. Lung Cancer 2014; 83(2):133–8.

78. France BD, Lewis RA, Sharma ML, et al. Cordotomy in mesothelioma-related pain: a systematic review. BMJ Support Palliat Care 2014;4(1):19–29.

Section 4: Pneumothorax

Pneumothorax
Classification and Etiology

Nai-Chien Huan, MBBS, MRCP[a], Calvin Sidhu, MBBS, FRACP[b,c],
Rajesh Thomas, MBBS, PhD, FRACP[c,d],*

KEYWORDS

- Pneumothorax • Smoking • Primary pneumothorax • Secondary pneumothorax
- Diffuse cystic lung disease

KEY POINTS

- Pneumothorax can develop because of diverse etiologies; in many cases, no specific cause may be identified.
- Tension pneumothorax is a pathophysiologic, not a radiologic, diagnosis.
- Patients with primary spontaneous pneumothorax may have lung abnormalities that are not apparent on chest radiographs. Tobacco smoking is the most important risk factor.
- Chronic obstructive pulmonary disease is the most common underlying lung disorder associated with secondary spontaneous pneumothorax.Recurrent pneumothorax is common in diffuse cystic lung diseases.
- The exact pathogenetic mechanisms of spontaneous pneumothorax development are unknown. An interplay between lung-related abnormalities and environmental factors is likely in most cases.

INTRODUCTION

Pneumothorax is a common clinical problem worldwide.[1] Pneumothorax is defined as presence of air in the pleural cavity. It can develop secondary to diverse etiologies including traumatic, inflammatory, infective, malignant, genetic, and hormonal causes; in many cases, the lung appears normal and there may be no recognizable underlying lung abnormality. The severity of clinical manifestations in a patient with pneumothorax ranges from asymptomatic to life-threatening, and may be disproportionate to pneumothorax size. In this review, we provide an overview of the historical perspective, epidemiology, classification, and etiology of pneumothorax. We also explore current knowledge and understanding of underlying risks and pathophysiologic mechanisms that lead to development of pneumothorax.

HISTORICAL PERSPECTIVE

Pneumothorax has been long recognized since the days of Hippocrates (circa 460–370 BC). Ancient Greek physicians would listen to a "succussion splash," elicited by vigorously shaking the patient's chest, to diagnose the presence of a hydropneumothorax. The native Americans had learned that a single arrow into the chest of a North American bison could quickly incapacitate it during hunting. Unlike most mammals, the bison has a single pleural cavity because of an incomplete

Funding: R. Thomas has received career research fellowship funding from National Health and Medical Research Council, Australia and Cancer Council Western Australia, Australia.
Declaration of interest: The authors have nothing to disclose.
[a] Department of Pulmonology, Serdang Hospital, Kajang, Malaysia; [b] Edith Cowan University, Perth, Australia; [c] Department of Respiratory Medicine, Sir Charles Gairdner Hospital, Perth, Australia; [d] School of Medicine, University of Western Australia, Perth, Australia
* Corresponding author.
E-mail address: rajesh.thomas@health.wa.gov.au

Clin Chest Med 42 (2021) 711–727
https://doi.org/10.1016/j.ccm.2021.08.007
0272-5231/21/© 2021 Elsevier Inc. All rights reserved.

mediastinum, making it vulnerable to bilateral tension pneumothoraces following a penetrating injury in one hemithorax (**Fig. 1**).

The term "pneumothorax" (a Greek composite word derived from "pneuma – air" and "thorax – chest") was first coined in 1803 by Jean Marc Gaspard Itard,[2] a French physician and student of Rene Laennec (1781–1826). Laennec[3] would later describe the clinical and anatomic details of pneumothorax in 1819. Most cases of pneumothorax were initially believed to be secondary to pulmonary tuberculosis.[4] Kjaergaad[5] in 1932 provided the first modern description of primary spontaneous pneumothorax (PSP) wherein he made a clear distinction of "pneumothorax simple" (ie, pneumothorax in young patients with no apparent lung disease) versus pneumothorax secondary to pulmonary tuberculosis. This distinction was important because patients with pulmonary tuberculosis in those days would be confined long-term in sanitoriums.

EPIDEMIOLOGY
Incidence

The reported incidence of pneumothorax varies depending on study regions and may be lower than the real incidence because of underreporting and underdiagnosis in asymptomatic patients. Epidemiologic studies have shown an overall incidence of spontaneous pneumothorax of 16.8 per 100,000 population per year (24/100,000/year for males; 9.8/100,000/year for females) in England.[6] The incidence of spontaneous pneumothorax from Sweden (Stockholm, 1975–1984) was lower at 18/100,000/year in males and 6/100,000/year in females.[7] The age-adjusted incidence of PSP and secondary spontaneous pneumothorax (SSP) in the United States was 4.2 and 3.8 per 100,000 population per year, respectively.[8]

The peak incidence of spontaneous pneumothorax shows a clear bimodal distribution: PSP is most commonly seen in patients between 15 and 34 years and the incidence of SSP is highest in patients older than 55 years.[6] The incidence of patients with pneumothorax who need hospitalization is reported to be 11.1 per 100,000 population per year (16.6/100,000/year for males and 5.8/100,000/year for females).[6] The annual cost of spontaneous pneumothorax management in the United States is estimated to be $130 million.[9]

The incidence of asymptomatic pneumothorax is harder to assess. One retrospective study that reviewed 101,709 chest radiographs performed during routine medical check-ups of university students in Tokyo, Japan reported a pneumothorax incidence rate of 0.042% (0.050% in males vs 0.018% in females).[10] Although asymptomatic, 50% of these affected students had moderate-severe pneumothorax on chest radiograph (defined as lung collapse >10% of hemithorax).

Recurrence

Recurrence of pneumothorax following an initial episode is common; this necessitates pneumothorax management plans to consider the likelihood of recurrence and need for recurrence prevention interventions. The reported rates of recurrence following spontaneous pneumothorax is highly variable because of heterogeneities in protocols, population, treatment algorithms, and follow-up periods in different studies.[11] Long-term follow-up studies show PSP recurrence rate ranging between 16% and 52%.[11–14] One age-stratified longitudinal epidemiologic study from Taiwan reported a PSP recurrence rate of 23.7%[15] and a similar study from France had a PSP recurrence rate of 28%; most pneumothorax recurrence was seen in the first year following the index episode.[16] A recent systematic review (29 studies involving 13,548 patients) reported similar findings of overall PSP recurrence rate of 32% (29% 1-year recurrence)[14]; recurrence was three times more among females (odds ratio, 3.03) and smoking cessation reduced recurrence risk by four-fold (odds ratio, 0.26).

Recurrence is higher in SSP (40%–56% in different studies)[17,18] and occurs earlier, usually within 6 months of the initial episode.[19] The risk of multiple subsequent pneumothorax episodes, without prevention intervention, also remains.[12] In one retrospective study by Voge and Anthracite, 28% patients had a second episode, 23% had a third episode, and 14% developed a fourth episode of spontaneous pneumothorax.[20]

CLASSIFICATION OF PNEUMOTHORAX
Classification by Size

Several methods have been described to measure and classify pneumothorax size. Light index calculates pneumothorax size from the ratio of cubed diameters of collapsed lung and hemithorax on a chest radiograph (pneumothorax size [%] = 100 × [1 − average lung diameter^3/average hemithorax diameter^3]) and shows good correlation with the volume of air removed (**Fig. 2**).[21] Collin formula to estimate pneumothorax volume from a chest radiograph was derived based on helical computed tomography (CT) volumetrics[22] and uses three interpleural distances measured at specified points (a, b, and c); the estimated pneumothorax volume is calculated by formula

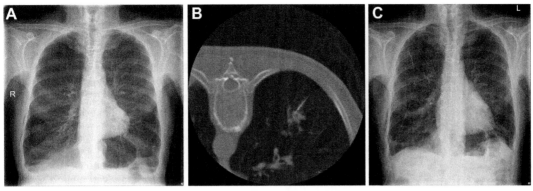

Fig. 1. Chest radiograph of a patient who developed bilateral pneumothorax (A) following computed tomography (CT)-guided lung biopsy of a right lower lobe nodule (B). Sternotomy wires from a previous coronary artery bypass graft are noted. The coronary artery bypass graft surgery resulted in communication between right and left pleural cavities across the mediastinum leading to bilateral pneumothorax following right lung biopsy. Chest radiograph performed 2 hours after placement of an intercostal catheter in the right pleural cavity shows improvement of pneumothorax on both sides (C).

$Y = 4.2 + (4.7 \times [a + b + c])$ (**Fig. 3**). CT scans using three-dimensional measurements are more accurate than chest radiographs in calculating pneumothorax size.

Several international guidelines recommend assessing pneumothorax size using chest radiograph measurements to guide treatment interventions. The Spanish Society of Pulmonology and Thoracic Surgery[23] classifies pneumothorax, based on morphologic and anatomic criteria, into (1) partial pneumothorax, when the visceral pleura is only partially detached from the chest wall, such as in isolated apical pneumothorax; (2) incomplete pneumothorax, when both visceral and parietal pleurae are fully separated from apex to base but without causing complete lung collapse; and (3) complete pneumothorax, for total lung collapse (**Fig. 4**). The American College of Chest Physicians (ACCP) pneumothorax guidelines classify pneumothorax size depending on the distance from the apex of the collapsed lung to the ipsilateral thoracic cupola.[9] This distance is greater than 3 cm with a large pneumothorax and less than 3 cm with a small pneumothorax (**Fig. 5**). This method can lead to overestimation of pneumothorax size with a predominantly apical pneumothorax. The British Thoracic Society (BTS) pneumothorax guidelines classify pneumothorax size based on the interpleural distance measured at the level of the hilum.[24] The interpleural distance is less than 2 cm in a small pneumothorax and correlates with a pneumothorax occupying less than 50% of the hemithorax volume (**Fig. 6**).[24,25] Interpleural distance of greater than 2 cm helps to identify a pneumothorax that could be drained safely by needle or chest drain decompression without causing lung injury.[26]

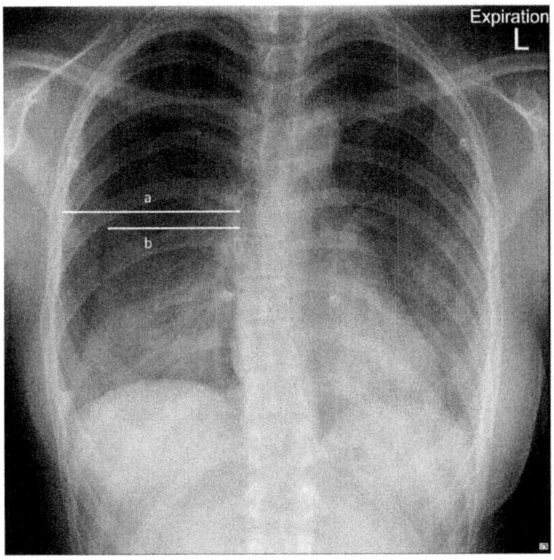

There is poor agreement between international guidelines and studies of pneumothorax size and management strategies. A study comparing the BTS, ACCP, and Belgian Society of Pulmonology guidelines showed agreement in only 47% of cases.[27] A different study showed that adherence in a UK hospital to the BTS guidelines was seen in 70% of PSP cases and to ACCP guidelines in 32%, and resulted in conflicting management recommendations depending on the guidelines used.[28] A pneumothorax typically resolves by 2% per day without intervention[29] and therefore, it was believed that a large pneumothorax is best treated by pleural drainage and rapid lung

Fig. 2. Light method to measure pneumothorax volume: Pneumothorax % = $100 \times [1-b^3/a^3]$.

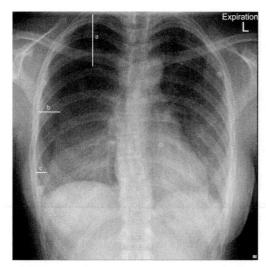

Fig. 3. Collin formula: Pneumothorax volume = $4.2 + [4.7 \times (a + b + c)]$.

re-expansion. However, precise measurements of pneumothorax size may not have as much clinical value as previously thought with increasing evidence suggesting that a symptom-driven management algorithm, rather than based on pneumothorax size alone, might be more beneficial.[30,31]

Classification by Pathophysiology and Etiology

Pneumothorax is classified by underlying etiology and pathophysiology; the clinical presentation, pneumothorax progress or resolution, likelihood of pneumothorax recurrence, and management strategies can vary significantly (**Box 1**).[24] Tension pneumothorax is a rare, life-threatening condition that develops when air trapped within the pleural cavity under positive pressure leads to cardiopulmonary compromise.[32] Traumatic pneumothorax

results from direct injury to the chest wall or lung. More commonly, pneumothorax occurs spontaneously without preceding injury or trauma. Spontaneous pneumothorax is broadly classified into PSP and SSP; PSP occurs in patients with "normal" lungs and no apparent abnormalities on chest radiographs, whereas SSP develops in patients who have underlying lung disease.[24]

Tension pneumothorax

It should be emphasized that tension pneumothorax is a pathophysiologic, and not a radiologic, diagnosis because patients with a large pneumothorax but without cardiopulmonary collapse often get misdiagnosed to have tension pneumothorax. Tension pneumothorax is rarely seen among spontaneously breathing patients with PSP[33] and SSP. It is more likely to occur among patients with traumatic pneumothorax and those receiving positive pressure mechanical ventilation[32]; the pneumothorax progresses rapidly because of ongoing positive pressure ventilation to cause cardiorespiratory collapse.[32,34] It is important to recognize tension pneumothorax because, unlike large PSP and SSP that usually do not require immediate drainage, tension pneumothorax requires emergency decompression.[34]

Traumatic pneumothorax

Pneumothorax caused by injuries to the chest or lung is classified as traumatic.[35] Traumatic pneumothorax may be iatrogenic, as a complication following medical procedures or interventions; and noniatrogenic, when caused by blunt or penetrating chest injuries, such as following motor vehicle accident trauma and falls (**Fig. 7**).[35,36] Greater than 10% of trauma patients may develop blunt chest injury-related pneumothorax that is associated with mortality rates of 5% to 20%[37] from life-threatening hemothorax, tension pneumothorax, and damage to surrounding major organs, such as the thoracic aorta.[35] Chest wall defects

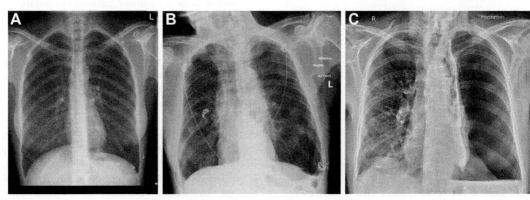

Fig. 4. Left partial left pneumothorax (*A*). Left incomplete pneumothorax (*B*). Left complete pneumothorax (*C*).

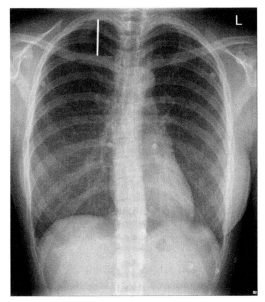

Fig. 5. The ACCP pneumothorax guidelines classify pneumothorax size based on lung apex-cupola distance of <3 cm (small pneumothorax) or >3 cm (large pneumothorax).

from penetrating chest injuries allows external air to be entrained into the pleural space during inspiration leading to open traumatic pneumothorax.[35] Noniatrogenic traumatic pneumothorax often

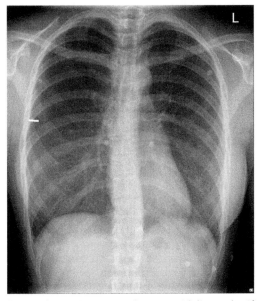

Fig. 6. The BTS pneumothorax guidelines classify pneumothorax size based on interpleural distance of <2 cm (small pneumothorax) or >2 cm (large pneumothorax). Interpleural distance of >2 cm helps to identify a pneumothorax that could be drained safely by needle or chest drain decompression without causing lung injury.

requires management by thoracic and/or trauma surgeons.

Iatrogenic pneumothorax develops following complications from medical interventions, such as transbronchial lung biopsy, transthoracic needle aspiration,[38,39] lung cryobiopsy,[40,41] central vascular catheter insertion,[42] pacemaker insertion,[43] thoracentesis,[44] and barotrauma in mechanically ventilated patients (**Fig. 8**).[36] Iatrogenic pneumothorax may be difficult to identify in intubated patients who develop barotrauma; the subtle deep sulcus sign on supine chest radiographs in these patients should be carefully looked for, otherwise delayed diagnosis of pneumothorax can result in significant morbidity and even death. Rare cases of iatrogenic pneumothorax associated with chest acupuncture,[45,46] colonoscopy,[47] breast augmentation,[48] and radiofrequency ablation (**Fig. 9**) have also been reported.

The overall prevalence of iatrogenic pneumothorax varies depending on the nature, frequency, and setting of medical interventions being performed. One study reported a 1.36% prevalence of iatrogenic pneumothorax related to invasive medical interventions, 57% of which were emergency procedures.[36] The most common causes of iatrogenic pneumothorax are central venous catheter insertions, thoracentesis, and mechanical ventilation.[49] Iatrogenic pneumothorax is more prevalent in teaching hospitals compared with nonteaching hospitals in the United States,[50] accounting for 56% of all pneumothorax cases among inpatients.[49]

Procedure-, patient-, and operator-related factors mainly determine the likelihood of iatrogenic pneumothorax (**Box 2**).

Primary spontaneous pneumothorax

Patients with PSP may have underlying risk factors and lung abnormalities that are not initially apparent on chest radiographs. Tobacco smoking is the single most important risk factor for PSP.[26,30] Up to 88% of patients with PSP are smokers in large-scale observational studies.[7] A smoker, compared with nonsmokers, has a 9-fold risk in females and a 22-fold risk in males of developing PSP with a strong dose-response link between the number of cigarettes smoked and pneumothorax risk.[7] Cannabis smoking also increases risk of developing spontaneous pneumothorax[30,51,52] and is associated with development of emphysematous changes and bullous lung disease.[30,51] Height and male sex are both important risk factors for PSP.[8] PSP is three- to six-fold more common in men than in women.[8,33] It is hypothesized that in tall men, pleural blebs may develop because of greater mechanical stretching of lung

> **Box 1**
> **Classification of pneumothorax by pathophysiology**
>
> 1. Tension pneumothorax
> 2. Traumatic pneumothorax
>   a. Iatrogenic pneumothorax
>   b. Noniatrogenic pneumothorax
> 3. Spontaneous pneumothorax
>   a. Primary spontaneous pneumothorax
>   b. Secondary spontaneous pneumothorax

tissue in the apex during growth or because the lung tissue in the apex grows faster than accompanying vasculature and outstrips its blood supply.[53]

Secondary spontaneous pneumothorax

SSP can occur in association with many primary lung diseases[33] and systemic conditions with lung involvement. Compared with PSP, patients with SSP are typically older.[6] The BTS pneumothorax guidelines recommended including patients older than 50 years and/or those with significant smoking history as having SSP, even when the chest radiograph appears normal, in view of their high likelihood of having underlying lung pathology.[24] Dyspnea is the most common presenting feature in SSP unlike with PSP, where patients commonly present with chest pain.[33] Patients with SSP can rapidly develop cyanosis,

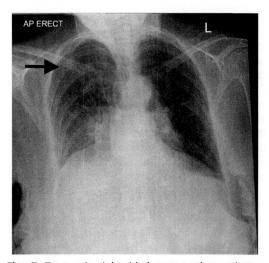

Fig. 7. Traumatic right-sided pneumothorax in an elderly woman with displaced rib fractures (*arrow*) following a fall.

hypoxemia, hypercapnia, and respiratory failure because of poor lung reserve.[33]

Air enters the pleural cavity via various routes including (1) alveolar and visceral pleural rupture causing an alveolopleural fistula, such as with emphysema and necrotizing pneumonia; (2) via the lung interstitium; and (3) via the mediastinal pleura causing a pneumomediastinum.[33]

Chronic obstructive pulmonary disease Chronic obstructive pulmonary disease (COPD) is the most frequent lung disease associated with SSP.[33,54] Data from a large English hospital database that recorded all admissions for spontaneous pneumothorax showed that 61% of cases were caused by COPD and predominantly affected males (73% vs 27% females)[6]; the proportion of COPD as a cause for pneumothorax also increased by 9% between 1968 and 2016. Another study reported that 80% of all spontaneous pneumothoraces requiring inpatient treatment were caused by COPD, interstitial lung disease, and malignancy.[55]

The most common mechanism for development of spontaneous pneumothorax in patients with COPD is by rupture of emphysematous blebs and bullae.[53] Patients with COPD, especially in the presence of significant air-trapping and lung hyperinflation, are also at increased risk of iatrogenic pneumothorax from procedures, such as central vascular catheter insertion, trans-thoracic lung biopsy, and transbronchial lung biopsy.[53]

Tuberculosis Pulmonary tuberculosis is the most common cause for SSP in endemic areas.[56] Spontaneous pneumothorax occurs when a tuberculous cavity ruptures into the pleural space or from direct tuberculous invasion and necrosis of lung parenchyma and visceral pleura.[53] A long-term follow-up study of 872 patients treated for spontaneous pneumothorax in Gran Canaria, Spain found the pneumothorax was tuberculosis-related in 5.4%[57]; this may be higher in tuberculosis-endemic areas. It is estimated that 0.6% to 1.4% of patients with pulmonary tuberculosis will develop SSP during the course of their treatment.[58,59] Tuberculosis-related pneumothorax can lead to empyema, acute respiratory failure, cachexia, and persistent bronchopleural fistula.[60] The overall burden of tuberculosis-related pneumothorax is likely to be significant because of the high incidence of tuberculosis worldwide.

Other pulmonary infections SSP can develop with typical and atypical pulmonary infections. Common bacterial pneumoniae secondary to *Klebsiella*, *Staphylococcus*, *Pseudomonas*, and

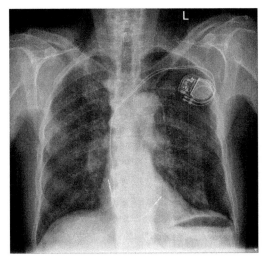

Fig. 8. Chest radiograph showing left-sided iatrogenic pneumothorax that developed 2 hours following permanent pacemaker insertion.

anaerobic organisms may result in unilateral SSP,[54] caused by direct invasion and necrosis of lung and visceral pleura (**Fig. 10**). Pneumothorax associated with *Pneumocystis jirovecii* pneumonia (PCP) is commonly bilateral.[61–63] Patients with HIV[64] infection and PCP are particularly at risk of developing a pneumothorax (9% vs 2%–4% of non-HIV patients with PCP).[62,63] An aspergilloma can rupture into the pleural cavity to cause pneumothorax.[65,66] The novel corona virus 2019 (COVID-19) infection is also associated with pneumothorax (incidence of 1%); the 28-day survival in this cohort was not significantly different to COVID-19 patients without.[67]

Diffuse cystic lung disease Diffuse cystic lung disease (DCLD) is group of heterogenous lung diseases with diverse pathophysiologic

mechanisms and characteristic lung cyst patterns on high-resolution CT (HRCT) imaging. The diseases are individually rare but collectively form a significant minority. They are broadly classified based on their underlying etiology into (1) neoplastic, such as lymphangioleiomyomatosis (LAM) and pulmonary Langerhans cell histiocytosis (PLCH); (2) developmental, such as Birt-Hogg-Dube (BHD) syndrome and neurofibromatosis; (3) lymphoproliferative, such as lymphocytic interstitial pneumonia; (4) infectious, such as *P jirovecii* and staphylococcal pneumonia; and (5) smoking-related, such as smoking-related PLCH.[68] DCLDs with overlapping features may be included in multiple categories.

The characteristic cystic patterns of different DCLDs are often diagnostic. The cysts develop following inflammatory or infiltrative destruction and/or replacement of alveolar septa, small airways and blood vessels in the secondary lung lobules. Spontaneous pneumothorax, often recurrent, is the presenting manifestation in greater than 50% of cases in many DCLDs; early diagnosis of DCLDs at this stage has therapeutic implications in cases where the natural disease course is modifiable with pharmacologic and nonpharmacologic interventions, such as sirolimus in LAM and smoking cessation in PLCH.

Lymphangioleiomyomatosis LAM is caused by infiltration of the lung by smooth muscle cells that are growth-activated by mutations in the tuberous sclerosis genes and spread through blood and lymphatics.[69,70] Infiltration and destruction of airways, lymphatics, and blood vessels by the smooth muscle cells lead to the formation of thin-walled, uniformly distributed lung cysts (**Fig. 11**A, B).[71] Cyst rupture results in recurrent pneumothorax. LAM is often not recognized to be the cause for pneumothorax in young patients

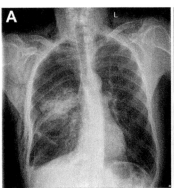
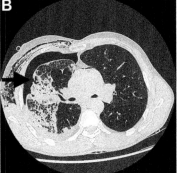
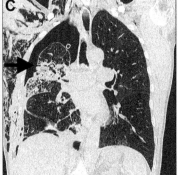

Fig. 9. Chest radiograph showing iatrogenic right-sided pneumothorax following radiofrequency ablation (RFA) of right upper lobe tumor (*A*). CT scan of chest (axial and coronal views) shows a bronchopleural fistula and breach of visceral pleura (*arrows*) caused by RFA leading to iatrogenic pneumothorax (*B, C*).

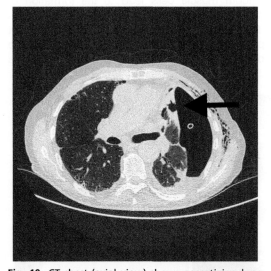

Fig. 10. CT chest (axial view) shows necrotizing lung abscess with bronchopleural fistula (arrow) in the left upper lobe causing spontaneous pneumothorax.

and without an HRCT scan, pneumothorax in patients with early LAM may be misdiagnosed as PSP.

LAM can occur either as part of the tuberous sclerosis complex LAM or sporadically in patients without tuberous sclerosis; the latter almost always develops in females of childbearing age.[72] In addition to spontaneous pneumothorax, LAM is associated with angiomyolipoma (**Fig. 11C**),[73] lymphangiomyoma, chylous ascites, and chylous pleural effusions. LAM is diagnosed based on the characteristic cystic pattern on CT, without needing a lung biopsy, when it is associated with tuberous sclerosis, angiomyolipoma, or chylothorax,[74] or when the serum vascular endothelial growth factor (VEGF)-D level is greater than 800 pg/mL.[75]

Pulmonary Langerhans cell histiocytosis PLCH is most commonly seen in young smokers; 10% to 20% of patients with PLCH develop a spontaneous pneumothorax.[76,77] PLCH is characterized by peribronchiolar accumulation of Langerhans cells that are specialized dendritic cells regulating mucosal airway immunity and activated by cigarette smoke–induced cytokine mediation.[78,79] The characteristic HRCT pattern is of nodular and cystic abnormalities, predominantly in the upper and middle lung zones (**Fig. 12**). The bizarrely shaped cysts are different to the uniform, thin-walled cysts seen with most other DCLDs. Smoking cessation and avoidance of second-hand smoke may result in stabilization and resolution of PLCH.

Birt-Hogg-Dube Syndrome BHD is an autosomal-dominant disorder characterized by the triad of hair follicle and renal tumors, and pulmonary cysts that typically manifest in the fourth to fifth decade.[80] Patients with BHD have a 50-fold risk of developing pneumothorax compared with the general population[81] and a 75% pneumothorax recurrence rate.[82] BHD may be more common than initially believed with studies reporting 5% to 10% prevalence in young adults presenting with pneumothorax.[83,84] Cyst rupture results in pneumothorax formation; however, pneumothorax in the absence of cysts is also reported.[85] BHD is caused by mutations in the FLCN gene, which encodes folliculin, a tumor suppressor protein. Cyst formation in BHD occurs following activation of the mTOR pathway causing adhesion protein defects that damage the alveolar-septal junction.[86] The characteristic pattern in BHD is of variably sized, round-lentiform-shaped, thin-walled cysts with a predominantly basal and subpleural distribution (**Fig. 13A–C**).[87] Renal tumors are seen in greater than 25% of patients with BHD and require

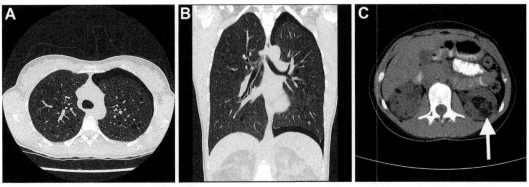

Fig. 11. CT chest axial (*A*) and coronal (*B*) views showing characteristic thin-walled uniformly shaped and distributed cysts of LAM in a young female presenting with recurrent left-sided pneumothorax. CT abdomen (*C*) shows a left-sided angiomyolipoma (arrow) in the same patient.

active screening and surveillance. BHD should be suspected in young patients with spontaneous pneumothorax, skin lesions resembling folliculomas (**Fig. 13**D, E), and renal tumors and in those with a similar family history.

Other rare inherited and genetic disorders, such as neurofibromatosis and Ehlers-Danlos syndrome, with characteristic DCLD patterns on HRCT are also associated with high risk of spontaneous pneumothorax and recurrence (**Fig. 14**).

Pneumothorax in women of childbearing age The overall incidence of pneumothorax is lower among females; however, there are unique conditions that present with recurrent spontaneous pneumothorax and occur only, or predominantly, in women

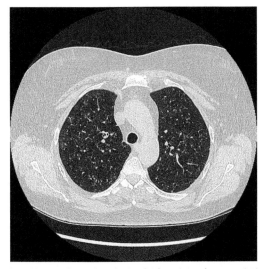

Fig. 12. CT chest (axial view) showing characteristic nodules and bizarrely shaped cysts, predominantly in the upper and middle lung zones, in a young smoker with PLCH.

of childbearing age.[88,89] Based on clinical and pathologic findings, pneumothorax in women of childbearing age is classified into three groups: (1) catamenial pneumothorax (with or without endometriosis), (2) endometriosis-related noncatamenial pneumothorax (pneumothorax occurring outside the menstrual period but with pathologic findings of endometriosis), and (3) idiopathic pneumothorax (noncatamenial and nonendometriosis with no underlying cause identified).[90]

Catamenial pneumothorax is associated with the menstrual cycle and typically occurs within 72 hours before and after the onset of menstrual period. Catamenial pneumothorax is likely underdiagnosed; a study of menstruating women undergoing surgery for spontaneous pneumothorax found a catamenial cause in 30%.[91] It is usually unilateral, predominantly on the right side, and associated with thoracic and/or extrathoracic endometriosis.[92,93] Pneumothorax develops when endometrial tissue in the lung and visceral pleura ruptures. The endometrial tissue is thought to reach the lung and pleura by intra-abdominal migration, micrometastatic seeding, or lymphovascular spread. Endometriosis-related pneumothorax can also develop following rupture of pelvic endometriosis and transgenital or transdiaphragmatic tracking up of air through diaphragmatic defects into the pleural space.[94] Single or multiple fenestrations are present in the tendinous part of the diaphragm and nodules are seen on the diaphragmatic/visceral pleura (**Fig. 15**A–E). The diaphragmatic defects may be missed at the time of surgery unless carefully searched for; without plication of the diaphragmatic defects, pneumothorax can recur in patients with extrathoracic endometriosis.

The correlation between development of pneumothorax to menstrual periods is not always

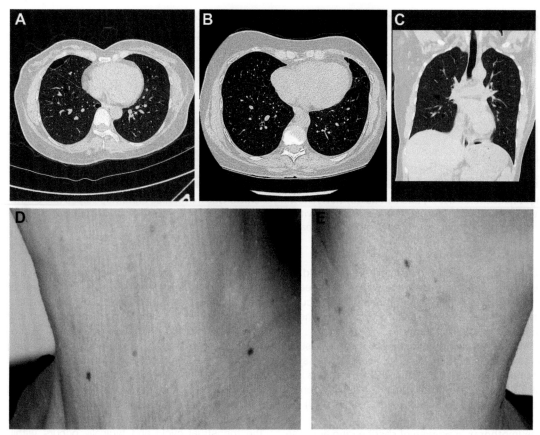

Fig. 13. CT chest axial (*A, B*) and coronal (*C*) views show round, lentiform-shaped, thin-walled cysts with a predominantly basal and subpleural distribution in a patient with BHD. BHD is associated with skin lesions formed by folliculomas (*D, E*).

apparent and the diagnosis of thoracic endometriosis may only be made when endometrial nodules are seen at the time of surgery. The nodules have glandular cells, endometrial stroma, and hemosiderin-laden macrophages and test positive for estrogen and progesterone receptors. CD10 staining on the resected specimen is useful to identify endometriosis tissue following resection.

Another important diagnosis to consider in young females presenting with recurrent pneumothorax is LAM (described previously). [95]

Miscellaneous causes Pressure swings secondary to changes in atmospheric pressure during thunderstorms and with high altitude,[96] air pollution,[97] exposure to loud music,[98] playing musical instruments, and blowing of balloons[99] have been reported to cause spontaneous pneumothorax. Anorexia nervosa has been found to be associated with pneumothorax. The risk of developing subsequent contralateral spontaneous pneumothorax is higher among underweight patients; malnutrition of pneumocytes may be a possible mechanism leading to

pneumothorax development.[100,101] A higher blood level of aluminum has been noted among patients with spontaneous pneumothorax[102] leading to the postulation that aluminum might play a role in formation of subpleural blebs and bullous lesions and pneumothorax development.[102]

PATHOGENESIS

The exact pathogenesis and mechanisms of spontaneous pneumothorax remain unclear. Although it was believed earlier that PSP occurs in patients with no underlying lung abnormalities, several factors have been identified that predispose to pneumothorax development. An interplay of lung-related abnormalities, such as subpleural blebs (**Fig. 16**A–C) and bullae (**Fig. 16**D),[26,103] visceral pleural porosity,[104] emphysema-like changes (ELCs),[105] chronic small airway inflammation,[104,106] and abnormal levels of matrix metalloproteinases (MMP),[107,108] and environmental factors, such as smoking, is now thought to lead to pneumothorax development and recurrence.

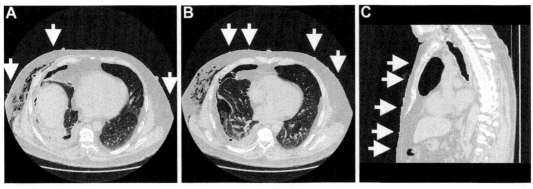

Fig. 14. CT chest axial (*A, B*) and sagittal (*C*) views showing skin neurofibroma nodules (*arrows*) in a patient with neurofibromatosis and presenting with spontaneous right-sided pneumothorax.

Blebs, Bullae, and Pleural Porosity

Pleural blebs and bullae are demonstrated in patients with PSP using advanced imaging techniques, such as CT and fluorescein-enhanced autofluorescence during thoracic surgery. Resected lung specimens show features of inflammation, disruption or absence of mesothelial cells, and presence of micropores measuring 10 to 20 μm in diameter.[104] How these then lead to pleural bleb and bullae formation is unknown.[30]

It is also unclear whether these lesions are solely responsible for air leak development[109,110]; multiple factors are likely involved. Air leak from ruptured blebs and bullae is not always present (3.6%–73%) during surgery for spontaneous pneumothorax.[111] Pneumothorax recurrence is high (up to 20%) when only bullectomy, and no surgical pleurodesis, is performed.[112,113] Additional to visible blebs or bullae, the pleura may also be abnormal with diffuse "pleural porosity." Fluorescein-enhanced autofluorescence assessment during thoracoscopy in patients with PSP can reveal abnormal areas of fluorescein leakage on the visceral pleura even in areas that appeared normal on white-light inspection.[112]

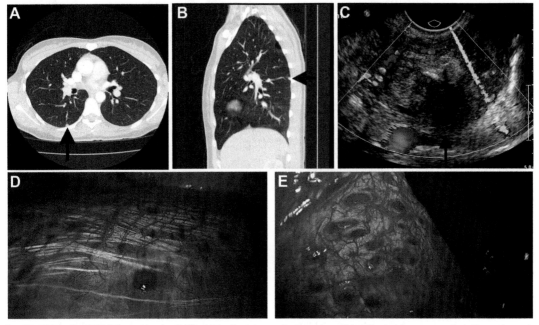

Fig. 15. CT chest axial (*A*) and sagittal (*B*) views showing subpleural nodules (*arrows*) representing thoracic endometriosis in a patient with catamenial pneumothorax. Ultrasound confirmed the presence of pelvic endometriosis (*C*). Multiple reddish-brown endometrial nodules were seen on the diaphragmatic pleura during video-assisted thoracoscopic surgery (*D, E*).

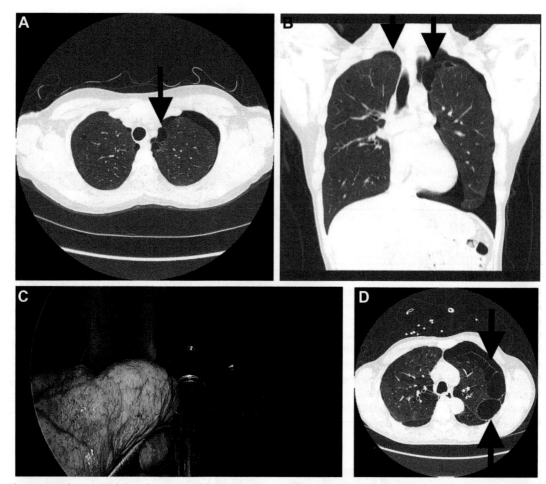

Fig. 16. CT chest axial (*A*) and coronal (*B*) views showing bilateral apical blebs (*arrows*). An apical bleb is seen on direct visualization during video-assisted thoracoscopic surgery (*C*). CT chest (axial view) shows multiple large left upper lobe bullae (*arrows*) and spontaneous secondary pneumothorax (*D*).

Emphysema-like changes

ELCs are low density areas that are seen separate to pleural blebs and bullae on CT lung imaging in patients with PSP and believed to be caused by early gas trapping and inflammation.[114] The mean lung density on lung parenchymal density assessment with CT is lower among patients with PSP and worse in smokers compared with control subjects.[105] Changes of emphysema have also been observed in resected lung tissue in PSP.[105]

Matrix Metalloproteinase

MMPs are a family of zinc-dependent enzymes involved in wound healing, tissue remodeling, and angiogenesis.[115,116] Various types of MMPs (eg, MMP-2 and MMP-9) are produced by bronchial epithelial cells, alveolar macrophages, and type-II pneumocytes[117]; overexpressions of

MMP-2, MMP-7, and MMP-9 has been noted in patients presenting with pneumothorax[107,108,118] and may be independent risk factors.[108] It is not clear if cigarette smoking–related oxidative changes and inflammation influence MMP levels.[108]

Chronic Small Airway Inflammation

Chronic small airway inflammatory changes are present in the lungs of patients with spontaneous pneumothorax; it is unclear whether these inflammatory changes are simply smoking-related abnormalities or if they actually contribute to pneumothorax development. Histologic findings of postinflammatory fibrosis, chronic bronchiolitis with pigmented macrophages and focal emphysema, and respiratory bronchiolitis have been noted in wedge resection specimens of patients with recurrent or persistent spontaneous pneumothorax.[104,106,119]

FUTURE DIRECTIONS

Significant gaps in knowledge remain regarding classification, pathogenesis, management, and outcomes of pneumothorax. The current pneumothorax classification of spontaneous pneumothorax into PSP and SSP, based on clinical and radiologic findings, is simplistic. With improved understanding of the underlying pathogenetic mechanisms, the distinction between PSP and SSP as separate entities rather than the ends of a continual disease spectrum has blurred. An "ideal" future classification system should take into consideration (1) patient risk factors and pathogenetic mechanisms, (2) underlying lung disease and abnormalities on high-resolution imaging of the lung, (3) patient symptoms and severity, and (4) improved risk stratifications to guide interventions and recurrence prevention. The role of ELCs, hormonal markers and biomarkers, such as CD10 levels in women of childbearing age, and MMP-9 in pneumothorax development and recurrence are important areas of research. Advancements in imaging technology and artificial intelligence algorithms may offer novel applications to improve diagnosis and risk stratification in the future.

CLINICS CARE POINTS

- Patients with primary spontaneous pneumothorax may have underlying risk factors and lung abnormalities that are not easily apparent on initial chest imaging.

- Tension pneumothorax is a pathophysiologic, NOT a radiologic, diagnosis.

- Tobacco smoking is the an important risk factor for both primary and secondary spontaneous pneumothorax.

- Recurrent spontaneous pneumothorax is a common presenting manifestation in diffuse cystic lung diseases.

- An interplay between lung-related abnormalities and environmental factors is the likely pathogenetic mechanisms of spontaneous pneumothorax in most cases.

REFERENCES

1. Light RW. Pleural diseases. 3rd edition. Baltimore: Williams & Wilkins; 1995.
2. Itard JMG. Dissertation sur le pneumothorax, ou les congestions gazeuses qui se forment dans la poitrine. Paris: De l'imprimerie des Sourds-Muets; 1803.
3. Laennec RTH. De l'auscultation médiate: ou traité du diagnostic des maladies des poumons et du coeur. Paris: Brosson et Chaudé; 1819.
4. Hyde B, Hyde L. Spontaneous pneumothorax: contrast of the benign idiopathic and the tuberculous types. Ann Intern Med 1950;33(6): 1373–7.
5. Kjaergaad H. Spontaneous pneumothorax in the apparently healthy. Acta Med Scand 1932;43: 1–159.
6. Gupta D, Hansell A, Nichols T, et al. Epidemiology of pneumothorax in England. Thorax 2000;55(8): 666–71.
7. Bense L, Eklund G, Wiman L-G. Smoking and the increased risk of contracting spontaneous pneumothorax. Chest 1987;92(6):1009–12.
8. Melton LJ, Hepper NGG, Offord KP. Incidence of spontaneous pneumothorax in Olmsted County, Minnesota—1950 to 1974. Am Rev Respir Dis 1979;120(6):1379–82.
9. Baumann MH, Strange C, Heffner JE, et al. Management of spontaneous pneumothorax: an American College of Chest Physicians Delphi consensus statement. Chest 2001;119(2):590–602.
10. Mitani A, Hakamata Y, Hosoi M, et al. The incidence and risk factors of asymptomatic primary spontaneous pneumothorax detected during health check-ups. BMC Pulm Med 2017;17(1):1–6.
11. Schramel FM, Postmus PE, Vanderschueren RG. Current aspects of spontaneous pneumothorax. Eur Respir J 1997;10(6):1372–9.
12. Sadikot R, Greene T, Meadows K, et al. Recurrence of primary spontaneous pneumothorax. Thorax 1997;52(9):805–9.
13. Olesen WH, Lindahl-Jacobsen R, Katballe N, et al. Recurrent primary spontaneous pneumothorax is common following chest tube and conservative treatment. World J Surg 2016;40(9):2163–70.
14. Walker SP, Bibby AC, Halford P, et al. Recurrence rates in primary spontaneous pneumothorax: a systematic review and meta-analysis. Eur Respir J 2018;52(3).
15. Huang YH, Chang PY, Wong KS, et al. An age-stratified longitudinal study of primary spontaneous pneumothorax. J Adolesc Health 2017;61(4): 527–32.
16. Bobbio A, Dechartres A, Bouam S, et al. Epidemiology of spontaneous pneumothorax: gender-related differences. Thorax 2015;70(7):653–8.
17. Lippert H, Lund O, Blegvad S, et al. Independent risk factors for cumulative recurrence rate after first spontaneous pneumothorax. Eur Respir J 1991; 4(3):324–31.
18. Videm V, Pillgram-Larsen J, Ellingsen O, et al. Spontaneous pneumothorax in chronic

obstructive pulmonary disease: complications, treatment and recurrences. Eur J Respir Dis 1987;71(5):365–71.

19. Baumann MH. Management of spontaneous pneumothorax. Clin Chest Med 2006;27(2):369–81.

20. Voge V, Anthracite R. Spontaneous pneumothorax in the USAF aircrew population: a retrospective study. Aviat Space Environ Med 1986;57(1): 939–49.

21. Light RW. Pleural diseases. Baltimore, MD: Lippincott Williams & Wilkins; 2007.

22. Collins CD, Lopez A, Mathie A, et al. Quantification of pneumothorax size on chest radiographs using interpleural distances: regression analysis based on volume measurements from helical CT. AJR Am J Roentgenol 1995;165(5):1127–30.

23. Rivas de Andrés JJ, Jiménez López MF, Molins López-Rodó L, et al. [Guidelines for the diagnosis and treatment of spontaneous pneumothorax]. Arch Bronconeumol 2008;44(8):437–48.

24. MacDuff A, Arnold A, Harvey J. Management of spontaneous pneumothorax: British Thoracic Society Pleural Disease Guideline 2010. Thorax 2010; 65(Suppl 2):ii18–31.

25. Henry M, Arnold T, Harvey J. BTS guidelines for the management of spontaneous pneumothorax. Thorax 2003;58(Suppl 2):ii39.

26. Bintcliffe OJ, Hallifax RJ, Edey A, et al. Spontaneous pneumothorax: time to rethink management? Lancet Respir Med 2015;3(7):578–88.

27. Kelly A-M, Druda D. Comparison of size classification of primary spontaneous pneumothorax by three international guidelines: a case for international consensus? Respir Med 2008;102(12): 1830–2.

28. Yoon J, Sivakumar P, O'Kane K, et al. A need to reconsider guidelines on management of primary spontaneous pneumothorax? Int J Emerg Med 2017;10(1):1–3.

29. Kelly A-M, Weldon D, Tsang AY, et al. Comparison between two methods for estimating pneumothorax size from chest X-rays. Respir Med 2006;100(8): 1356–9.

30. Tschopp J-M, Bintcliffe O, Astoul P, et al. ERS task force statement: diagnosis and treatment of primary spontaneous pneumothorax. Eur Respir J 2015;46(2):321–35.

31. Brown SGA, Ball EL, Perrin K, et al. Conservative versus interventional treatment for spontaneous pneumothorax. N Engl J Med 2020;382(5):405–15.

32. Noppen M, de Keukeleire T. Pneumothorax. Respiration 2008;76(2):121–7.

33. Noppen M. Spontaneous pneumothorax: epidemiology, pathophysiology and cause. Eur Respir Rev 2010;19(117):217–9.

34. Roberts DJ, Leigh-Smith S, Faris PD, et al. Clinical presentation of patients with tension

pneumothorax: a systematic review. Ann Surg 2015;261(6):1068–78.

35. Galvagno SM, Nahmias JT, Young DA. Advanced trauma life support® Update 2019: management and applications for adults and special populations. Anesthesiology 2019;37(1): 13–32.

36. Celik B, Sahin E, Nadir A, et al. Iatrogenic pneumothorax: etiology, incidence and risk factors. Thorac Cardiovasc Surg 2009;57(05):286–90.

37. Battle CE, Hutchings H, Evans PA. Risk factors that predict mortality in patients with blunt chest wall trauma: a systematic review and meta-analysis. Injury 2012;43(1):8–17.

38. Huang Y, Huang H, Li Q, et al. Transbronchial lung biopsy and pneumothorax. J Thorac Dis 2014; 6(Suppl 4):S443.

39. Galli JA, Panetta NL, Gaeckle N, et al. Pneumothorax after transbronchial biopsy in pulmonary fibrosis: lessons from the multicenter COMET trial. Lung 2017;195(5):537–43.

40. Dhooria S, Sehgal IS, Aggarwal AN, et al. Diagnostic yield and safety of cryoprobe transbronchial lung biopsy in diffuse parenchymal lung diseases: systematic review and meta-analysis. Respir Care 2016;61(5):700–12.

41. Gershman E, Fruchter O, Benjamin F, et al. Safety of cryo-transbronchial biopsy in diffuse lung diseases: analysis of three hundred cases. Respiration 2015;90(1):40–6.

42. Tsotsolis N, Tsirgogianni K, Kioumis I, et al. Pneumothorax as a complication of central venous catheter insertion. Ann Transl Med 2015;3(3).

43. Kirkfeldt RE, Johansen JB, Nohr EA, et al. Pneumothorax in cardiac pacing: a population-based cohort study of 28 860 Danish patients. Europace 2012;14(8):1132–8.

44. Gordon CE, Feller-Kopman D, Balk EM, et al. Pneumothorax following thoracentesis: a systematic review and meta-analysis. Arch Intern Med 2010; 170(4):332–9.

45. Corado SC, Santos MG, Quaresma L, et al. Pneumothorax after acupuncture. BMJ Case Rep 2019;12(6):e228770.

46. Ying X, Wang P, Xu P, et al. Pneumothorax associated with acupuncture: a systematic review and analysis. J Altern Complement Med 2016;4(4):17–25.

47. Gupta A, Hammad Zaidi KH. Pneumothorax after colonoscopy–a review of literature. Clin Endosc 2017;50(5):446.

48. Senthilkumaran S, Balamurugan N, Menezes RG, et al. Bilateral pneumothorax following breast augmentation: beware and be aware. Indian J Plast Surg 2012;45(3):579.

49. Kogos A, Alakhras M, Hossain Z, et al. Iatrogenic pneumothorax: etiology, morbidity, and mortality. Chest 2004;126(4):893S.

50. John J, Seifi A. Incidence of iatrogenic pneumo-thorax in the United States in teaching vs. non-teaching hospitals from 2000 to 2012. J Crit Care 2016;34:66–8.

51. Johnson MK, Smith RP, Morrison D, et al. Large lung bullae in marijuana smokers. Thorax 2000; 55(4):340–2.

52. Wu T-c, Tashkin DP, Djahed B, et al. Pulmonary hazards of smoking marijuana as compared with tobacco. N Engl J Med 1988;318(6):347–51.

53. Light RW, Lee YCG. Pneumothorax in adults: epidemiology and etiology. In: UpToDate (proceed-ings), Light RW (Ed), UpToDate, Waltham, MA. 2020.

54. Chen C-H, Liao W-C, Liu Y-H, et al. Secondary spontaneous pneumothorax: which associated conditions benefit from pigtail catheter treatment? Am J Emerg Med 2012;30(1):45–50.

55. Hallifax RJ, Goldacre R, Landray MJ, et al. Trends in the incidence and recurrence of inpatient-treated spontaneous pneumothorax, 1968-2016. JAMA 2018;320(14):1471–80.

56. Shamaei M, Tabarsi P, Pojhan S, et al. Tuberculosis-associated secondary pneumothorax: a retrospec-tive study of 53 patients. Respir Care 2011;56(3): 298–302.

57. Freixinet JL, Caminero JA, Marchena J, et al. Spon-taneous pneumothorax and tuberculosis: long-term follow-up. Eur Respir J 2011;38(1):126–31.

58. Ihm HJ, Hankins JR, Miller JE, et al. Pneumothorax associated with pulmonary tuberculosis. J Thorac Cardiovasc Surg 1972;64(2):211–9.

59. Blanco-Perez J, Bordón J, Pi L, et al. Pneumo-thorax in active pulmonary tuberculosis: resur-gence of an old complication? Respir Med 1998; 92(11):1269–73.

60. Saad SB, Melki B, El Gharbi LD, et al. Pneumo-thorax tuberculeux: prise en charge diagnostique et thérapeutique. Revue de Pneumologie Clinique 2018;74(2):81–8.

61. Radhi S, Alexander T, Ukwu M, et al. Outcome of HIV-associated *Pneumocystis* pneumonia in hospi-talized patients from 2000 through 2003. BMC Infect Dis 2008;8(1):1–10.

62. Afessa B. Pleural effusions and pneumothoraces in AIDS. Curr Opin Pulm Med 2001;7(4):202–9.

63. Rivero A, Perez-Camacho I, Lozano F, et al. Etiol-ogy of spontaneous pneumothorax in 105 HIV-infected patients without highly active antiretroviral therapy. Eur J Radiol 2009;71(2):264–8.

64. Grams ST, von Saltiel R, Mayer AF, et al. Assess-ment of the reproducibility of the indirect ultra-sound method of measuring diaphragm mobility. Clin Physiol Funct Imaging 2014;34(1):18–25.

65. Nonga BN, Jemea B, Pondy AO, et al. Unusual life-threatening pneumothorax complicating a ruptured complex aspergilloma in an immunocompetent patient in Cameroon. Case Rep Surg 2018;2018.

66. Zhang W, Hu Y, Gao J, et al. Pleural aspergillosis complicated by recurrent pneumothorax: a case report. J Med Case Rep 2010;4(1):1–4.

67. Martinelli AW, Ingle T, Newman J, et al. COVID-19 and pneumothorax: a multicentre retrospective case series. Eur Respir J 2020;56(5).

68. Gupta N, Vassallo R, Wikenheiser-Brokamp KA, et al. Diffuse cystic lung disease. Part I. Am J Re-spir Crit Care Med 2015;191(12):1354–66.

69. Henske EP, McCormack FX. Lymphangioleiomyo-matosis: a wolf in sheep's clothing. J Clin Invest 2012;122(11):3807–16.

70. McCormack FX, Travis WD, Colby TV, et al. Lym-phangioleiomyomatosis: calling it what it is: a low-grade, destructive, metastasizing neoplasm. Am J Respir Crit Care Med 2012;186(12):1210–2.

71. Ferrans V, Yu Z-X, Nelson W, et al. Lymphangioleio-myomatosis (LAM) a review of clinical and morpho-logical features. J Nippon Med Sch 2000;67(5): 311–29.

72. Crino PB, Nathanson KL, Henske EP. The tuberous sclerosis complex. N Engl J Med 2006;355(13): 1345–56.

73. Ryu JH, Hartman TE, Torres VE, et al. Frequency of undiagnosed cystic lung disease in patients with sporadic renal angiomyolipomas. Chest 2012; 141(1):163–8.

74. Johnson SR, Cordier J-F, Lazor R, et al. European Respiratory Society guidelines for the diagnosis and management of lymphangioleiomyomatosis. Eur Respir J 2010;35(1):14–26.

75. Young LR, VanDyke R, Gulleman PM, et al. Serum vascular endothelial growth factor-D prospectively distinguishes lymphangioleiomyomatosis from other diseases. Chest 2010;138(3):674–81.

76. Vassallo R, Ryu JH, Schroeder DR, et al. Clinical outcomes of pulmonary Langerhans'-cell histiocy-tosis in adults. N Engl J Med 2002;346(7):484–90.

77. Mendez JL, Nadrous HF, Vassallo R, et al. Pneumo-thorax in pulmonary Langerhans cell histiocytosis. Chest 2004;125(3):1028–32.

78. Tazi A, Bonay M, Bergeron A, et al. Role of granulocyte-macrophage colony stimulating factor (GM-CSF) in the pathogenesis of adult pulmonary histiocytosis X. Thorax 1996;51(6):611–4.

79. Tazi A, Moreau J, Bergeron A, et al. Evidence that Langerhans cells in adult pulmonary Langerhans cell histiocytosis are mature dendritic cells: impor-tance of the cytokine microenvironment. The J Im-munol 1999;163(6):3511–5.

80. Kunogi M, Kurihara M, Ikegami TS, et al. Clinical and genetic spectrum of Birt–Hogg–Dube syn-drome patients in whom pneumothorax and/or mul-tiple lung cysts are the presenting feature. J Med Genet 2010;47(4):281–7.

81. Zbar B, Alvord WG, Glenn G, et al. Risk of renal and colonic neoplasms and spontaneous pneumothorax in the Birt-Hogg-Dube syndrome. Cancer Epidemiol Biomarkers Prev 2002;11(4):393–400.

82. Toro JR, Pautler SE, Stewart L, et al. Lung cysts, spontaneous pneumothorax, and genetic associations in 89 families with Birt-Hogg-Dubé syndrome. Am J Respir Crit Care Med 2007; 175(10):1044–53.

83. Johannesma PC, Reinhard R, Kon Y, et al. Prevalence of Birt–Hogg–Dubé syndrome in patients with apparently primary spontaneous pneumothorax. Eur Respir J 2015;45(4):1191–4.

84. Ren HZ, Zhu CC, Yang C, et al. Mutation analysis of the FLCN gene in Chinese patients with sporadic and familial isolated primary spontaneous pneumothorax. Clin Genet 2008;74(2):178–83.

85. Onuki T, Goto Y, Kuramochi M, et al. Radiologically indeterminate pulmonary cysts in Birt-Hogg-Dubé syndrome. Ann Thorac Surg 2014;97(2):682–5.

86. Kumasaka T, Hayashi T, Mitani K, et al. Characterization of pulmonary cysts in Birt–Hogg–Dubé syndrome: histopathological and morphometric analysis of 229 pulmonary cysts from 50 unrelated patients. Histopathology 2014;65(1):100–10.

87. Tobino K, Hirai T, Johkoh T, et al. Differentiation between Birt–Hogg–Dubé syndrome and lymphangioleiomyomatosis: quantitative analysis of pulmonary cysts on computed tomography of the chest in 66 females. Eur J Radiol 2012;81(6): 1340–6.

88. Alifano M, Legras A, Rousset-Jablonski C, et al. Pneumothorax recurrence after surgery in women: clinicopathologic characteristics and management. Ann Thorac Surg 2011;92(1):322–6.

89. Alifano M, Roth T, Broe SC, et al. Catamenial pneumothorax: a prospective study. Chest 2003;124(3): 1004–8.

90. Legras A, Mansuet-Lupo A, Rousset-Jablonski C, et al. Pneumothorax in women of child-bearing age: an update classification based on clinical and pathologic findings. Chest 2014;145(2):354–60.

91. Rousset-Jablonski C, Alifano M, Plu-Bureau G, et al. Catamenial pneumothorax and endometriosis-related pneumothorax: clinical features and risk factors. Humanit Rep 2011;26(9):2322–9.

92. Joseph J, Sahn SA. Thoracic endometriosis syndrome: new observations from an analysis of 110 cases. Am J Med 1996;100(2):164–70.

93. Haga T, Kurihara M, Kataoka H, et al. Clinical-pathological findings of catamenial pneumothorax: comparison between recurrent cases and non-recurrent cases. Ann Thorac Cardiovasc Surg 2013;20(3):202–6.

94. Visouli AN, Zarogoulidis K, Kougioumtzi I, et al. Catamenial pneumothorax. J Minim Invasive Gynecol 2014;6(Suppl 4):S448.

95. McCormack FX, Gupta N, Finlay GR, et al. Official American Thoracic Society/Japanese Respiratory Society clinical practice guidelines: lymphangioleiomyomatosis diagnosis and management. Am J Respir Crit Care Med 2016; 194(6):748–61.

96. Alifano M, Parri SNF, Bonfanti B, et al. Atmospheric pressure influences the risk of pneumothorax: beware of the storm! Chest 2007;131(6):1877–82.

97. Bertolaccini L, Alemanno L, Rocco G, et al. Air pollution, weather variations and primary spontaneous pneumothorax. J Thorac Dis 2010;2(1):9.

98. Noppen M, Verbanck S, Harvey J, et al. Music: a new cause of primary spontaneous pneumothorax. Thorax 2004;59(8):722–4.

99. Shiferaw Dejene FA, Jack K, Anthony A. Pneumothorax, music and balloons: a case series. Ann Thorac Med 2013;8(3):176.

100. Huang T-W, Lee S-C, Cheng Y-L, et al. Contralateral recurrence of primary spontaneous pneumothorax. Chest 2007;132(4):1146–50.

101. Biffl WL, Narayanan V, Gaudiani JL, et al. The management of pneumothorax in patients with anorexia nervosa: a case report and review of the literature. Patient Saf Surg 2010;4(1):1–4.

102. Han S, Sakinci U, Kose SK, et al. The relationship between aluminum and spontaneous pneumothorax; treatment, prognosis, follow-up? Interactive cardiovascular and thoracic surgery. Interact Cardiovasc Thorac Surg 2004;3(1):79–82.

103. Mitlehner W, Friedrich M, Dissmann W. Value of computer tomography in the detection of bullae and blebs in patients with primary spontaneous pneumothorax. Respiration 1992;59(4):221–7.

104. Ohata M, Suzuki H. Pathogenesis of spontaneous pneumothorax: with special reference to the ultrastructure of emphysematous bullae. Chest 1980; 77(6):771–6.

105. Bintcliffe OJ, Edey AJ, Armstrong L, et al. Lung parenchymal assessment in primary and secondary pneumothorax. Ann Am Thorac Soc 2016; 13(3):350–5.

106. Lichter I, Gwynne J. Spontaneous pneumothorax in young subjects: a clinical and pathological study. Thorax 1971;26(4):409–17.

107. Chen C-K, Chen P-R, Huang H-C, et al. Overexpression of matrix metalloproteinases in lung tissue of patients with primary spontaneous pneumothorax. Respiration 2014;88(5):418–25.

108. Huang Y-F, Chiu W-C, Chou S-H, et al. Association of MMP-2 and MMP-9 expression with recurrences in primary spontaneous pneumothorax. Kaohsiung J Med Sci 2017;33(1):17–23.

109. Baumann MH. Do blebs cause primary spontaneous pneumothorax?: Pro: blebs do cause primary spontaneous pneumothorax. J Bronchol Interv Pulmonol 2002;9(4):313–8.

110. Noppen M. Do blebs cause primary spontaneous pneumothorax?: Con: blebs do not cause primary spontaneous pneumothorax. J Bronchol Interv Pulmonol 2002;9(4):319–23.

111. Noppen M. Management of primary spontaneous pneumothorax. Curr Opin Pulm Med 2003;9(4): 272–5.

112. Noppen M, Dekeukeleire T, Hanon S, et al. Fluorescein-enhanced autofluorescence thoracoscopy in patients with primary spontaneous pneumothorax and normal subjects. Am J Respir Crit Care Med 2006;26–30.

113. Linde K, Clausius N, Ramirez G, et al. Are the clinical effects of homoeopathy placebo effects? A meta-analysis of placebo-controlled trials. Lancet 1997;350(9081):834–43.

114. Hallifax R, Walker S, Marciniak S. Pneumothorax: how to predict, prevent and cure. Pleural disease (ERS monograph). Sheffield, UK: European Respiratory Society; 2020. p. 193–210.

115. Ohbayashi H. Matrix metalloproteinases in lung diseases. Curr Protein Pept Sci 2002;3(4):409–21.

116. Cathcart J, Pulkoski-Gross A, Cao J. Targeting matrix metalloproteinases in cancer: bringing new life to old ideas. Genes Dis 2015;2(1):26–34.

117. Chakrabarti S, Patel KD. Matrix metalloproteinase-2 (MMP-2) and MMP-9 in pulmonary pathology. Exp Lung Res 2005;31(6):599–621.

118. Chiu W-C, Lee Y-C, Su Y-H, et al. Correlation of matrix metalloproteinase-2 and-9 expression with recurrences in primary spontaneous pneumothorax patients. J Thorac Dis 2016;8(12): 3667.

119. Cottin V, Streichenberger N, Gamondes J, et al. Respiratory bronchiolitis in smokers with spontaneous pneumothorax. Eur Respir J 1998;12(3): 702–4.

Management of Pneumothorax

Andrew DeMaio, MD[a], Roy Semaan, MD[b],*

KEYWORDS

- Pneumothorax • Needle aspiration • Tube thoracostomy • Conservative management
- Thoracoscopic surgery

KEY POINTS

- Spontaneous pneumothorax is a relatively common condition and may present with a wide variety of severity.
- Treatment of pneumothorax is based on symptoms, size, and the presence of underlying lung disease.
- Conservative management of primary spontaneous pneumothorax is a reasonable alternative for patients with limited symptoms and ability to follow-up.
- When tube thoracostomy is chosen, small-bore catheters ($\leq$14F) are preferred in a majority of cases including patients on mechanical ventilation.

INTRODUCTION

Pneumothorax is a common medical condition defined as the accumulation of air in the pleural space. It can be encountered in both the emergency department and inpatient medical setting, presenting in a wide variety of clinical presentations, ranging from asymptomatic, when incidentally detected on an imaging study, to life-threatening with hemodynamic and respiratory compromise secondary to tension physiology.

Pneumothorax is divided into 2 main categories: traumatic and spontaneous. Traumatic pneumothorax may be due to blunt or penetrating trauma or may be iatrogenic from medical procedures associated with visceral pleural injury. Classically, spontaneous pneumothorax has been divided into primary (ie, in the absence of underlying lung disease) and secondary (ie, associated with underlying lung disease) etiologies.[1] Although an arbitrary distinction, this is often clinically relevant as secondary spontaneous pneumothorax (SSP) is often not well-tolerated owing to limited cardiopulmonary reserve.[2]

In general, treatment depends on severity of symptoms (including dyspnea and chest pain), the size of the pneumothorax, and clinical features (including need for supplemental oxygen). Guidelines define size in various ways. For example, the American College of Chest Physicians defines a large pneumothorax as one where the apex-to-cupola distance is at least 3 cm.[3] Meanwhile, the British Thoracic Society guidelines define a large pneumothorax as one where the interpleural distance at the level of the hilum is at least 2 cm[4] (**Fig. 1**).

PRIMARY SPONTANEOUS PNEUMOTHORAX

Because patients are often young and otherwise healthy, primary spontaneous pneumothorax (PSP) may present with minimal or absent symptoms. Guidelines suggest that symptoms, rather than the size of the pneumothorax, should be the primary determinant of treatment.[4] Size is associated with the rate of resolution if treated conservatively and should be considered when choosing therapy. The risk of recurrence of PSP varies

[a] Interventional Pulmonology, Johns Hopkins Hospital, Sheikh Zayed Cardiovascular Critical Care Tower, 1800 Orleans Street, Suite 7125L, Baltimore, MD 21287, USA; [b] Interventional Pulmonology, University of Pittsburgh Medical Center, Montefiore Hospital, NW628, 3459 Fifth Avenue, Pittsburgh, PA 15213, USA
* Corresponding author.
E-mail address: semaanrw2@upmc.edu

Clin Chest Med 42 (2021) 729–738
https://doi.org/10.1016/j.ccm.2021.08.008
0272-5231/21/Published by Elsevier Inc.

chestmed.theclinics.com

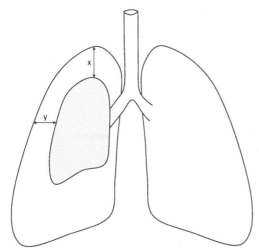

Fig. 1. Varying definitions of pneumothorax size. x = apex-to-cupola distance; y = interpleural distance at the hilum. Large pneumothorax: x > 3 cm (American College of Chest Physicians); y > 2 cm (British Thoracic Society).

widely across the literature, frequently cited as between 16% and 52%.[5] A recent meta-analysis suggested a recurrence rate of 32%, with a large majority of these occurring within the first year.[6] Although many factors may influence treatment for pneumothorax and will be discussed further, personalizing treatment based on risk of recurrence has been suggested as a way to optimize treatment for this broad clinical entity.

First Episode

Three options exist after the first episode of PSP: conservative management, simple aspiration, and tube thoracostomy. An algorithm suggesting management of PSP is shown in **Fig. 2**.

Conservative management

PSP may not cause significant respiratory symptoms, and tension pneumothorax from PSP is extremely rare.[7] Meanwhile, needle aspiration or chest tube insertion can be painful and is associated with a small but finite risk of complications including injury to surrounding organs (0.2%), malposition (0.6%), empyema (0.2%), and drain blockage (8.1%).[8] Thus, if a patient does not report dyspnea and the pneumothorax is small, conservative therapy is the preferred management strategy.[4] Conservative therapy may also be chosen in select patients with a large pneumothorax with minimal symptoms.

The administration of supplemental oxygen by face mask has been shown to increase the resorption of a pneumothorax by up to 4-fold.[9] Thus, administration by face mask at 10 L/min is suggested with an observation period of 4 to 6 hours followed by a repeat chest radiograph. If the pneumothorax remains stable or decreases in size and the patient does not report any significant symptoms, intervention may be deferred. Risk factor modification should also be pursued. Patients should be discouraged from airline travel or underwater diving until at least 1 week after radiographic resolution of spontaneous pneumothorax and 2 weeks after a traumatic pneumothorax.[10] Smoking is associated with the risk of recurrence of PSP,[11] and cessation should be strongly encouraged, because those who quit smoking had a 4-fold decreased risk of recurrence in a recent meta-analysis.[6] Even when managed conservatively, short-term follow-up with a thoracic specialist and repeat imaging should be arranged to ensure complete re-expansion of the lung.

A recent trial randomized 316 patients to conservative versus interventional treatment of moderate-to-large PSP, defined as occupying at least 32% of the hemithorax as calculated by the Collins method.[12,13] Although 15.4% of the patients assigned to the conservative treatment group underwent interventions for pneumothorax for prespecified reasons, the primary outcome of lung re-expansion within 8 weeks was not significantly different between the conservative and interventional groups (94.4% vs 98.5%). The trial concluded that conservative management of PSP resulted in a lower risk of serious adverse events or recurrence than interventional management.

Aspiration

Simple aspiration has been shown to be effective in up to 70% of patients with PSP[14–16] and may be associated with a decrease in the hospital length of stay.[17] Expertise with aspiration varies, and studies have shown poor compliance with guidelines suggesting aspiration as first-line intervention, possibly related to the ease and availability of small-bore chest tube insertion.[18,19] Further, studies have suggested a higher success rate of small-bore chest tube placement versus needle aspiration.[20] When performed, aspiration should proceed until 2.5 L of air is aspirated or increased resistance is encountered.[4] If no resistance is noted by 2.5 L, further lung re-expansion is unlikely to occur owing to the presence of persistent air leak. Depending on symptoms and size of pneumothorax, a tube thoracostomy may be considered.

Tube thoracostomy

When intervention is desired for significant symptoms, or needle aspiration fails, tube thoracostomy should be pursued. This procedure has been

Primary spontaneous pneumothorax (PSP)

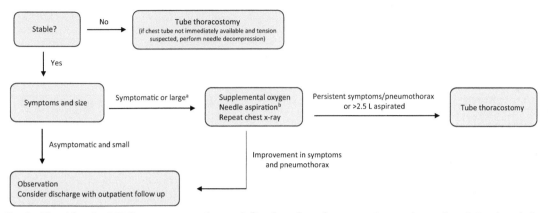

Fig. 2. Algorithm for PSP. [a]Large pneumothorax defined as >3 cm from apex to cupola or >2 cm interpleural distance at the level of the hilum. [b]Depending on local resources and expertise, pleural vent with ambulatory management or small-bore (≤14F) chest tube with hospital admission is an appropriate alternative.

considered the standard treatment and allows for the detection of an air leak after placement.

Small-bore versus large-bore chest tube In general, small-bore (≤14F) chest tubes are preferred to large-bore (>14F) chest tubes for the management of pneumothorax.[4,21] Specifically, a recent meta-analysis suggested that small-bore catheters are associated with similar success rates and a decreased incidence of complications, as well as a decreased length of drainage, versus large-bore chest tubes.[22] Several studies have shown decreased pain with small-bore chest tubes.[23,24] Further, most patients on mechanical ventilation are able to be managed with small-bore chest tubes.[25]

There are several instances when a large-bore chest tube may be more effective, such as when a large air leak is present or viscous fluid must be drained in addition to air. For example, 1 study showed a significantly decreased success rate of small-bore versus large-bore chest tubes (43% vs 88%; $P < .0001$) in mechanically ventilated patients with pneumothorax owing to barotrauma.[26] Additionally, large-bore chest tubes may be beneficial in unstable trauma patients and those with large volume air leaks related to bronchopleural fistula.[27] Finally, large-bore chest tubes placed by blunt dissection may be safer to place than small-bore chest tubes by the Seldinger technique in several instances. For example, in case of a small pneumothorax on mechanical ventilation or in previously instrumented pleural spaces, finger thoracostomy can ensure there is no pleurodesis at the access site and avoid needle injury to the lung parenchyma and intraparenchymal tube placement.

Suction or water seal? There is a theoretic risk that perpetuating flow through a visceral pleural defect with the use of suction may delay healing when compared with a water seal. However, objective data to prove this theory are lacking. Although some authors have suggested a shorter duration of air leak when chest tubes are placed to water seal after pulmonary resection,[28,29] other investigators have revealed no difference.[30] A recent meta-analysis revealed no difference in air leak duration, hospital length of stay, or occurrence of prolonged air leak after pulmonary surgery when comparing use of suction or water seal after pulmonary resection.[31]

The British Thoracic Society guidelines suggest against the routine use of suction after tube thoracostomy, citing the risk of re-expansion edema.[4,7] If the lung does not completely re-expand after 24 to 48 hours, suction may be considered to aid in visceral–parietal pleural apposition. However, other investigators suggest an initial period of suction to ensure pleural apposition, followed by a water seal when the lung has expanded. To the best of our knowledge, there are no data to indicate which strategy is superior. To prevent drain blockage, the tube should be flushed with 10 mL of sterile saline every 8 to 12 hours.[25] A sample algorithm for chest tube management after placement in PSP is shown is show in **Fig. 3**.

Ambulatory management

The Randomized Ambulatory Management of Primary Pneumothorax (RAMPP) trial recently evaluated the role of ambulatory management of PSP with an 8F pleural vent (Rocket Medical PLC, Watford, UK) versus standard management, which may include aspiration or insertion of tube

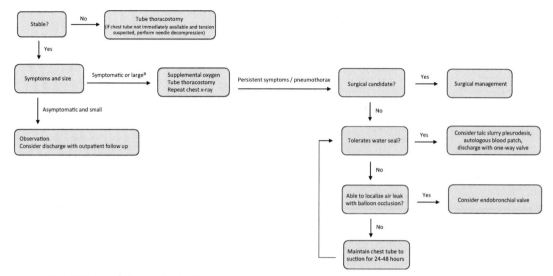

Fig. 3. Management of chest tube in PSP.

thoracostomy attached to underwater seal and admission to the hospital.[32] There was a significantly shorter hospital length of stay for patients managed with the pleural vent versus standard care. Those randomized to the pleural vent were at an increased risk of adverse events, including a 3% rate of enlarging pneumothorax requiring tube thoracostomy and 2% device malfunction. Although early results are promising, further studies are needed to define the role of the ambulatory management of PSP.

Recurrent Spontaneous Pneumothorax

Recurrence of spontaneous pneumothorax confers an increased risk of subsequent pneumothorax. One study suggested a 33% chance of recurrence after PSP and a 61% of second recurrence if treated conservatively.[33] Thus, in the case of recurrent spontaneous pneumothorax, tube thoracostomy should be placed if symptomatic and definitive management should be considered to reduce further risk of recurrence.

In addition to patients with recurrent PSP, definitive management may be considered for several groups: those in at-risk professions (eg, airline personnel, divers), a persistent air leak lasting more than 3 days, and bilateral pneumothorax or hemopneumothorax.[34] Definitive management strategies for pneumothorax are discussed elsewhere in this article.

SECONDARY SPONTANEOUS PNEUMOTHORAX
Conservative Management

In contrast with PSP, SSP is a potentially life-threatening event; patients with this condition are

at risk of increased symptoms and morbidity given the limited cardiopulmonary reserve in this patient population.[2] Further, SSP is associated with higher rates of recurrence (around 45%) and persistent air leak than PSP.[35,36] Thus, conservative management is not frequently used.

Ambulatory Management

A recent study evaluating ambulatory management of SSP with tube thoracostomy and underwater seal suggested safety using a 12F chest tube connected to an underwater seal. However, the overall length of stay was not shortened compared with standard management. The 8F pleural vent had a high failure rate (46%) and is not suggested in the ambulatory management of SSP.[37] Further trials are needed before this strategy is adopted routinely.

Treatment of the Underlying Disorder

Several underlying disorders contribute to the pathophysiology of pneumothorax, often through the formation of cysts or emphysema. Chronic obstructive pulmonary disease is the most common cause of SSP. Other disorders that are often associated with an increased risk of pneumothorax include cystic fibrosis, Birt–Hogg–Dube syndrome, lymphangioleiomyomatosis, pulmonary Langerhans cell histiocytosis, and catamenial pneumothorax. When SSP occurs, treatment of the underlying disorder should also be pursued to the extent possible. For example, catamenial pneumothorax is thought to be due to thoracic endometriosis, which causes cyclical pneumothorax within 3 days of menstruation.[38] Ectopic endometrial tissue is hormone responsive and in theory may be controlled with the administration of oral contraceptive pills or gonadotropin-releasing hormone agonists. However, a large case series suggests that recurrent pneumothorax occurs in 50% of patients treated with medical therapy alone at 6 months, and only 5% of patients treated with surgical therapy.[39] Thus, thoracoscopic surgery is important for both the diagnosis and management of this condition. Several authors have suggested the removal of the endometrial implants, repair of the diaphragmatic defects, and mechanical pleurodesis during thoracoscopic procedure in addition to postprocedural hormone therapy to minimize the risk of recurrence.[38]

Tube Thoracostomy and Definitive Management

In the case of recurrent SSP, tube thoracostomy and definitive management to mitigate risk of recurrence is suggested. Candidacy for operative approaches should be considered first, because the recurrence rates with either thoracoscopy or thoracotomy are lower than other methods.[4] For those unwilling or unfit for surgery, pleurodesis may also be achieved with the use of a sclerosant delivered through a chest tube. **Fig. 4** outlines the algorithm for management of a SSP.

TRAUMATIC PNEUMOTHORAX

Pneumothorax may also be caused by trauma, both blunt and penetrating, and iatrogenic causes. In fact, iatrogenic pneumothorax is seen more commonly than spontaneous pneumothorax.[40] Iatrogenic pneumothorax may be related to transthoracic needle aspiration, central line placement, pacemaker placement, bronchoscopic lung biopsies, thoracentesis, and pleural biopsy.[7]

Classically, chest tube placement has been recommended for all traumatic pneumothorax, owing to the fear that the pneumothorax may enlarge and contribute to an increased risk of tension physiology owing to hypovolemia from hemorrhage in many traumas. Occult pneumothorax, defined as a pneumothorax not seen on chest radiograph but visualized on computed tomography (CT) imaging, has been increasingly recognized in trauma.[41] However, more recent studies have suggested that observation in most occult pneumothorax is safe,[42,43] even in select patients requiring mechanical ventilation.[44]

DEFINITIVE MANAGEMENT

At the initial episode, indications for definitive management of pneumothorax include prolonged air leak (>72 hours), failure of lung re-expansion,

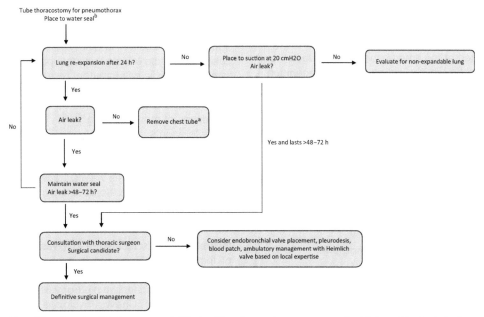

Fig. 4. Algorithm for chest tube removal. [a]If significant symptoms or suspected intermittent air leak, consider clamping chest tube for 4 hours followed by repeat chest radiograph before removal. [b]Alternatively, suction may be considered at chest tube placement, although has occasionally been associated with re-expansion pulmonary edema.

bilateral pneumothorax, tension pneumothorax, or the presence of single large bulla (**Box 1**).[4,34,45] Definitive management should also be considered with occupational hazards (eg, aircraft personnel or scuba divers). Additionally, definitive management is suggested in case of recurrence of pneumothorax, because studies have shown, that after the first recurrence, the likelihood of second recurrence ranges from 62% to 83%.[46]

Video-Assisted Thoracoscopic Surgery Versus Thoracotomy

Surgical approaches provide the most definitive treatment of pneumothorax and provide the lowest recurrence rates. The goals include resection of any abnormal lung parenchyma including visible bullae and obliteration of the pleural space. This process was originally described with open thoracotomy, but is now most commonly performed using thoracoscopic approaches.[4] Although thoracotomy has the lowest recurrence rate (1%–2%) for pneumothorax, it is not commonly performed owing to postoperative pain and recovery time. A meta-analysis suggested a 4-fold increased risk of recurrence with thoracoscopic surgery versus open surgery in recurrent pneumothorax.[47] However, recurrence rates with thoracoscopic surgery remain low (around 5%) and international guidelines recommend thoracoscopic surgery as the preferred approach owing to decreased bleeding, less postoperative pain, and a shorter postoperative hospital stay.[3,4,34,48,49] Often, additional procedures including chemical or mechanical pleurodesis are performed at the time of surgery to reduce recurrence, although it is not clear which technique is superior.

Box 1
Indications for definitive management of pneumothorax

Indications for surgical management in PSP

Prolonged air leak (>72 hours)

Failure of lung re-expansion

Bilateral or tension pneumothorax

Hemopneumothorax

Presence of single large bulla

Occupation at risk (eg, aircraft personnel, scuba diver)

Recurrent pneumothorax (ipsilateral or contralateral)

Increasingly, authors have questioned whether definitive management (including surgery) should be pursued after a first episode of PSP because the rates of recurrence are approximately 30% after a first episode.[46,50] Several studies have evaluated the use of a CT-based scoring system to predict the recurrence of pneumothorax.[51–55] Unfortunately, the results have been conflicting and a recent meta-analysis suggested that CT-based scores could not predict the recurrence of pneumothorax.[6] A recent trial associated a larger air leak, as measured by a digital air leak measurement device, with a prolonged hospital stay and an increased risk of treatment failure.[56] This finding suggests that early digital air leak measures may help to identify patients at high risk of failure or recurrence to undergo risk mitigation strategies at the first episode.

Pleurodesis

Mechanical Mechanical pleural abrasion during thoracotomy was first described in 1941 to decrease recurrence of pneumothorax.[57] This is most commonly achieved with the use of a scratch pad but has also been reported using Nd-YAG laser.[58] Although commonly performed, mechanical pleurodesis remains controversial as some trials have shown increased complications (mostly bleeding) and no decrease in recurrence of pneumothorax.[59,60]

Chemical A variety of agents have been used for pleurodesis including talc,[61] tetracycline,[36] bleomycin,[62] iodine,[63] and others.[64,65] Talc has shown the highest success rates up to 90%[66] and is frequently the agent of choice.[67] It is safe, with occasional adverse effects including pain, fever, and rarely a systemic inflammatory response. Reports of respiratory distress related to its use are thought to be related to older ungraded talc preparations and doses of more than 5 g.[68,69]

These agents may be delivered during surgical procedure (eg, talc poudrage) or via chest tube (via slurry). It is important to note that the efficacy of chemical pleurodesis via a surgical approach is higher than via a tube thoracostomy,[4] so this procedure should always be considered first if the patient is fit and willing to undergo surgery.

Pleurectomy This technique involves the removal of the parietal pleura and is another method to obliterate the pleural space. It is considered an alternative to mechanical pleurodesis in the American College of Chest Physicians guidelines.[3] Retrospective studies have suggested that pleurectomy has similar recurrence rate to pleurodesis.[70] The optimal surgical treatment of pneumothorax has not yet been determined, and many different approaches are followed based on local expertise. Further information will be obtained from randomized clinical trials evaluating wedge resection versus partial parietal pleurectomy in PSP (NCT01855464).

Resection

Wedge resection If any abnormal areas in the apical segment of the upper lobe are identified, they are often resected. Even if clear bullae cannot be clearly identified thoracoscopically, some surgeons may perform a wedge resection in the apical segment of the upper lobe and the superior segment of the lower lobe.[71] This is because abnormal pleural porosity may be detected in the absence of gross abnormality on CT scan or white light thoracoscopic inspection of the pleural surface.[72]

Endobronchial valves

Bronchoscopic valves have been used for the treatment of persistent air leaks, typically in those who are not candidate for surgery.[73–78] To be effective, the leak must be localized to a lobe, segment, or subsegment of the lung using balloon occlusion, with resolution or significant improvement of the air leak. This process also depends on whether patients have a complete fissure and if collateral ventilation is present. If balloon occlusion can localize and significantly decrease or stop a leak, valves may be placed in those segments. Typically, the valves are removed after about 6 weeks, when the visceral pleural defect has had time to heal.

Ambulatory chest tube with pneumostat

In patients who are unwilling or unfit to undergo surgery, he or she may be discharged home with a chest tube attached to a 1-way valve. There is extensive clinical experience with these valves, which have been used for more than 50 years.[79] Patients discharged with a chest tube and Heimlich valve must be able to access medical care and require close outpatient follow-up. Potential issues with this strategy include clogging or dislodgement of the tube, which may not be recognized by the patient.

FUTURE DIRECTIONS

Pneumothorax is a broad clinical condition with variety of severity. Several recent studies have evaluated less invasive management strategies for pneumothorax, including conservative or outpatient management. Future studies may help to identify who is most at risk for recurrence and direct earlier definitive management strategies, including thoracoscopic surgery, to those patients.

CLINICS CARE POINTS

- Initial management of a primary spontaneous pneumothorax does not always necessitate tube thoracostomy and can be managed conservatively if the patient is stable and asymptomatic.
- Pigtail chest tubes should almost always be chosen over large bore chest tubes for pneumothorax due to equivalent efficacy as well as significantly less patient discomfort.
- Newer technologies such as endobronchial valve placement should be considered for SSP alongside classic therapies such as slurry or thoracoscopic pleurodesis.

REFERENCES

1. Feller-Kopman D, Light R. Pleural disease. N Engl J Med 2018;378(8):740–51.
2. Sahn SA, Heffner JE. Spontaneous pneumothorax. N Engl J Med 2000;342(12):868–74.
3. Baumann MH, Strange C, Heffner JE, et al. Management of spontaneous pneumothorax: an American College of Chest Physicians Delphi consensus statement. Chest 2001;119(2):590–602.
4. MacDuff A, Arnold A, Harvey J, et al. Management of spontaneous pneumothorax: British Thoracic Society Pleural Disease Guideline 2010. Thorax 2010; 65(Suppl 2):ii18–31.
5. Schramel FM, Postmus PE, Vanderschueren RG. Current aspects of spontaneous pneumothorax. Eur Respir J 1997;10(6):1372–9.
6. Walker SP, Bibby AC, Halford P, et al. Recurrence rates in primary spontaneous pneumothorax: a systematic review and meta-analysis. Eur Respir J 2018;52(3).
7. Light RW. Pleural diseases. 6th edition. Philadelphia: Wolters Kluwer/Lippincott Williams & Wilkins Health; 2013. p. xiii,504.
8. Havelock T, Teoh R, Laws D, et al. Pleural procedures and thoracic ultrasound: British Thoracic Society Pleural Disease Guideline 2010. Thorax 2010; 65(Suppl 2):ii61–76.
9. Northfield TC. Oxygen therapy for spontaneous pneumothorax. Br Med J 1971;4(5779):86–8.
10. Ahmedzai S, Balfour-Lynn IM, Bewick T, et al. Managing passengers with stable respiratory disease planning air travel: British Thoracic Society recommendations. Thorax 2011;66(Suppl 1):i1–30.
11. Sadikot RT, Greene T, Meadows K, et al. Recurrence of primary spontaneous pneumothorax. Thorax 1997;52(9):805–9.

12. Brown SGA, Ball EL, Perrin K, et al. Conservative versus interventional treatment for spontaneous pneumothorax. N Engl J Med 2020;382(5):405–15.

13. Collins CD, Lopez A, Mathie A, et al. Quantification of pneumothorax size on chest radiographs using interpleural distances: regression analysis based on volume measurements from helical CT. AJR Am J Roentgenol 1995;165(5):1127–30.

14. Noppen M, Alexander P, Driesen P, et al. Manual aspiration versus chest tube drainage in first episodes of primary spontaneous pneumothorax: a multicenter, prospective, randomized pilot study. Am J Respir Crit Care Med 2002;165(9):1240–4.

15. Ayed AK, Chandrasekaran C, Sukumar M. Aspiration versus tube drainage in primary spontaneous pneumothorax: a randomised study. Eur Respir J 2006;27(3):477–82.

16. Thelle A, Gjerdevik M, SueChu M, et al. Randomised comparison of needle aspiration and chest tube drainage in spontaneous pneumothorax. Eur Respir J 2017;49(4).

17. Zhu P, Xia H, Sun Z, et al. Manual aspiration versus chest tube drainage in primary spontaneous pneumothorax without underlying lung diseases: a meta-analysis of randomized controlled trials. Interact Cardiovasc Thorac Surg 2019;28(6): 936–44.

18. Mendis D, El-Shanawany T, Mathur A, et al. Management of spontaneous pneumothorax: are British Thoracic Society guidelines being followed? Postgrad Med J 2002;78(916):80–4.

19. Packham S, Jaiswal P. Spontaneous pneumothorax: use of aspiration and outcomes of management by respiratory and general physicians. Postgrad Med J 2003;79(932):345–7.

20. Carson-Chahhoud KV, Wakai A, van Agteren JE, et al. Simple aspiration versus intercostal tube drainage for primary spontaneous pneumothorax in adults. Cochrane Database Syst Rev 2017;9: CD004479.

21. Light RW. Pleural controversy: optimal chest tube size for drainage. Respirology 2011;16(2):244–8.

22. Chang SH, Kang YN, Chiu HY, et al. A Systematic review and meta-analysis comparing pigtail catheter and chest tube as the initial treatment for pneumothorax. Chest 2018;153(5):1201–12.

23. Rahman NM, Pepperell J, Rehal S, et al. Effect of opioids vs NSAIDs and larger vs smaller chest tube size on pain control and pleurodesis efficacy among patients with malignant pleural effusion: the TIME1 randomized clinical trial. JAMA 2015; 314(24):2641–53.

24. Akowuah E, Ho EC, George R, et al. Less pain with flexible fluted silicone chest drains than with conventional rigid chest tubes after cardiac surgery. J Thorac Cardiovasc Surg 2002;124(5):1027–8.

25. Yarmus L, Feller-Kopman D. Pneumothorax in the critically ill patient. Chest 2012;141(4):1098–105.

26. Lin YC, Tu CY, Liang SJ, et al. Pigtail catheter for the management of pneumothorax in mechanically ventilated patients. Am J Emerg Med 2010;28(4): 466–71.

27. Ritchie M, Brown C, Bowling M. Chest tubes: indications, sizing, placement, and management. Clin Pulm Med 2017;24(1):37–53.

28. Cerfolio RJ, Bass C, Katholi CR. Prospective randomized trial compares suction versus water seal for air leaks. Ann Thorac Surg 2001;71(5):1613–7.

29. Marshall MB, Deeb ME, Bleier JI, et al. Suction vs water seal after pulmonary resection: a randomized prospective study. Chest 2002;121(3):831–5.

30. Alphonso N, Tan C, Utley M, et al. A prospective randomized controlled trial of suction versus non-suction to the under-water seal drains following lung resection. Eur J Cardiothorac Surg 2005; 27(3):391–4.

31. Zhou J, Chen N, Hai Y, et al. External suction versus simple water-seal on chest drainage following pulmonary surgery: an updated meta-analysis. Interact Cardiovasc Thorac Surg 2019;28(1):29–36.

32. Hallifax RJ, McKeown E, Sivakumar P, et al. Ambulatory management of primary spontaneous pneumothorax: an open-label, randomised controlled trial. Lancet 2020;396(10243):39–49.

33. Kuzucu A, Soysal O, Ulutas H. Optimal timing for surgical treatment to prevent recurrence of spontaneous pneumothorax. Surg Today 2006;36(10): 865–8.

34. Tschopp JM, Bintcliffe O, Astoul P, et al. ERS task force statement: diagnosis and treatment of primary spontaneous pneumothorax. Eur Respir J 2015; 46(2):321–35.

35. Chee CB, Abisheganaden J, Yeo JK, et al. Persistent air-leak in spontaneous pneumothorax–clinical course and outcome. Respir Med 1998;92(5):757–61.

36. Light RW, O'Hara VS, Moritz TE, et al. Intrapleural tetracycline for the prevention of recurrent spontaneous pneumothorax. Results of a Department of Veterans Affairs cooperative study. JAMA 1990; 264(17):2224–30.

37. Walker SP, Keenan E, Bintcliffe O, et al. Ambulatory management of secondary spontaneous pneumothorax: a randomised controlled trial. Eur Respir J 2021;57(6):2003375.

38. Alifano M. Catamenial pneumothorax. Curr Opin Pulm Med 2010;16(4):381–6.

39. Joseph J, Sahn SA. Thoracic endometriosis syndrome: new observations from an analysis of 110 cases. Am J Med 1996;100(2):164–70.

40. Despars JA, Sassoon CS, Light RW. Significance of iatrogenic pneumothoraces. Chest 1994;105(4): 1147–50.

41. Ball CG, Kirkpatrick AW, Feliciano DV. The occult pneumothorax: what have we learned? Can J Surg 2009;52(5):E173–9.

42. Walker SP, Barratt SL, Thompson J, et al. Conservative management in traumatic pneumothoraces: an observational study. Chest 2018;153(4):946–53.

43. Moore FO, Goslar PW, Coimbra R, et al. Blunt traumatic occult pneumothorax: is observation safe?–results of a prospective, AAST multicenter study. J Trauma 2011;70(5):1019–23 [discussion: 23–5].

44. Clements TW, Sirois M, Parry N, et al. OPTICC: a multicentre trial of Occult Pneumothoraces subjected to mechanical ventilation: the final report. Am J Surg 2021;221(6):1252–8.

45. Shields' general thoracic surgery. 8th edition. Philadelphia: Wolters Kluwer Health/Lippincott Williams & Wilkins; 2019. p. 2512.

46. Schnell J, Beer M, Eggeling S, et al. Management of spontaneous pneumothorax and post-interventional pneumothorax: German S3 guideline. Respiration 2019;97(4):370–402.

47. Barker A, Maratos EC, Edmonds L, et al. Recurrence rates of video-assisted thoracoscopic versus open surgery in the prevention of recurrent pneumothoraces: a systematic review of randomised and non-randomised trials. Lancet 2007;370(9584):329–35.

48. Goto T, Kadota Y, Mori T, et al. Video-assisted thoracic surgery for pneumothorax: republication of a systematic review and a proposal by the guideline committee of the Japanese association for chest surgery 2014. Gen Thorac Cardiovasc Surg 2015;63(1):8–13.

49. Tschopp JM, Rami-Porta R, Noppen M, et al. Management of spontaneous pneumothorax: state of the art. Eur Respir J 2006;28(3):637–50.

50. Cardillo G, Ricciardi S, Rahman N, et al. Primary spontaneous pneumothorax: time for surgery at first episode? J Thorac Dis 2019;11(Suppl 9):S1393–7.

51. Martinez-Ramos D, Angel-Yepes V, Escrig-Sos J, et al. [Usefulness of computed tomography in determining risk of recurrence after a first episode of primary spontaneous pneumothorax: therapeutic implications]. Arch Bronconeumol 2007;43(6):304–8.

52. Ouanes-Besbes L, Golli M, Knani J, et al. Prediction of recurrent spontaneous pneumothorax: CT scan findings versus management features. Respir Med 2007;101(2):230–6.

53. Casali C, Stefani A, Ligabue G, et al. Role of blebs and bullae detected by high-resolution computed tomography and recurrent spontaneous pneumothorax. Ann Thorac Surg 2013;95(1):249–55.

54. Primavesi F, Jager T, Meissnitzer T, et al. First episode of spontaneous pneumothorax: CT-based scoring to select patients for early surgery. World J Surg 2016;40(5):1112–20.

55. Park S, Jang HJ, Song JH, et al. Do blebs or bullae on high-resolution computed tomography predict ipsilateral recurrence in young patients at the first episode of primary spontaneous pneumothorax? Korean J Thorac Cardiovasc Surg 2019;52(2):91–9.

56. Hallifax RJ, Laskawiec-Szkonter M, Rahman NM, et al. Predicting outcomes in primary spontaneous pneumothorax using air leak measurements. Thorax 2019;74(4):410–2.

57. Tyson M, Crandall W. The surgical treatment of recurrent idiopathic spontaneous pneumothorax. J Thorac Surg 1941;10:566–70.

58. Torre M, Grassi M, Nerli FP, et al. Nd-YAG laser pleurodesis via thoracoscopy. Endoscopic therapy in spontaneous pneumothorax Nd-YAG laser pleurodesis. Chest 1994;106(2):338–41.

59. Min X, Huang Y, Yang Y, et al. Mechanical pleurodesis does not reduce recurrence of spontaneous pneumothorax: a randomized trial. Ann Thorac Surg 2014;98(5):1790–6 [discussion: 6].

60. Ling ZG, Wu YB, Ming MY, et al. The effect of pleural abrasion on the treatment of primary spontaneous pneumothorax: a systematic review of randomized controlled trials. PLoS One 2015;10(6):e0127857.

61. Genofre EH, Marchi E, Vargas FS. Inflammation and clinical repercussions of pleurodesis induced by intrapleural talc administration. Clinics (Sao Paulo) 2007;62(5):627–34.

62. Ong KC, Indumathi V, Raghuram J, et al. A comparative study of pleurodesis using talc slurry and bleomycin in the management of malignant pleural effusions. Respirology 2000;5(2):99–103.

63. Mohsen TA, Zeid AA, Meshref M, et al. Local iodine pleurodesis versus thoracoscopic talc insufflation in recurrent malignant pleural effusion: a prospective randomized control trial. Eur J Cardiothorac Surg 2011;40(2):282–6.

64. Chen JS, Hsu HH, Chen RJ, et al. Additional minocycline pleurodesis after thoracoscopic surgery for primary spontaneous pneumothorax. Am J Respir Crit Care Med 2006;173(5):548–54.

65. Tsuboshima K, Wakahara T, Matoba Y, et al. Pleural coating by 50% glucose solution reduces postoperative recurrence of spontaneous pneumothorax. Ann Thorac Surg 2018;106(1):184–91.

66. Kennedy L, Sahn SA. Talc pleurodesis for the treatment of pneumothorax and pleural effusion. Chest 1994;106(4):1215–22.

67. Sahn SA. Talc should be used for pleurodesis. Am J Respir Crit Care Med 2000;162(6):2023–4 [discussion: 6].

68. Janssen JP, Collier G, Astoul P, et al. Safety of pleurodesis with talc poudrage in malignant pleural effusion: a prospective cohort study. Lancet 2007;369(9572):1535–9.

69. Maskell NA, Lee YC, Gleeson FV, et al. Randomized trials describing lung inflammation after pleurodesis with talc of varying particle size. Am J Respir Crit Care Med 2004;170(4):377–82.

70. Ocakcioglu I, Kupeli M. Surgical treatment of spontaneous pneumothorax: pleural abrasion or pleurectomy? Surg Laparosc Endosc Percutan Tech 2019; 29(1):58–63.

71. Sugarbaker DJ. Sugarbaker's adult chest surgery. 3rd edition. New York: McGraw Hill Education; 2020.

72. Noppen M, Stratakos G, Verbanck S, et al. Fluorescein-enhanced autofluorescence thoracoscopy in primary spontaneous pneumothorax. Am J Respir Crit Care Med 2004;170(6):680–2.

73. Ferguson JS, Sprenger K, Van Natta T. Closure of a bronchopleural fistula using bronchoscopic placement of an endobronchial valve designed for the treatment of emphysema. Chest 2006;129(2): 479–81.

74. Wood DE, Cerfolio RJ, Gonzalez X, et al. Bronchoscopic management of prolonged air leak. Clin Chest Med 2010;31(1):127–33.

75. Schiavon M, Marulli G, Zuin A, et al. Endobronchial valve for secondary pneumothorax in a severe emphysema patient. Thorac Cardiovasc Surg 2011;59(8):509–10.

76. Gillespie CT, Sterman DH, Cerfolio RJ, et al. Endobronchial valve treatment for prolonged air leaks of the lung: a case series. Ann Thorac Surg 2011; 91(1):270–3.

77. Fischer W, Feller-Kopman D, Shah A, et al. Endobronchial valve therapy for pneumothorax as a bridge to lung transplantation. J Heart Lung Transpl 2012;31(3):334–6.

78. Travaline JM, McKenna RJ Jr, De Giacomo T, et al. Treatment of persistent pulmonary air leaks using endobronchial valves. Chest 2009;136(2):355–60.

79. Heimlich HJ. Valve drainage of the pleural cavity. Dis Chest 1968;53(3):282–7.

Section 5: Minimally Invasive Definitive Pleural Intervention

Indwelling Pleural Catheters

Audra J. Schwalk, MD, MBA[a],*, David E. Ost, MD, MPH[b]

KEYWORDS

- Indwelling pleural catheter • Tunneled pleural catheter • Malignant pleural effusion
- Nonmalignant pleural effusion • Pleurodesis

KEY POINTS

- Indwelling pleural catheters may be used in the management of recurrent, symptomatic malignant and nonmalignant pleural effusions and are the treatment of choice for nonexpandable lung.
- Indwelling pleural catheters and thoracoscopic or chest tube chemical pleurodesis both improve patient symptoms of breathlessness and health-related quality of life to a similar extent.
- Indwelling pleural catheter placement plus pleural sclerosant administration may be both a palliative and cost-effective treatment option for patients with an expandable lung.
- Many indwelling pleural catheter-related infectious complications can be managed without catheter removal.

INTRODUCTION

Pleural effusion is a common clinical problem estimated to affect 1.5 million people in the United States each year.[1] A large proportion are either nonmalignant or related to infection,[2] but malignant pleural effusions (MPEs) may also lead to significant health care resource use with an estimated 150,000 cases annually.[3,4] Lung cancer is the leading cause of MPE and is present in up to 15% of patients at diagnosis, with an even greater proportion of patients developing MPE at some point in the course of their disease.[5] MPE can complicate almost any cancer[6] and may also develop as the primary manifestation of a disease, as is the case with malignant mesothelioma.

After the identification of a symptomatic pleural effusion, a thoracentesis is typically performed for cytologic and laboratory evaluation of pleural fluid, as well as for assessment of symptom improvement and lung re-expansion. Despite initial drainage, more than one-half of MPEs will recur within 90 days.[7] Recurrent effusions may cause significant dyspnea, cough, and chest discomfort,

resulting in a poor quality of life for these patients. A definitive pleural procedure is recommended for patients with recurrent, symptomatic MPE,[3,6,8] except in cases of slow fluid reaccumulation, an expected rapid and marked response to treatment, or a very short life expectancy. Several options are available for the definitive management of MPE.

Indwelling pleural catheters (IPCs) are one option for definitive MPE management. IPCs are being placed with increasing frequency since their introduction more than 30 years ago[9] and the body of evidence pertaining to their use continues to grow. Initially, observational studies and retrospective reviews comprised the majority of publications, but several larger, randomized controlled trials (RCTs) are now available. Many compare IPC placement to chemical pleurodesis, either thoracoscopic or via chest tube, but the primary outcomes between studies are inconsistent, making direct comparison of results difficult. Until recently, most of the available literature on IPCs pertained to patient selection, indications, and postprocedural outcomes; however, guidelines

[a] Division of Pulmonary and Critical Care, The University of Texas Southwestern Medical Center, Professional Office Building II, 5939 Harry Hines Boulevard, Dallas, TX 75390, USA; [b] Department of Pulmonary Medicine, The University of Texas MD Anderson Cancer Center, Unit 1462, 1515 Holcombe Boulevard, Houston, TX 77030, USA
* Corresponding author.
E-mail address: Audra.schwalk@utsouthwestern.edu

Clin Chest Med 42 (2021) 739–750
https://doi.org/10.1016/j.ccm.2021.08.009
0272-5231/21/© 2021 Elsevier Inc. All rights reserved.

and expert panel recommendations regarding postinsertion IPC management are now available. This review summarizes the latest, high-quality evidence and recommendations for IPC use.

THERAPEUTIC OPTIONS

Before discussing IPCs in greater detail, it is important to review available options for the management of recurrent, symptomatic MPE. Historically, definitive treatment involved a surgical procedure and hospitalization, with a median length of stay ranging from 5 to 10 days depending on the specific procedure performed.[5] Thoracoscopic talc pleurodesis may be performed by an interventional pulmonologist in an endoscopy suite using one access port with local anesthesia and moderate sedation. A video-assisted thoracoscopic surgery (VATS) pleurodesis procedure, however, is usually performed by a thoracic surgeon in an operating room. This procedure is more invasive because it typically requires multiple access ports, a double-lumen endotracheal tube, and general anesthesia. Both procedures allow for biopsy of the parietal pleura, evaluation of full lung re-expansion, lysis of simple adhesions, and adequate instillation of pleural sclerosants, but VATS may allow for improved visualization of the pleura given the lung is fully deflated.[5] VATS also provides the ability to perform complementary procedures such as mechanical abrasion, lysis of more complex adhesions, decortication for treatment of nonexpandable lung, and parietal pleurectomy, which may be beneficial in certain clinical scenarios.[5] VATS is typically reserved for patients with good functional status who are deemed acceptable surgical candidates, but for those not meeting these criteria, alternative treatment methods are typically pursued.

Chest tube drainage followed by pleurodesis with a sclerosing agent is another option for the management of recurrent, symptomatic MPE. This method may be an option for patients who are not surgical candidates or for patients who already have a chest tube in place; however, similar to VATS pleurodesis, it requires an inpatient hospital stay of several days.[10–13]

IPCs are now commonly being offered as an alternative to surgical pleurodesis and other definitive procedures.[9,14] This change is likely secondary to the ease of placement and lack of need for hospitalization and sedation,[9,10] while still providing improvement in symptoms.[15] IPC placement may be performed by a variety of practitioners, such as pulmonologists, surgeons, and interventional radiologists. The administration of talc and other sclerosants through an IPC is also a viable treatment option in some patients and has been the focus of recent publications.[16]

PREPROCEDURE PLANNING

Patients with a recurrent pleural effusion that experience symptom improvement after initial pleural fluid drainage should be considered for IPC placement or other definitive treatment.[3,6,8] Preprocedure counseling pertaining to IPC placement, home drainage procedures, and catheter-related care should be routine.[17] Patients should provide their informed consent, demonstrate an adequate understanding of the IPC and potential complications, and also have a reliable caregiver available to assist in catheter drainage and routine care before consideration of IPC placement. Insurance often covers IPC drainage bottles and related supplies, but this factor should also be confirmed before catheter placement to avoid any interruptions in patient care.

PROCEDURAL APPROACH

Several IPC options are available and the decision to use one catheter over another depends on local availability as well as patient and provider preference. Each of the catheters have slight differences, but all are made of soft silicone and have multiple fenestrations to allow for the drainage of pleural fluid. The Merit Medical Aspira pleural drainage system is designed to drain pleural fluid with low pressure via gravity,[18] whereas the PleurX and Rocket pleural drainage systems are designed to drain pleural fluid via a vacuum bottle.[19,20]

The details of IPC placement may vary between institutions and depending on what specific catheter is being placed, but generally are quite similar. One approach to IPC placement is provided in **Box 1**. Videos for PleurX, Aspira, and Rocket catheter placement may be viewed at: https://www.bd.com/en-us/company/video-gallery?video=903266637001 (procedure begins at 3:46 minutes), https://www.myaspira.com/videos/ (insertion of a peritoneal catheter, although similar kit contents and technique), and https://sales.rocketmedical.com/products/indwelling-drainage-catheters, respectively.

Complications during IPC placement are rare but should be recognized because they can occur in 2.8% to 6% of procedures. Complications are similar to those encountered with any pleural procedure and include pneumothorax (generally not clinically significant because these usually arise from the entry of atmospheric air as opposed to visceral pleural injury and there will now be a catheter in the pleural space), bleeding, subcutaneous

Box 1
Outlined procedure for IPC placement

1. Place the patient in a semirecumbent position. Other positions are acceptable depending on patient tolerance and expected insertion site.

2. Secure the patient's ipsilateral arm above the head or across the chest to fully expose the potential pleural entry site.

3. Identify the optimal site for IPC insertion and exit with the use of ultrasound examination and mark these sites. When possible, avoid areas of skin with evidence of active infection or malignant skin infiltration.

4. Clean the pleural entry and exit sites as well as the surrounding chest wall.

5. Don sterile personal protective equipment and prepare the IPC insertion kit.

6. Use the filter straw to prepare syringes with 1% lidocaine and then anesthetize the skin, subcutaneous tissue and parietal pleura with the 22G or 25G needles.

7. Advance the guidewire introducer with needle in the anesthetized area, while applying suction, until pleural fluid is aspirated.

8. Hold the needle and syringe stable and advance the guidewire introducer into the pleural space until it is flush against the patient's skin. Remove the needle. Pleural fluid may drain out of the guidewire introducer at this point.

9. Insert the J-tip wire through the guidewire introducer and into the pleural space.

10. Remove the guidewire introducer, leaving the guidewire in place.

11. Use the scalpel to make an approximate 1-cm incision around the wire in the patient's skin and subcutaneous tissue. This is the pleural entry site. Make a second incision approximately 5 cm from the pleural entry site. This will serve as the catheter exit site.

12. Attach the metal tunneler to the fenestrated end of the pleural catheter and tunnel the catheter under the skin and subcutaneous tissue, entering at the catheter exit site and directing the tunneler toward the pleural entry site. Pass the tunneler out through the pleural entry site (where the guidewire is located). Pull the tunneler through the pleural entry site until the catheter cuff is just under the skin at the catheter exit site. Once in position, remove the metal tunneler from the catheter.

13. Advance the peel-away introducer over the wire and into the pleural space.

14. Remove the central dilator and the wire while leaving the peel away sheath in place. Pleural fluid may drain out of the peel away sheath at this point.

15. Insert the fenestrated end of the catheter through the peel away sheath and into the pleural space.

16. Peel away the sheath while advancing the catheter into the pleural space using a thumb.

17. Ensure the catheter is inserted fully into the pleural space and feel for any evidence of a kinked catheter.

18. Attach the catheter tip to the specialized drainage bottle or suction using the appropriate adapter with access tip. Drain the pleural space. This process ensures that the catheter is functioning well after placement and allows for any necessary troubleshooting while the patient is in the procedure area.

19. Remove the access tip and drainage line and place the specialized cap on the end of the catheter.

20. Use the 2-0 silk, straight needle suture to secure the IPC to the skin.

21. Use the 4-0 absorbable, curved needle suture to close the insertion site incision.

22. Place the foam catheter pad on the skin and coil the catheter on top of it, then cover with gauze.

23. Use the provided self-adhesive dressing for optimal coverage and catheter protection.

emphysema, pain, and unintended mispositioning of the catheter (**Fig. 1**).[21] Postprocedure chest radiography is often obtained to document proper IPC placement and the patient is typically discharged the same day.

POSTPROCEDURE RECOVERY AND MANAGEMENT

IPC drainage can be performed by a variety of people, including the patient, spouse or other caregivers, and medical providers. Routine IPC education is again provided before discharge and is typically accomplished with hands-on training, in addition to instructional videos and handbooks provided by the IPC manufacturer.

A specific follow-up schedule for patients with an IPC has not been established given the lack of formal studies pertaining to this topic. Regular follow-up is recommended, even in the absence of catheter-related concerns, with the frequency being determined on an individual basis.[4] The

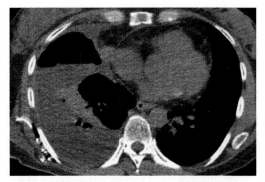

Fig. 1. A malpositioned IPC as seen outside the pleural space in this chest computed tomography image. This catheter was replaced without significant long-term complications.

hope is that potential complications or concerns are identified and addressed early in the process. It is important to acknowledge that many patients with cancer report a substantial time burden related to treatment and follow-up appointments[22]; therefore,

personalized decision-making should be used when determining the optimal follow-up plan.

Drainage protocols and algorithms for IPC removal vary between institutions. General recommendations are to decrease drainage frequency when output decreases to less than a certain volume, often 50 to 100 mL.[14] One example of a conservative IPC drainage and removal algorithm is provided in **Fig. 2**. The reported incidence of successful pleurodesis allowing IPC removal is variable, but seems to be less than 50%.[15,23,24] Before removal, patients should be made aware of the potential need for future pleural interventions because up to 10% of pleural effusions may recur after IPC removal.[15,25]

CONSIDERATIONS
Nonexpandable Lung

An IPC may be placed in almost any patient and allows for regular home drainage of pleural fluid with resultant improvement in symptoms and quality of

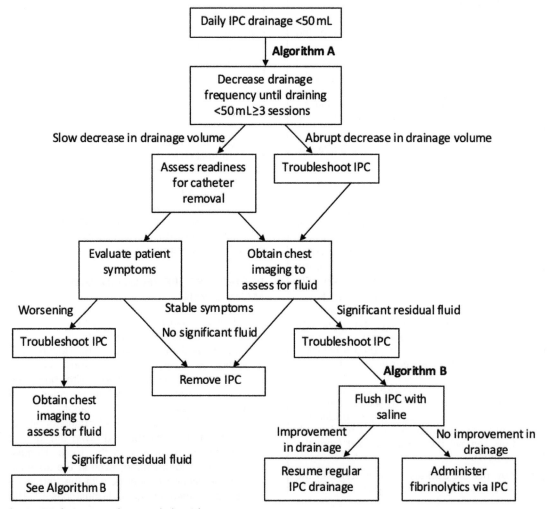

Fig. 2. IPC drainage and removal algorithm.

life.[10,15,23,24] Specific patient populations may benefit more from IPC placement when compared with other definitive management approaches. In patients with a nonexpandable lung, where adequate apposition of the parietal and visceral pleura are not achieved after pleural fluid drainage, guidelines recommend the placement of an IPC over chemical pleurodesis.[6–8] One of the first publications to report the use of IPCs for MPE and nonexpandable lung was by Pien and colleagues in 2001,[26] when they described their experience with 11 patients, 3 of whom had previously been treated with radiation therapy, attempted talc pleurodesis, or decortication without successful resolution of symptoms. Although the specific details regarding how symptom and radiographic improvement were determined were not provided, all patients were reported to have symptomatic benefit in cough, dyspnea, and exercise tolerance.[26] Several larger observational studies on the use of IPC for patients with nonexpandable lung have since been published, each reporting various patient outcomes, including symptom improvement, pleurodesis rate, median survival after IPC placement, and complications.[27–32] It is difficult to directly compare results from these studies because the units of measurement for the outcomes are quite variable, but most studies report symptomatic improvement in the majority of patients. More recent RCTs have shown improvement in dyspnea and quality of life that is comparable with that achieved in patients with a fully expandable lung after talc pleurodesis.[10] It should also be noted that, in the AMPLE-2 trial, approximately 50% of patients with a nonexpandable lung achieved pleurodesis at 6 months.[23] In addition to patients with a nonexpandable lung, IPC placement may be the best treatment strategy for those with interconnected pleural loculations, especially if deemed a poor surgical candidate.[7]

Failed Pleurodesis Procedure

A pleurodesis procedure may be unsuccessful in up to 30% of patients[33]; therefore, further interventions may be necessary in a good proportion of these patients.[27] IPCs are often placed at the time of a talc poudrage procedure. This practice allows for continuous pleural fluid drainage after the procedure, facilitating visceral and parietal apposition and hopefully improving the chance of successful pleurodesis, while also serving as a back-up therapy in the event that pleurodesis fails.[9,34,35] This strategy may shorten hospital length of stay because a standard chest tube is not required and patients can continue regular drainage after hospital discharge.[34,35]

Other Clinical Considerations

IPC placement is a straightforward procedure that is performed using local anesthesia without the need for sedation. It provides a good alternative treatment option for patients unable or unwilling to undergo a surgical procedure, as well as for patients wishing to minimize hospitalization.[10–13] Patients with a very short life expectancy, however, may be best managed with repeat thoracentesis and other supportive measures, rather than an IPC or pleurodesis procedure.[25]

After a discussion of viable treatment options, patient preference should take priority. Swimming, submerging in bath water, diving, or otherwise performing activities that may result in soaking of the IPC dressing are not recommended for some of the IPCs owing to fears of an increased risk of infection; however, there are no data to support this supposition. If the patient is interested in performing these activities, it may be necessary to discuss alternative methods for symptom management.

GOALS

Given that MPE is generally considered a poor prognostic factor,[8] the main goals for treatment are palliation of symptoms, limiting unnecessary pleural procedures, and minimizing the need for hospitalization, as well as decreasing the hospital length of stay when required. Historically, pleurodesis rates have been the focus of many early IPC studies. More recent publications, however, emphasize patient-centered outcomes such as dyspnea, quality of life, complications, and hospital length of stay.[10–12,23] It is from these studies that we know IPCs improve patient symptoms, but are only associated with modest improvements in quality-adjusted lifedays and utility. The greatest improvements are seen in patients with worse baseline shortness of breath and those who pursue systemic chemotherapy or localized radiation after placement.[15] There are also potential disadvantages to treatment with an IPC, including complications, cost, and the need for regular drainage procedures. These issues further highlight the need for a thorough discussion regarding patient preferences and expected outcomes during individualized management of an MPE.

CLINICAL OUTCOMES
Pleurodesis Rates

Because IPC use is increasing and drainage may be performed at the convenience of the patient, investigations to identify optimal drainage regimens have been conducted. Two RCTs, ASAP (Impact of Aggressive vs Standard Drainage Regimen Using a Long Term IPC) and AMPLE-2 (Australasian Malignant PLeural Effusion-2) evaluated patient outcomes with various drainage regimens. The ASAP trial compared daily with every other day drainage of the same volume of fluid,[24] whereas the AMPLE-2 study compared daily with symptom-guided IPC drainage.[23] Both studies defined pleurodesis as pleural fluid drainage of less than 50 mL on 3 consecutive drainage attempts and improved radiographic scores, but the ASAP trial also specified a lack of patient symptoms.[23,24] Each study determined that daily IPC drainage was more likely to result in either complete or partial pleurodesis after IPC placement, with associated fewer catheter-days, when compared with a less aggressive drainage regimen, although pleurodesis rates were not the primary outcome in the AMPLE-2 trial.[23,24] Most cases of pleurodesis and catheter removal occurred in the first 60 days after placement.[23,24] If IPC removal is a patient priority, then an aggressive drainage regimen should be used, but in instances when this is not a strong consideration, symptom-guided drainage is reasonable.[4]

The pleurodesis rates of IPC in conjunction with pleural sclerosants has also been evaluated. Bhatnagar and colleagues[16] randomized patients to IPC plus talc slurry or placebo and found those treated with IPC plus talc slurry achieved pleurodesis at a significantly higher rate, at least during the initial follow-up period. A small study evaluating the safety of silver nitrate–coated IPCs also reported high pleurodesis rates with a median time to pleurodesis of 4 days. No formal conclusions can be drawn from this study given the small sample size, but results from a larger, multicenter RCT should be available in the near future.[36]

Whereas patient-centered outcomes should be a priority when managing recurrent MPE, pleurodesis rates are important from a cost perspective. A recent analysis evaluating the cost effectiveness of various drainage regimens and IPC plus talc administration determined daily IPC drainage was not cost effective in any clinical scenario.[37] Symptom-guided IPC drainage was most cost effective for patients with a life expectancy of less than 4 months or an expected probability of pleurodesis greater than 20%.[37] Considering individual patient-related factors such as life expectancy and desire to minimize catheter-days, IPC plus pleural sclerosant administration may provide a palliative and cost-effective option for the treatment of recurrent, symptomatic MPE.[37]

The optimal IPC drainage regimen in patients with a nonexpandable lung is less clear than in those with a fully expandable lung because of a lack of formal studies evaluating this topic. Approximately one-third of the patients included in the AMPLE-2 trial had nonexpandable lung. Although patients with a nonexpandable lung had an overall lower pleurodesis rate than patients whose lungs expanded, aggressive IPC drainage was still associated with a higher pleurodesis rate when compared with symptom-guided drainage in patients with nonexpandable lung.[23] Although this data may provide insight as to the effect of daily drainage on patients with a nonexpandable lung, it should be interpreted with caution because it was obtained after a post hoc analysis of very few patients. If catheter removal is a priority, then an aggressive IPC drainage strategy can be considered, even in the setting of a nonexpandable lung, but in patients who experience significant discomfort with daily drainage, this regimen is not recommended.[4]

Chemical pleurodesis rates are variable and depend on the sclerosing agent as well as the underlying method of instillation.[25,38] IPC-related pleurodesis rates are typically lower when compared with chemical or surgical pleurodesis performed as a slurry via chest tube or via poudrage, but as discussed elsewhere in this article, patient-centered outcomes, rather than the achievement of pleurodesis, may be the best measures of successful MPE management.[15,25]

Symptomatic Improvement

Although it is now well-established that IPCs provide symptomatic improvement in patients with MPE,[15,23,24] many studies have sought to determine if there is a significant difference in improvement when compared with that achieved with chemical pleurodesis. The TIME2 (Second Therapeutic Intervention in Malignant Effusion) RCT evaluated whether IPCs were more effective at relieving dyspnea than chest tube placement and talc slurry pleurodesis as measured on a 100-mm visual analog scale. Both groups experienced an improvement in dyspnea and there was no significant difference between the 2 groups at 3 months, but at 6 months patients with an IPC had less dyspnea than patients who underwent talc pleurodesis.[10] A second, smaller RCT compared IPC with talc pleurodesis with the primary end point being improvement in the baseline Modified Borg Score. Again, dyspnea improved in both groups after the intervention, but the magnitude of improvement was not significantly different between the 2 groups.[12] Two other RCTs evaluated both dyspnea and quality of life improvement in patients with IPC compared with chemical pleurodesis.[11,13]

Whereas the measurements of breathlessness and quality of life were different in the 2 studies, both reported high baseline breathlessness scores and poor quality of life that improved after the respective interventions. Putnam and colleagues[13] noted that patients with IPC had significantly improved Borg scores after exercise at 30 days when compared with the doxycycline pleurodesis group, but this difference was not sustained throughout the follow-up period. No other significant between group differences were identified in breathlessness or quality of life in either study.[11,13] One propensity-matched observational study compared symptom palliation in patients with IPC versus VATS talc pleurodesis. Although the long-term follow-up was poor, no significant difference in Eastern Cooperative Oncology Group performance status was identified.[39] A review of the available data shows that IPC placement leads to an improvement in breathlessness and quality of life comparable with that achieved with chemical pleurodesis. In addition, the combination of IPC plus talc slurry administration further improves patient breathlessness and quality of life scores at various timepoints when compared with IPC alone.[16] The usefulness of other pleural sclerosants in conjunction with IPCs is currently being evaluated.

IPC drainage regimens have also been evaluated for their effect on symptom improvement. In the AMPLE-2 study comparing daily versus symptom-guided drainage, there was no significant difference in the mean daily breathlessness or quality of life as measured on a 100-mm visual analog scale between the 2 groups; however, patients in the daily drainage group reported a better quality of life than patients in the symptom-guided group as measured by the EuroQoL-5 Dimensions-5 Levels.[23] Similar improvements in both the Karnofsky Performance Score and the RAND 36-Item Short Form Health Survey scores were obtained in the ASAP trial comparing daily versus 3 times a week drainage.[24] IPC drainage regimen does not seem to have a significant effect on breathlessness, but there are conflicting data on whether quality of life is impacted by drainage strategy.

Health Care Resource Use

Patients with MPE spend a substantial amount of time in the hospital, and decreased hospitalization rates and shorter lengths of stay are a priority for many, especially near the end of their life.[11] Two RCTs have compared IPC placement with chemical pleurodesis and evaluated hospital length of stay as the primary study outcome. The AMPLE (Australasian Malignant PLeural Effusion) trial found that, in those treated with an IPC, there

was a significant decrease in total hospitalization days within the first year after the initial procedure, including the initial hospitalization. Putnam and colleagues[13] also determined that the initial hospital length of stay was significantly shorter for the IPC group when compared with the pleurodesis group. Two other studies have evaluated hospital length of stay in patients undergoing IPC placement versus talc pleurodesis as a secondary outcome and also found an IPC shortens the duration of the initial hospitalization.[10,12] A smaller observational study came to the same conclusion as these larger RCTs when comparing IPC versus VATS talc pleurodesis.[39] Overall, it is clear from the literature that IPC placement is associated with fewer hospitalization days when compared with chemical pleurodesis using either chest tubes or thoracoscopy.

Although the need for additional procedures has not been the primary outcome of any available study, IPC placement is associated with a significantly decreased need for ipsilateral pleural fluid drainage when compared with either chest tube or thoracoscopic chemical pleurodesis, and this difference becomes more evident the longer patients are followed.[11,12,39,40]

From a health care cost perspective, the initial hospitalization required for thoracoscopic or chest tube pleurodesis is more costly, but a comparison with IPC requires consideration of life expectancy and total cost over the life of the patient to manage the problem of MPE. For patients with a shorter expected survival duration, the total costs of IPC strategies may be lower, whereas for those expected to live longer, chemical pleurodesis may prove to be less expensive because the cost for supplies related to continued IPC use would be less.[37] These cost considerations must be balanced against any differences in quality-adjusted survival.[37] Individual patient preferences strongly impact perceived utility and quality of life, so cost-effectiveness analysis should be applied appropriately and with caution, making sure to take into account individual level factors for each decision.

Survival

From the available data, there does not seem to be a difference in mortality between patients with IPC versus those treated with chemical pleurodesis for recurrent, symptomatic MPE.[40]

Nonmalignant Pleural Effusion

The cause of nonmalignant pleural effusions (NMPEs) is quite variable, but congestive heart failure, hepatic hydrothorax, chylothorax, and end-stage renal disease are the most common. Management of the underlying disease process is the mainstay of treatment, but symptomatic NMPEs may persist despite optimal management. It should also be noted that patients with advanced heart and liver disease who have pleural effusions may have similar mortality rates to patients with MPE.[41,42] Whereas IPCs were initially designed for treatment of MPE, their use in patients with NMPEs is increasing. Older publications included patients with a variety of etiologies for their NMPE and are composed primarily of low-quality non-RCTs. Newer studies, however, have evaluated the safety and efficacy of IPCs for NMPEs from specific etiologies. This finding is important because the efficacy and complication rates of IPCs varies significantly based on the underlying cause of the effusion.

Complication rates of IPCs when used for hepatic hydrothorax are indeed higher than with MPE. Shojaee and colleagues[43] published a multicenter retrospective evaluation of IPC use in patients with refractory hepatic hydrothorax. No specific information regarding symptom improvement was provided, but 28% of patients experienced pleurodesis, allowing for IPC removal. However, the observed infection rate in this population was 10% with an associated 2.5% mortality rate.[43] Other studies of drainage procedures for patients with hepatic hydrothorax have reported even higher infection rates ranging from 16% with IPCs up to almost 50% with chest tube placement and hospitalization.[44,45] Infectious complications are not the only concern with IPC use for hepatic hydrothorax. Electrolyte disorders, renal failure, and protein loss are other things to consider when placing an IPC for treatment of refractory hepatic hydrothorax. In contrast with hepatic hydrothorax, IPCs are generally well-tolerated and associated with a relatively low risk of infection in patients with congestive heart failure, with most studies reporting empyema rates between 0% and 4%.[45] Pleurodesis rates in patients with congestive heart failure–related effusions may also be higher compared with those with hepatic hydrothorax.[46] Reported pleurodesis rates range from 25% to 44% and even higher when combined with talc administration.[45,47]

Only small case series are available for IPC use in patients with chylothorax or end-stage renal disease–related NMPEs; therefore, we cannot draw strong conclusions. Potechin and colleagues[48] reported the outcomes of 8 patients with end-stage renal disease–related pleural effusions treated with IPC and found that all patients experienced significant improvement in dyspnea with 37.5%, achieving pleurodesis allowing for successful IPC removal. No cases of empyema or other serious complications were reported. Small retrospective case series describing the use of IPC for refractory chylothorax report pleurodesis rates up to 64% with no significant infectious or nutritional complications reported.[49,50] Because the use of IPCs for NMPEs may continue to increase over time, well-designed RCTs will be necessary to determine how suitable they are for long-term use in specific patient populations.

COMPLICATIONS

Despite all the highlighted benefits of IPCs, there are potential complications. The most common long-term complications include a nondraining catheter, tract metastasis, and infection, but each of these are relatively rare occurrences. Removal of an IPC in response to any complication occurs in fewer than 10% of patients.[25]

A nondraining catheter may be a sign of successful pleurodesis, but may also be related to catheter malfunction, an issue reported to occur in 5% to 14% of patients.[4] Evaluation of the pleural space with chest imaging as well as a review of patient symptoms is indicated when catheter drainage ceases, especially when it occurs suddenly. Catheter malfunction is likely in the presence of a persistent pleural effusion and respiratory symptoms. Occlusion of the IPC with a fibrin clot may occur and symptomatic pleural loculations may also develop. Flushing the IPC with saline is the recommended first step for treatment of catheter malfunction. If pleural fluid drainage does not improve after the saline flush, administration of intrapleural fibrinolytics may be indicated. Several studies have evaluated the use of intrapleural fibrinolytics via IPC for the treatment of symptomatic pleural loculations, with a variety of medications and dosages being reported.[4,51,52] Most studies show fibrinolytic administration may be successful in improving IPC drainage after a dwell time of 60 to 120 minutes, but many patients will require repeat administration.[4] Alteplase is the most commonly reported fibrinolytic, usually at a dose of 2 to 10 mg. A recent consensus statement from Gilbert and colleagues recommends alteplase to reestablish IPC patency, whereas guidelines from Miller and colleagues do not recommend any particular fibrinolytic or dose.[4,14] Although reported to occur in less than 3% of patients with a nondraining catheter, bleeding is the most common complication of fibrinolysis and, therefore, individual bleeding risk must be considered before use.[4,51,52]

Infections, particularly empyema, are the most worrisome potential complications associated with IPC use. Cellulitis and exit site infections occur slightly more frequently, but pleural space infections are reported to occur in less than 5% of patients with an IPC for MPE.[4,7] The largest study evaluating clinical outcomes of patients with IPC-related pleural infections reported an associated mortality rate of 6%, suggesting that the outcomes are much better than previously reported.[53] Recent guidelines and expert panel recommendations for the management of IPC-related infectious complications are now available.[4,14] Specific recommendations depend on the individual process (**Table 1**), but despite previous notions, removal of an IPC is often not required.

Cellulitis, exit site, and tunnel tract infections can usually be managed with outpatient antibiotics that adequately cover skin pathogens, although longer courses of treatment may be necessary for tunnel tract infections. When a pleural space infection is suspected, pleural fluid cultures should be obtained, although the ideal method for obtaining the fluid (via the catheter or a thoracentesis) has not been evaluated formally. Broad spectrum intravenous antibiotics, including consideration of anaerobic coverage, should be started while awaiting culture results. Continuous or increased frequency of pleural fluid drainage should also be

Table 1
Summary of IPC infectious complications and management recommendations[4,14]

Type of Infectious Complication	Recommended Management	Indications for IPC Removal
Cellulitis Erythema, warmth, edema and pain of the skin and immediate subcutaneous tissue Exit site Purulent drainage at the catheter skin exit site Erythema, edema, induration and tenderness may be present Localized within 2 cm of the exit site Tunnel tract Erythema, edema, induration and tenderness greater than 2 cm along the catheter tract	Antibiotic therapy Adequate coverage of typical skin pathogens Outpatient management usually sufficient Longer duration of treatment may be necessary for tunnel tract infections	Failure of antibiotics to resolve the infection

Pleural space
 Either:
  Purulent material draining from the catheter
  Clinical symptoms of infection and positive pleural fluid Gram stain or culture
  Clinical symptoms of infection and apparent infectious pleural fluid based on lactate dehydrogenase, glucose, or pH
	Obtain pleural fluid for microbiological studies
	Attempt continuous or increased frequency drainage of IPC
	Consider instillation of fibrinolytics and DNase via IPC if inadequate drainage
	Administer broad spectrum antibiotics initially and de-escalate based on microbiological studies
		Concomitant tunnel tract and pleural space infection
		Inadequate pleural drainage despite fibrinolytic administration
		Lack of clinical improvement despite aggressive care

Data from Miller RJ, Chrissian AA, Lee YCG, et al. AABIP Evidence-informed Guidelines and Expert Panel Report for the Management of Indwelling Pleural Catheters. *J Bronchology Interv Pulmonol.* 2020;27(4):229-245 and Gilbert CR, Wahidi MM, Light RW, et al. Management of Indwelling Tunneled Pleural Catheters: A Modified Delphi Consensus Statement. *Chest.* 2020;158(5):2221-2228.

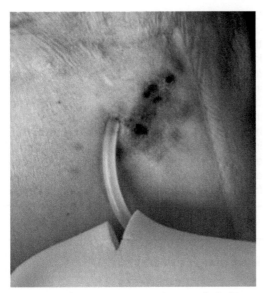

Fig. 3. Tunnel tract metastases diagnosed via biopsy after no significant improvement was seen with antibiotic therapy. (Photo courtesy of Dr. Horiana Grosu.)

initiated. If drainage is incomplete or significant loculations are present, intrapleural fibrinolytics and DNase are recommended in an attempt to prevent the need for lung decortication. There are several instances where the removal of an IPC and the placement of a chest tube may be necessary. These circumstances include concomitant tunnel tract and pleural space infection, poor pleural fluid drainage despite fibrinolytic administration, or a poor clinical response to aggressive treatment.[4,14] Historically, there have been concerns that patients actively treated with chemotherapy may be at increased risk of IPC-related infectious complications, but current evidence suggests otherwise.[4,54] There are currently no recommendations for prophylactic IPC removal before chemotherapy administration or to withhold placement in preparation for systemic treatment.[4]

Tunnel tract metastasis is an uncommon occurrence seen in less than 5% of patients with an IPC (**Fig. 3**). It is thought to occur from migration of tumor cells from the pleural space through the subcutaneous tissue and is most common in patients with mesothelioma. Diagnosis can be obtained with a percutaneous biopsy and treatment generally consists of localized radiation.[21]

SUMMARY

The breadth of knowledge regarding IPCs has increased substantially in the last decade. Available research has established that IPCs are effective at improving patient symptoms and

minimizing hospitalization rates and lengths of stay, but are associated with a risk of potential complications. Fortunately, recent research has shown that the complication rates are relatively low, albeit not negligible. Pleurodesis rates achieved with IPCs are lower when compared with chemical or surgical pleurodesis, but IPCs are associated with a decreased need for repeat pleural procedures and similar quality of life.

Understanding individual patient preferences and utilities is essential when determining optimal management for a recurrent, symptomatic pleural effusion and this information should influence treatment decisions. The future of MPE management likely lies in combined therapies, such as IPC plus a pleural sclerosant, at least in patients whose lung expands with drainage. This combination therapy may provide more optimal benefits than each individual procedure, although further research is needed. Effective pleurodesis and subsequent IPC removal is important, especially in regard to cost effectiveness and burden of catheter-related care, but future research should ideally focus on patient-centered outcomes.[15] Consistency of measurements between studies would also allow for a more direct comparison of results and add to the current body of knowledge.

CLINICS CARE POINTS

- IPCs improve baseline breathlessness and quality of life, while also decreasing hospital length of stay when compared with chest tube and thoracoscopic pleurodesis.
- IPC-related infectious complications contribute to less patient morbidity and mortality than previously believed.
- Well-designed RCTs emphasizing patient-centered outcomes should be the focus of future IPC studies.

DISCLOSURE

A.J. Schwalk has no relevant disclosures. D.E. Ost has worked as a consultant for Becton Dickinson.

REFERENCES

1. Light RW. Pleural effusions. Med Clin North Am 2011;95(6):1055–70.
2. Wrightson JM, Davies HE, Lee GY. Pleural effusion, empyema and pneumothorax. In: Spiro S,

Silvestri G, Agusti A, editors. Clinical respiratory medicine. 4th edition. Elsevier; 2012. p. 818–36.

3. Antony V, Loddenkemper R, Astoul P, et al. Management of malignant pleural effusions. Am J Respir Crit Care Med 2000;162:1987–2001.

4. Miller RJ, Chrissian AA, Lee YCG, et al. AABIP evidence-informed guidelines and expert panel report for the management of indwelling pleural catheters. J Bronchol Interv Pulmonol 2020;27(4):229–45.

5. Koegelenberg CFN, Shaw JA, Irusen EM, et al. Contemporary best practice in the management of malignant pleural effusion. Ther Adv Respir Dis 2018;12. 1753466618785098.

6. Roberts ME, Neville E, Berrisford RG, et al, Group BTSPDG. Management of a malignant pleural effusion: British Thoracic Society pleural disease guideline 2010. Thorax 2010;65(Suppl 2):ii32–40.

7. Feller-Kopman DJ, Reddy CB, DeCamp MM, et al. Management of malignant pleural effusions. An Official ATS/STS/STR clinical practice guideline. Am J Respir Crit Care Med 2018;198(7):839–49.

8. Bibby AC, Dorn P, Psallidas I, et al. ERS/EACTS statement on the management of malignant pleural effusions. Eur Respir J 2018;52(1):1800349.

9. Ost DE, Niu J, Zhao H, et al. Quality gaps and comparative effectiveness of management strategies for recurrent malignant pleural effusions. Chest 2018;153(2):438–52.

10. Davies HE, Mishra EK, Kahan BC, et al. Effect of an indwelling pleural catheter vs chest tube and talc pleurodesis for relieving dyspnea in patients with malignant pleural effusion: the TIME2 randomized controlled trial. JAMA 2012;307(22):2383–9.

11. Thomas R, Fysh ETH, Smith NA, et al. Effect of an indwelling pleural catheter vs talc pleurodesis on hospitalization days in patients with malignant pleural effusion: the AMPLE randomized clinical trial. JAMA 2017;318(19):1903–12.

12. Boshuizen RC, Vd Noort V, Burgers JA, et al. A randomized controlled trial comparing indwelling pleural catheters with talc pleurodesis (NVALT-14). Lung Cancer 2017;108:9–14.

13. Putnam JB, Light RW, Rodriguez RM, et al. A randomized comparison of indwelling pleural catheter and doxycycline pleurodesis in the management of malignant pleural effusions. Cancer 1999;86:1992–9.

14. Gilbert CR, Wahidi MM, Light RW, et al. Management of indwelling tunneled pleural catheters: a modified Delphi consensus statement. Chest 2020; 158(5):2221–8.

15. Ost DE, Jimenez CA, Lei X, et al. Quality-adjusted survival following treatment of malignant pleural effusions with indwelling pleural catheters. Chest 2014; 145(6):1347–56.

16. Bhatnagar R, Keenan EK, Morley AJ, et al. Outpatient talc administration by indwelling pleural catheter for malignant effusion. N Engl J Med 2018;378(14):1313–22.

17. Gilbert CR, Lee HJ, Akulian JA, et al. A quality improvement intervention to reduce indwelling tunneled pleural catheter infection rates. Ann Am Thorac Soc 2015;12(6):847–53.

18. Medical M. Aspira Drainage System Clinician Product Brochure 2019.

19. Patient information - PleurX system BD. 2021. Available at: https://www.bd.com/en-us/offerings/capabilities/interventional-specialties/peritoneal-and-pleural-drainage/about-the-pleurx-drainage-system/patient-information-pleurx-system. Accessed March 5, 2021.

20. Plc. RM. IPC indwelling drainage catheters - pleural & peritoneal. 2011-2019. Available at: https://sales.rocketmedical.com/products/indwelling-drainage-catheters. Accessed March 5, 2021.

21. Chalhoub M, Saqib A, Castellano M. Indwelling pleural catheters: complications and management strategies. J Thorac Dis 2018;10(7):4659–66.

22. Henry DH, Viswanathan HN, Elkin EP, et al. Symptoms and treatment burden associated with cancer treatment: results from a cross-sectional national survey in the U.S. Support Care Cancer 2008; 16(7):791–801.

23. Muruganandan S, Azzopardi M, Fitzgerald DB, et al. Aggressive versus symptom-guided drainage of malignant pleural effusion via indwelling pleural catheters (AMPLE-2): an open-label randomised trial. Lancet Respir Med 2018;6(9):671–80.

24. Wahidi MM, Reddy C, Yarmus L, et al. Randomized trial of pleural fluid drainage frequency in patients with malignant pleural effusions. The ASAP trial. Am J Respir Crit Care Med 2017;195(8):1050–7.

25. Fortin M, Tremblay A. Pleural controversies: indwelling pleural catheter vs. pleurodesis for malignant pleural effusions. J Thorac Dis 2015;7(6):1052–7.

26. Pien GW, Gant MJ, Washam CL, et al. Use of an implantable pleural catheter for trapped lung syndrome in patients with malignant pleural effusion. Chest 2001;119(6):1641–6.

27. Bazerbashi S, Villaquiran J, Awan MY, et al. Ambulatory intercostal drainage for the management of malignant pleural effusion: a single center experience. Ann Surg Oncol 2009;16(12):3482–7.

28. Warren WH, Kalimi R, Khodadadian LM, et al. Management of malignant pleural effusions using the Pleur(x) catheter. Ann Thorac Surg 2008;85(3):1049–55.

29. Qureshi RA, Collinson SL, Powell RJ, et al. Management of malignant pleural effusion associated with trapped lung syndrome. Asian Cardiovasc Thorac Ann 2008;16(2):120–3.

30. Sioris T, Sihvo E, Salo J, et al. Long-term indwelling pleural catheter (PleurX) for malignant pleural effusion unsuitable for talc pleurodesis. Eur J Surg Oncol 2009;35(5):546–51.

31. van den Toorn LM, Schaap E, Surmont VF, et al. Management of recurrent malignant pleural effusions with a chronic indwelling pleural catheter. Lung Cancer 2005;50(1):123–7.

32. Efthymiou CA, Masudi T, Thorpe JA, et al. Malignant pleural effusion in the presence of trapped lung. Five-year experience of PleurX tunnelled catheters. Interact Cardiovasc Thorac Surg 2009;9(6):961–4.

33. Dresler CM, Olak J, Herndon JE 2nd, et al. Phase III intergroup study of talc poudrage vs talc slurry sclerosis for malignant pleural effusion. Chest 2005; 127(3):909–15.

34. Boujaoude Z, Bartter T, Abboud M, et al. Pleuroscopic pleurodesis combined with tunneled pleural catheter for management of malignant pleural effusion- a prospective observational study. J Bronchol Interv Pulmonol 2015;22:237–43.

35. Reddy C, Ernst A, Lamb C, et al. Rapid pleurodesis for malignant pleural effusions: a pilot study. Chest 2011;139(6):1419–23.

36. Bhatnagar R, Zahan-Evans N, Kearney C, et al. A novel drug-eluting indwelling pleural catheter for the management of malignant effusions. Am J Respir Crit Care Med 2018;197(1):136–8.

37. Shafiq M, Simkovich S, Hossen S, et al. Indwelling pleural catheter drainage strategy for malignant effusion: a cost-effectiveness analysis. Ann Am Thorac Soc 2020;17(6):746–53.

38. Bhatnagar R, Piotrowska HEG, Laskawiec-Szkonter M, et al. Effect of thoracoscopic talc poudrage vs talc slurry via chest tube on pleurodesis failure rate among patients with malignant pleural effusions: a randomized clinical trial. JAMA 2019;323(1):60–9.

39. Freeman RK, Ascioti AJ, Mahidhara RS. A propensity-matched comparison of pleurodesis or tunneled pleural catheter in patients undergoing diagnostic thoracoscopy for malignancy. Ann Thorac Surg 2013;96(1):259–63 [discussion 263–4].

40. Iyer NP, Reddy CB, Wahidi MM, et al. Indwelling pleural catheter versus pleurodesis for malignant pleural effusions. A systematic review and meta-analysis. Ann Am Thorac Soc 2019;16(1):124–31.

41. Walker SP, Morley AJ, Stadon L, et al. Nonmalignant pleural effusions: a prospective study of 356 consecutive unselected patients. Chest 2017; 151(5):1099–105.

42. DeBiasi EM, Pisani MA, Murphy TE, et al. Mortality among patients with pleural effusion undergoing thoracentesis. Eur Respir J 2015;46(2):495–502.

43. Shojaee S, Rahman N, Haas K, et al. Indwelling tunneled pleural catheters for refractory hepatic hydrothorax in patients with cirrhosis: a multicenter study. Chest 2019;155(3):546–53.

44. Liu LU, Haddadin HA, Bodian CA, et al. Outcome analysis of cirrhotic patients undergoing chest tube placement. Chest 2004;126(1):142–8.

45. Bramley K, DeBiasi E, Puchalski J. Indwelling pleural catheter placement for nonmalignant pleural effusions. Semin Respir Crit Care Med 2018;39(6): 713–9.

46. Aboudara M, Maldonado F. Indwelling pleural catheters for benign pleural effusions: what is the evidence? Curr Opin Pulm Med 2019;25(4):369–73.

47. Majid A, Kheir F, Fashjian M, et al. Tunneled pleural catheter placement with and without talc poudrage for treatment of pleural effusions due to congestive heart failure. Ann Am Thorac Soc 2016;13(2):212–6.

48. Potechin R, Amjadi K, Srour N. Indwelling pleural catheters for pleural effusions associated with end-stage renal disease: a case series. Ther Adv Respir Dis 2015;9(1):22–7.

49. DePew ZS, Iqbal S, Mullon JJ, et al. The role for tunneled indwelling pleural catheters in patients with persistent benign chylothorax. Am J Med Sci 2013;346(5):349–52.

50. Jimenez CA, Mhatre AD, Martinez CH, et al. Use of an indwelling pleural catheter for the management of recurrent chylothorax in patients with cancer. Chest 2007;132(5):1584–90.

51. Thomas R, Piccolo F, Miller D, et al. Intrapleural fibrinolysis for the treatment of indwelling pleural catheter-related symptomatic loculations: a multicenter observational study. Chest 2015;148(3): 746–51.

52. Vial MR, Ost DE, Eapen GA, et al. Intrapleural fibrinolytic therapy in patients with nondraining indwelling pleural catheters. J Bronchol Interv Pulmonol 2016;23(2):98–105.

53. Fysh ETH, Tremblay A, Feller-Kopman D, et al. Clinical outcomes of indwelling pleural catheter-related pleural infections: an international multicenter study. Chest 2013;144(5):1597–602.

54. Mekhaiel E, Kashyap R, Mullon J, et al. Infections associated with tunnelled indwelling pleural catheters in patients undergoing chemotherapy. J Bronchol Interv Pulmonol 2013;20:299–303.

Medical Thoracoscopy

Sameer K. Avasarala, MD[a], Robert J. Lentz, MD[b,c],
Fabien Maldonado, MD, FCCP[b,c],*

KEYWORDS

- Medical thoracoscopy • Pleuroscopy • Pleurodesis • Pleural effusion • Malignant mesothelioma
- Pneumothorax

KEY POINTS

- Medical thoracoscopy is a minimally invasive diagnostic and therapeutic procedure for a variety of pleural diseases.
- It has a high diagnostic yield in the evaluation and management of exudative pleural effusions, especially in malignant pleural effusion and tubercular pleuritis.
- Medical thoracoscopy can be performed with the use of local anesthesia, usually combined with intravenous medications for moderate sedation.
- Both rigid and semirigid thoracoscopes can be used, approaches are similar, but equipment differs greatly.
- In a subset of patients with pleural disease, invasive management strategy discussions are best undertaken in a multidisciplinary manner.

INTRODUCTION

Medical thoracoscopy (or pleuroscopy; MT) is a commonly performed diagnostic and therapeutic procedure in which the pleural space is visualized using a thoracoscope. It is mainly a diagnostic procedure, although some therapeutic applications do exist. In the United States, it is primarily performed by pulmonologists with interventional pulmonology (IP) training. The main indication for MT is the diagnosis of undiagnosed exudative pleural effusions. However, some therapeutic indications have been proposed, such as thoracoscopic talc poudrage pleurodesis and the management of complicated intrapleural infections. Introduced over a century ago, it remains a foundational intervention in pleural medicine, albeit underused. When applied to the right patient, it is a safe and effective procedure that can be performed in the endoscopy suite or the operating room.

HISTORY

The term "thoracoscopy" (or its derivatives) is found in French reference books as early as the 1840s.[1] Although cited in the literature, it is not clear if MT was being performed at that time. The first reported procedure that mirrors modern MT was published in 1866 by Samuel Gordon, and performed by an Irish urologist, Francis Cruise.[2] He reported using an endoscope inserted into a pleural fistula of an 11-year-old girl with chronic empyema.

The application of modern MT is credited to Hans Christian Jacobeus (1879–1937), a Swedish internist.[2] In 1910, 2 thoracoscopies were described in a series of endoscopic examinations.[3] A year later, a follow-up report of 35 cases was published. Jacobeus adapted a cystoscope for these procedures and performed them using local anesthesia (LA). Initial applications of this procedure were for the treatment of tuberculosis.

[a] Division of Pulmonary, Critical Care, and Sleep Medicine, University Hospitals, 11100 Euclid Avenue, Cleveland, OH 44106, USA; [b] Division of Allergy, Pulmonary and Critical Care Medicine, Department of Internal Medicine, Vanderbilt University Medical Center, T-1218 Medical Center North, 1161 21st Avenue South, Nashville, TN 37232, USA; [c] Division of Allergy, Pulmonary and Critical Care Medicine, Department of Thoracic Surgery, Vanderbilt University Medical Center, T-1218 Medical Center North, 1161 21st Avenue South, Nashville, TN 37232, USA
* Corresponding author. T-1218 Medical Center North, 1161 21st Avenue South, Nashville, TN 37232.
E-mail address: fabien.maldonado@vumc.org
Twitter: @SKAvasarala (S.K.A.); @RobJLentz (R.J.L.); @MaldonadoFabien (F.M.)

Clin Chest Med 42 (2021) 751–766
https://doi.org/10.1016/j.ccm.2021.08.010

Thoracoscopy was used for adhesiolysis to intentionally collapse infected lobes, which was the main treatment for tuberculosis at the time. The procedure became known as the Jacobeus Unverricht Operation.[4,5] Treatment of pulmonary tuberculosis was the most common application for MT until antituberculous medical therapy became established in the 1950s. After this period, the use of MT dramatically declined outside of a few expert centers in some countries of continental Europe: Germany, Austria, Holland, Italy, and France.[6]

Owing to the advancement of optics and video technology, modern MT resurged in the 1980s and 1990s. These same advances also propelled surgeon-led video-assisted thoracoscopic surgery (VATS). Although there is some overlap in indications and techniques between these procedures, they remain distinct. MT typically involves the introduction of a thoracoscope into the pleural space via a single small intercostal incision to inspect and perform biopsies of visible structures (biopsies are principally obtained of the parietal pleura). MT is most often facilitated by LA in a spontaneously breathing patient, and in fact, labeled as "local anesthetic thoracoscopy" in the United Kingdom. VATS, alternatively, is performed under general anesthesia, the lung in the hemithorax of interest is isolated from ventilation, and multiple incisions are used to permit insertion of an optical instrument as well as surgical instruments to facilitate a therapeutic intervention (eg, lobectomy). VATS indications are primarily therapeutic, whereas MT indications are primarily diagnostic. VATS requires single lung ventilation and the use of general anesthesia.[7] It should be noted that VATS can be performed in awake, spontaneously breathing patients, and MT can be performed with general anesthesia and lung isolation.

MT and VATS are best seen as complementary procedures and critical components of a necessarily multidisciplinary approach to complex pleural diseases. One misconception is that MT should be considered in patients who, for general medical reasons, are not suitable candidates for VATS. In our opinion, aside from rare situations, MT should be viewed as a minimally invasive technique offered to patients when conversion to VATS is not expected, and diagnosis can be made by biopsy of the parietal pleura (ie, tuberculosis and malignancy). Primary VATS, however, should be performed (in a diagnostic setting), when the visceral pleura/lung would need to be biopsied, the pleural space is complex with multiple adhesions, or there is a higher risk of needing to convert to thoracotomy. Such a conversion is rarely needed but does occasionally happen. A scenario like this highlights the need for a multidisciplinary approach in which general pulmonologists, IP, and thoracic surgery synergistically contribute to pleural disease management.

There are geographic variations in MT practice patterns. MT is more commonly performed outside of the United States. In a survey study that included responses from England, Scotland, and Wales, 95% of responding centers (n = 37) considered LA MT their preferred method for investigating pleural effusions of unclear etiology.[8] In a survey study conducted in India, 100 of the 105 respondents reported they performed MT. Most respondents were pulmonologists who used a rigid thoracoscope.[9]

COMMON INDICATIONS AND OUTCOMES

MT provides access sufficient for sampling of pleural fluid, visualization of the parietal and visceral pleura, biopsies of the parietal pleura, and a pathway to introduce agents to achieve pleurodesis. When indicated, MT may provide valuable diagnostic information or treatment options with little risk to patients.

The common indications for MT are evaluating exudative pleural effusions of unclear etiology, performing pleurodesis, diagnosis, and staging of malignant pleural mesothelioma (MPM), and in some selected cases, empyema management. It is essential to keep in mind that regardless of the indication, MT should only be performed when other simpler and safer diagnostic or therapeutic methods failed or cannot be performed (ie, thoracentesis with pleural fluid analysis [PFA]). As with any invasive procedure, careful analysis of a risk-benefit ratio should take place.

Exudative Pleural Effusion

The most common indication for MT is the evaluation of exudative effusions of unclear etiology.[10] When investigating a pleural effusion, a thoracentesis with PFA is widely considered the first diagnostic step in the management pathway. However, it is estimated that PFA can help establish the diagnosis of effusion in only 75% of patients.[11] In scenarios in which a PFA is not diagnostic, progression to MT may be able to provide a definitive diagnosis in up to 95% of patients.

There are many causes of pleural effusions including transudates (typically from heart, liver, or kidney disease), parapneumonic effusions, pleural space infections, and malignant pleural effusions (MPEs), among many more uncommon etiologies.[12] Often, a careful history and physical examination can help narrow the differential diagnosis. Laboratory and radiographic investigations also provide valuable information.[13] However, it often remains challenging to ascertain the diagnosis of an exudative pleural effusion.[11] These tend to be exudative effusions, particularly lymphocytic-predominant exudates, in which malignancy and tuberculosis account for most cases of unclear etiology (as the other prevalent cause of lymphocytic exudates, postcardiac surgery effusions, is typically clear based on medical history). For MPE, the sensitivity of pleural fluid cytology for identifying a malignancy is limited to 60%, although it varies based on cell type.[14] The sensitivity of pleural fluid cytology for breast cancer or pancreatic cancer is higher, whereas sensitivity for head and neck malignancy, sarcoma, or renal cancer is low.[15] Pleural fluid cytology diagnostic rates are also higher in lung adenocarcinomas versus lung squamous cell carcinomas.[12] When tumors with a low likelihood of positive pleural fluid cytology yield are suspected, MT may be considered as a first step in the diagnostic algorithm of unexplained exudative pleural effusions.

When clinical history and supporting investigations (including imaging and PFA) cannot solidify a diagnosis, a diagnostic MT is indicated. In addition to obtaining samples for PFA, MT allows for various tools to be used to biopsy the parietal pleural. Generally, samples are obtained from abnormal-looking pleura. Flexible forceps can be used via a semirigid thoracoscope, and rigid forceps can be used through a rigid thoracoscope. The diagnostic yield for MT in pleural diseases such as MPE and tuberculous pleural effusions is very high (91%–99%).[12,16] Importantly, it has been proven to be a safe procedure; morbidity (1.8%) and mortality (0.3%) rates are low.[16]

At times, the parietal pleura appears grossly normal. In this scenario, random biopsies are obtained from parietal pleura overlying ribs where there is minimal risk of disrupting an intercostal artery. The application of narrow-band imaging (NBI) has shown some promise and may assist in cases without gross visual abnormalities. In a case series of 100 patients, NBI was found to have a higher specificity for pathology (81.82%) when compared to white light thoracoscopy (27.27%).[17] NBI can be used to help identify optimal target biopsy sites.[18] Similarly, some data suggest autofluorescence MT has higher diagnostic sensitivity than white light MT (100% vs 92.8%), it has also been used to help identify parenchymal abnormalities.[19,20] These findings are important as it has been shown that MT proceduralists are not adept at predicting whether obvious pleural abnormalities are benign or malignant on a visual basis.[21] The role of intraprocedural rapid on-site cytologic examination is not clear for MT but is under active study.[22]

At times, samples obtained from flexible forceps are too small or unable to provide helpful information. In a scenario such as a fibrothorax or mesothelioma, obtaining biopsy samples with flexible forceps may be limited because of the presence of a scarred, thickened pleural surface. Additional tools can be used through the working channel of the semirigid thoracoscope. Cryobiopsies, for example, have been obtained from the pleural cavity. In a crossover study, Dhooria and colleagues reported that pleural cryobiopsies were larger when compared to flexible forceps biopsies (median size 7.0 mm vs 4.0 mm).[23] The procedure was also noted to be faster when performed with a cryoprobe. However, there were no differences in the diagnostic yield between the 2 tools. Patients in this study underwent semirigid thoracoscopy for undiagnosed pleural effusion and had both flexible forceps biopsies and cryobiopsies performed.[23] A meta-analysis of 7 observational studies (which included 311 cryobiopsies and 275 flexible forceps biopsies) showed similar diagnostic yields for both tools.[24] In addition to using a cryoprobe, various cutting and coagulation tools can be used to assist in obtaining biopsies in MT; data are limited to case reports and case series. The sample sizes are small and are limited to 2 to 20 patients per study.[25–27]

Much like using a cryoprobe, larger samples can be acquired with the more robust tools that are used with a rigid thoracoscope. Similar diagnostic adequacy of biopsy specimens between semirigid or rigid MT has been reported.[28,29] Other studies have reported conflicting data.[30] A randomized controlled trial (73 patients randomized in a 1:1 ratio) that compared semirigid MT and rigid MT in patients with undiagnosed exudative pleural effusions showed that the diagnostic yield of rigid MT was not superior to that of semirigid MT.[31]

The diagnostic yield of MT has also been compared to VATS. In a retrospective study that assessed MT and VATS pleural biopsies in patients with undiagnosed pleural effusions, MT was found to have similar diagnostic yield and safety compared to VATS.[32] Importantly, MT was noted to be associated with a shorter length of stay (median of 0 days vs 3 days) and a lower average cost per procedure ($2815 vs $7962) when compared with VATS.

In some parts of the world, TB is a common etiology of undiagnosed lymphocytic exudates. Based on a Chinese case series of 429%, 78% of unilateral non-MPE were due to tuberculosis.[33] Thoracoscopy continues to play an essential role in the management of TB pleural disease. The microbiological analysis of pleural fluid has poor sensitivity in TB pleuritis; one series estimates it is less than 18%.[34] While generally considered a last remaining indication for closed (blind) pleural biopsies, MT has outperformed closed pleural biopsies as a diagnostic tool in patients with TB pleuritis. A histopathological confirmation rate of 99% via MT acquired samples (333 cases of confirmed TB pleuritis) has been reproted.[16]

Pleurodesis

Pleurodesis by talc poudrage is a technique in which a pleural sclerosant is blown/insufflated into the pleural space to evenly coat the parietal and visceral pleural surfaces. Poudrage is a common indication for MT, it is a method that can be used for definitive treatment of primary spontaneous pneumothorax (PSP) or MPE. However, some still recommend lung resection of visceral pleural blebs and bullae (thus favoring surgical approaches) for PSP management. Recent evidence suggests no difference between a thoracoscopic approach and less invasive talc slurry for achieving pleurodesis in patients with MPE.[35] Although the invasiveness of the procedures varies, there is no definitive evidence to suggest a particular strategy of recurrence prevention in PSP.[36] There is no significant evidence that blebectomy offers any advantage over talc pleurodesis alone in the treatment of pneumothorax. Pleurodesis is usually undertaken in the setting of ipsilateral recurrence, an initial contralateral episode, or initial episodes in special occupations such as airline pilots.[37,38] Poudrage is also commonly performed in the setting of MPE, sometimes in conjunction with diagnostic MT. Talc is the most used sclerosant.

The European Respiratory Society's PSP Task Force Statement recommends pleurodesis be performed for the indications listed earlier.[36] MT with talc poudrage is one method of achieving pleurodesis. It has been shown to prevent recurrence in patients with PSP. In a prospective randomized control trial, 180 patients with PSPs were treated with either MT with talc instillation (n = 61) or pleural drainage (n = 47). The need for a second procedure and pneumothorax management was greater in the pleural drainage tube group (10/47, 21%) than the MT with talc installation group (1/61, 2%). In addition, a 5-year follow-up showed that recurrence was higher in the pleural drainage (24%) versus the thoracoscopic group (5%).[39]

Although talc pleurodesis has also been shown to be effective in MPE, in a Cochrane network meta-analysis of MPE management, talc poudrage was highly effective and resulted in fewer pleurodesis failures.[40] A multicenter randomized control trial of 330 patients who received either talc poudrage (via MT, 166 patients) or talc slurry (via chest drain, 164 patients) showed that both modalities had similarly low pleurodesis failure rates at 90 days. The failure rate in the poudrage group was 22%, and the failure rate in the talc slurry group was 24%.[35]

Talc poudrage is performed after entering the pleural space, draining the pleural effusion (if present), and performing a full inspection of the hemithorax. Poudrage is completed by insufflating sterile, graded talc in an even distribution across the pleural cavity. Typically, 2 to 5 gm are used to achieve pleurodesis in MPE. The dose used for the treatment of pneumothorax is less (1–2 gm). Insufflation devices consisting of a power-filled insufflation bulb attached to a cannula can be used to create the mist for evenly coating the surfaces of the parietal and visceral pleura in a controlled fashion.[41] Graded talc is used for these procedures. Large particles do not disseminate systemically and therefore do not result in inflammatory responses and acute respiratory distress syndrome previously described with nongraded talc. A large multicenter study of 558 patients using large-particle-graded talc showed a 0% frequency of acute respiratory distress syndrome development.[42]

Empyema and Complex Pleural Effusions

The presence of active suppuration within the pleural space, or a positive Gram stain/culture defines an empyema.[43] It is a serious condition, and morbidity and mortality remain high. Treatment strategies span a spectrum and include antibiotics in a combination of chest tube drainage (without or without intrapleural enzymatic therapy [IET]) or surgical management via VATS or an open thoracotomy. Defining the gold standard of treatment remains an area of active investigation. The American Association for Thoracic Surgery consensus guidelines for the management of empyema recommends VATS as the first-line approach in all patients with stage II acute empyema (class IIb recommendation, level B evidence).[44]

MT has limited application in the setting of empyema. Typically, conservative therapy (tube thoracostomy with or without IET) is followed by surgery if unsuccessful. Surgery is usually performed via VATS, but occasionally open thoracotomy may be required as well. Some data suggest that VATS is superior to tube thoracostomy for patients with empyema or complex pleural effusions: two different randomized controlled trials showed that early/immediate VATS was associated with a lower length of stay compared to an only tube thoracostomy approach.[45,46] These studies, however, were conspicuously underpowered, did not include patients treated with IET, and further research is needed to clarify these findings.

There have been several reports describing MT as a therapeutic option for the management of empyema. Success rates are reported to be between 75% and 91%.[47,48] These studies are limited by their retrospective nature and small sample size. MT was deemed successful in 91% of patients with empyema treated with MT on one retrospective study (n = 127). Six percent of patients required surgical pleurectomy.[47] Another retrospective study (n = 41) showed an MT success rate of 85.4%.[48] In this series, there was 94% success (31/33) in patients who had ultrasound features showing a free-flowing fluid or multiloculated fluid. There was only 50% success (4/8) in patients with an organized effusion. Kheir and colleagues reported the results of a randomized controlled trial that compared IET and MT in patients with pleural infection. Patients who underwent MT had a shorter medial length of stay (2 days) when compared with those who received IET (4 days).[49] The study, however, was criticized for comparing two treatments with inherently distinct lengths of inpatient treatment, which biased the primary endpoint in favor of MT.[50]

There are no published data that compare outcomes of MT versus VATS in patients with pleural space infections. It is critical to keep this in mind as MT is not considered the standard of care for empyema, and patient selection remains essential.

If MT is performed to treat a pleural space infection, it is believed that rigid thoracoscopy is better than semirigid thoracoscopy. The rigid thoracoscope tools allow for a more extensive lysis of adhesions. In a case series of 160 patients with empyema who were subjected to LA MT, 150 (93.7%) had either complete or partial radiographic resolution.[51] All patients in this study underwent rigid thoracoscopy.

In summary, the more complex the pleural space is, the less likely that MT will be useful. However, several publications regarding the effectiveness of rigid thoracoscopy for multiloculated empyema have been published. Their summative effectiveness is 287 of 311 (92.8%).[47,48,51]

Malignant Pleural Mesothelioma

The worldwide annual case rate of MPM is 30,000; its incidence is estimated to double over the next 20 years.[10] Within the United States, the incidence of MPM is falling.[52] The diagnosis is generally considered difficult if not impossible to make by PFA-derived cytology; pleural biopsies are usually required. Sensitivity for MPM via PFA varies widely.[4,53] Data suggest that pleural fluid cytology

has poor sensitivity for diagnosing MPM (20%–51%).[12,54,55] Even if PFA suggests MPM, biopsies provide useful information about histologic subtypes.[56] There are various ways to obtain pleural biopsies when investigating MPM: radiologically assisted percutaneous sampling, MT, and VATS.[57] Procedure site metastasis has to be kept in mind in patients with MPM, an incidence of 16% has been reported with thoracoscopy.[58]

MT has a high diagnostic yield for MPM; it is estimated to be greater than 95%.[59–61] To mitigate the risk of MPM seeding, the American Society of Clinical Oncology recommends limiting the number of ports used to obtain diagnostic biopsies a single or dual-port approach.[62] MT as a single port approach is commonly used. The thick fibrous lesions of MPM may limit the ability of the semirigid thoracoscope's flexible forceps to obtain adequate samples. Adjunct tools for imaging (fluorescence-guided) or sample acquisition (cryobiopsy or thermal modalities).[10]

PREPROCEDURE PLANNING

Before the decision to perform MT, a thorough patient evaluation must occur. The acquisition of a detailed medical and drug history and the performance of a physical examination is essential. Appropriate imaging must be reviewed. Available blood work such as a complete blood count and coagulation profile can provide helpful information. Several contraindications exist for MT (**Table 1**). The most important of which include the lack of pleural space. Obesity may make the procedure technically challenging.[63]

Although a large body of MT-specific data does not exist, most proceduralists follow the coagulation parameters and recommendations for anticoagulation and antiplatelet agents advised for obtained traditional transbronchial biopsies.[64]

PROCEDURE SPECIFICS
Environment

MT should be performed either in an endoscopy suite room or an operating room to mitigate the risk of infection.[65] This determination is based on institutional resources and anesthesia needs. There are no studies that address if prophylactic antibiotics are required for MT. However, it is suggested that a first-generation cephalosporin (such as cefazolin) is the appropriate prophylactic antibiotic choice for lung resection surgery.[66] Vancomycin is suggested as an alternative if there is a penicillin allergy or if there is a history of methicillin-resistant *Staphylococcus aureus*.[66] Its benefit in MT remains unknown.

Table 1
Contraindications to medical thoracoscopy

Relative	Absolute
Short life expectancy or poor functional status	Lack of safe access to the pleural space
Refractory cough	Inability to obtain informed consent from the patient or their surrogate
Coagulopathy	Evidence of infection at the planned access site
Hypersensitivity to local anesthesia or other medications that are being used	
Unstable hemodynamic or respiratory status	

Anesthesia

One of the advantages of MT is the ability to perform the procedure without the need for general anesthesia. The procedure itself can be performed with LA alone. Patient comfort can be enhanced using moderate sedation or monitored anesthetic care in conjunction with LA. A randomized control trial compared MT with lidocaine-based LA (n = 40) and MT with lidocaine LA and midazolam (n = 40). Those in the midazolam group showed more favorable scores measured by visual analog scale for both cough and pain at the end of MT.[67] Their scores for discomfort, fear, and willingness to repeat the procedure 24 hours after MT were also lower.[67] Another randomized study compared MT with midazolam or MT with propofol. The primary endpoint was intraprocedural mean oxygen saturation nadir. Patients randomized to the propofol group showed more episodes of hypoxemia and hypotension compared with the midazolam group.[68]

Anatomy

The most common access point for MT is the axillary triangle. The area is bounded superiorly by the axilla, anteriorly by the lower edge of the pectoralis major muscle, and posteriorly by the anterior edge of the latissimus dorsi muscle. The inferior border is typically the level of the nipple. Caution must be considered in scenarios in which the nipple level is lower than anatomically expected (pendulous breasts).

Special Access

Before positioning the patient, safe access to the pleural space must be ensured. Often, this is performed using a preprocedural ultrasound to identify a pleural effusion or findings consistent with a pneumothorax. A lack of lung sliding on ultrasound should give pause before MT. Unless there is a known pneumothorax, this finding may suggest pleurodesis and an inability to safely access the pleural space. In situations where access to the pleural space may be challenging (small pneumothorax or small pleural effusion), additional air can be entrained into the pleural space. Air entry will enlarge the pleural space and allow for safer access. Air entry can be performed in a variety of ways; one technique is a use of a Boutin Trocar (Novatech, La Ciotat, France) (**Fig. 1**). A pneumothorax can also be introduced via a special pneumothorax needle under pressure control.[69] In cases of extreme difficulty with creating a pneumothorax (secondary to adhesions), blunt dissection with the use of a finger or Kelly forceps can be considered. It is important to note that MT is contraindicated if the pleural space has been completely obliterated.

Procedural Steps

- The appropriate monitoring devices should be placed on the patient. When MT is being performed with moderate sedation or monitored anesthesia care, this typically includes telemetry leads for continuous monitoring, pulse oximetry probe, and noninvasive blood pressure monitoring. Adequate oxygenation should be assured, with supplemental oxygen being given as needed to maintain an acceptable pulse oximetry reading.
- The patient is positioned in a lateral decubitus position with the affected side up (**Fig. 2**). Their head should be comfortably resting on a pillow. The arm of the affected side should be placed above the patient's head with the help of the sling or similar device. The patient's dependent flank should be supported; a rolled sheet can be used. An axillary roll should be used to protect the brachial plexus

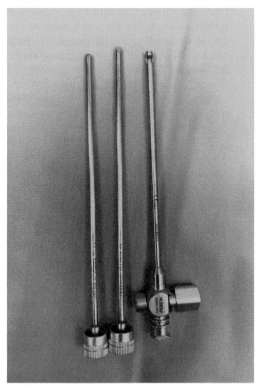

Fig. 1. In scenarios where the pleural space may be challenging to access because of a small pleural effusion or pneumothorax, adjunct tools can be used to gain access and enlarge the space. An example is the Boutin Trocar (Novatech, La Ciotat, France). This trocar can be used to puncture the parietal pleural and entrain air from the atmosphere to induce or enlarge a pneumothorax. This maneuver allows the lung to collapse toward the hilum, allowing for a larger window for safe pleural access.

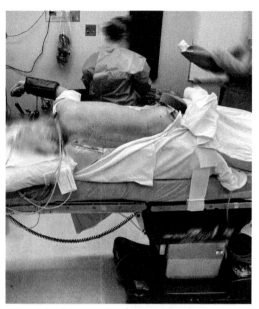

Fig. 2. The patient should be positioned with the affected side facing up. Their pressure points should be supported appropriately. The affected side's arm should be positioned in a manner that places it out of the surgical field. In this image, an arm supported is used to position the patient's right arm.

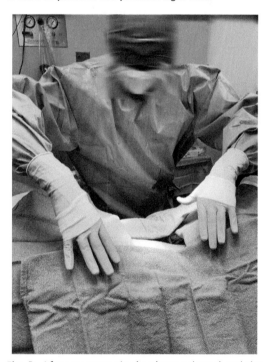

Fig. 3. After an entry site has been selected and the patient has been positioned appropriately, the site must be prepped in a similar manner to thoracic surgical procedures. The area should be cleaned according to local surgical site preparation recommendations. Ample drying time must be allowed before the area is draped.

of the recumbent side. It is vital to protect the patient's pressure contact points using padding between the knees and the lower legs. The operator stands on the ventral side of the patient's face.

- After proper positioning, the patient is prepared and draped based on local institutional recommendations (**Fig. 3**).
- Generous administration of LA (1% lidocaine without epinephrine) to pain-sensing structures of the entry site (skin, subcutaneous tissue, intercostal muscles, periosteum of the ribs, and parietal pleura) is of utmost importance. Care should be taken not to inject LA into local vascular structures such as the intercostal vessels.
- There are multiple ways to perform MT after the administration of LA. We outlined one approach in this text: MT with a semirigid thoracoscope under LA and monitored anesthesia

care in the operating room (**Fig. 4**). Similar steps are undertaken if a rigid thoracoscope is used, the thoracoscope equipment will differ.

○ After administering LA, a small 25-gauge needle is used to aspirate either air or fluid from the affected pleural space (**Fig. 5**). Once confirmed that pleural contents have been aspirated, it is safe to proceed with further dissection of the soft tissues. In situations of small pneumothoraxes or small pleural effusions, a Boutin Trocar or similar device can be used to induce or enlarge a pneumothorax for safe entry into the affected pleural space (**Fig. 1**). The technique of artificially inducing a pneumothorax has been described in the literature and thought to be safe.[70]

○ After the ability to safely access the pleural space has been confirmed, a scalpel is used to make a 1 cm incision that runs parrel with the selected intercostal space (**Fig. 6**). This incision should be deep enough to expose subcutaneous tissue. Once this depth has been reached, a Kelly forceps can start blunt dissection to expose the area further. Palpation with the forceps or finger should be undertaken to palpate the underlying rib. The forceps are then used to guide over the superior border of the rib, this plane of entry avoids injury to the neurovascular bundle that runs under the rib. The pleural space can then be

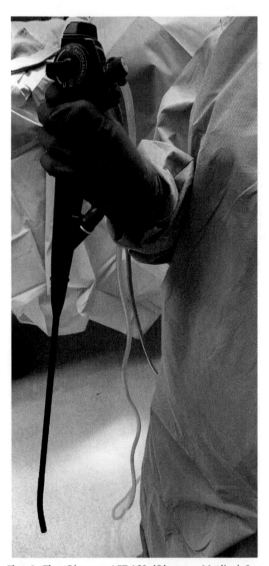

Fig. 4. The Olympus LFT-160 (Olympus Medical Systems Corporation, Tokyo, Japan) is a semirigid thoracoscope, which is commonly used for medical thoracoscopy. It required a single-entry site, an 8 mm inner diameter disposable trocar. Analogous to some flexible bronchoscopes, its insertion tube is narrow (7 mm), and it has a 2.8 mm working channel. It also features 160° upward and 130° downward angulation capability. This thoracoscope is also autoclavable.

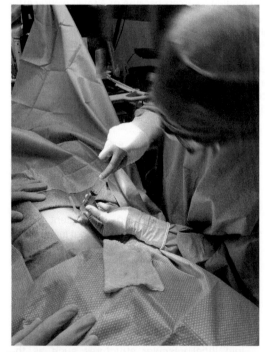

Fig. 5. Before making any incisions, the area of interest should be thoroughly anesthetized with local anesthesia. Small profile needles used to deliver local anesthesia to deeper structures should also be used to access the pleural space and confirm the location by aspirating abnormal contents.

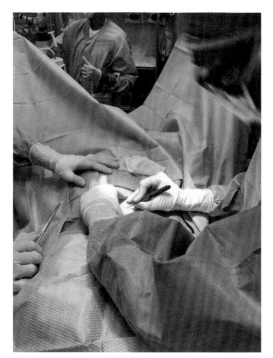

Fig. 6. Once an access area has been selected and appropriately anesthetized, a scalpel can be used to create a 1-cm incision for the trocar. This incision should run parrel with the ribs and be placed at the inferior border of the rib in the rib space of interest. The incision can be deepened with blunt dissection till resistance is lost; this indicates the visceral pleural has been violated.

entered bluntly using the forceps or a gloved finger, which is then used to sweep around the parietal pleural to ensure no adhesions are present. A trocar is usually inserted in corkscrew motion while holding the trocar handle firmly in the palm. While inserting the trocar, an extended index finger is used to limit the depth of insertion. Once the trocar is within the pleural cavity, the inner introducer can be removed. Typically, the inner cannula lies 1 to 3 cm within the pleural cavity. Removal of the inner cannula usually allows for additional confirmation of presence in the pleural space due to movement of air and/or fluid with the respiratory cycle. After removal of the inner cannula, the thoracoscope is inserted (**Fig. 7**).
○ The thoracoscope is inserted under direct visualization. The operator is standing on the ventral side of the patient, the pleural cavity is displayed on a monitor directly adjacent to the operator, or on the dorsal side of the patient such that the operator

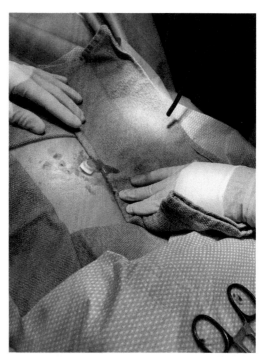

Fig. 7. The trocar is well seated into the affected pleural space; pleural fluid is seen escaping from the space in sync with the respiratory cycle. To visual the pleural cavity, the semirigid thoracoscope is inserted through the trocar.

can look straight ahead (**Fig. 8**). Depending on the indication, either pleural fluid, abnormal pleural, or septations will be seen (**Fig. 9**). If fluid is present, it can be

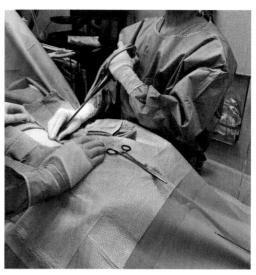

Fig. 8. Once the trocar has been successfully placed into the pleural space. The thoracoscope is used to drain and inspect the pleural cavity. The semirigid thoracoscope (pictured) can be maneuvered in a fashion that is like a flexible bronchoscope.

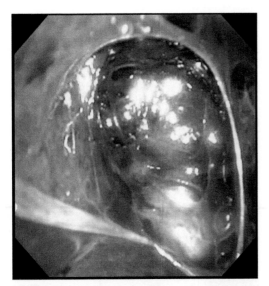

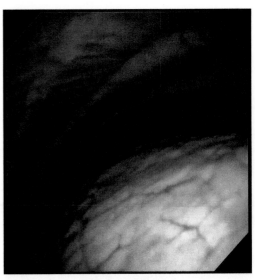

Fig. 9. In most scenarios, the thoracoscope is met with either pleural fluid (pleural effusion) or air (pneumothorax) after the parietal pleural is breached. At times, dense septations may make access and visualization of the pleural space a challenge. In this image, septations were seen immediately after the parietal pleural was penetrated. This scenario can be seen in conditions such as empyema or fibrothorax. A view can be established by carefully clearing these separations with the tools used with the thoracoscope. Callous breakdown of these septations could lead to bleeding if a vascular structure is present within the bands.

Fig. 10. The thoracoscope can be angled in various positions to perform a visual examination of the pleural space. In this image, the semirigid thoracoscope is flattened to the patient's body surface and pointed cephalad. This allows for visualization of the chest wall and visceral pleural (and associated underlying pulmonary parenchyma) toward the apex of the lung.

removed with a suction catheter or the use of the suction channel of a semirigid thoracoscope. While aspirating large volumes, care should be taken to ensure air can be entrained into the pleural space around the thoracoscope or suction catheter via the insertion trocar. This helps to eliminate the risk of inducing potentially injurious negative pleural pressures.

○ After clear visualization of the pleural cavity is obtained, a thorough inspection of the pleural space is completed (**Fig. 10**). Specific visual markers of the lung parenchyma can be used to assist with orientation. On the right side, the junction of the horizontal and oblique fissure serves as a landmark. In the left pleural space, an oblique fissure can be used as a marker for orientation. On either side, the diaphragm is easily visualized as it moves with respiration. Additional structures that can be seen include ribs, fat, intercostal muscles, blood vessels, and any nonfluid pathologic findings such as adhesions or pleural nodules. The mediastinal compartment can also be visualized.

○ Biopsies are typically obtained of normal or abnormal-appearing parietal pleura. Biopsies of the visceral pleura risk intraparenchymal hemorrhage and the creation of air leaks, while abnormalities on the diaphragmatic surface are quite mobile throughout the respiratory cycle making accurate biopsy slightly more challenging. When there is clear nodularity or other obvious parietal pleural abnormality present, these areas are biopsied. When no gross abnormalities are present, the parietal pleura is preferentially biopsied from regions with an overlying rib (which can be felt by biopsy forceps), to reduce the risk of inadvertent injury of intercostal vasculature. The parietal pleura is grasped, then the forceps are directed laterally in a "peeling" motion, which typically generates a long strip of parietal pleura (**Fig. 11**). It is thought that biopsies obtained via a peeling motion are less likely to cause bleeding than those obtained by a punching motion. Care should be taken to avoid biopsying the apices of the lungs, mediastinal pleural, and areas near the internal mammary artery. The operator should be comfortable with the use of coagulation forceps or coagulation electrodes to achieving hemostasis.

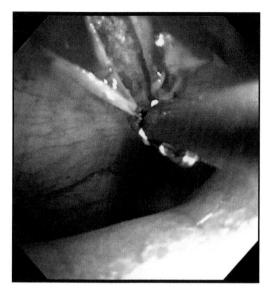

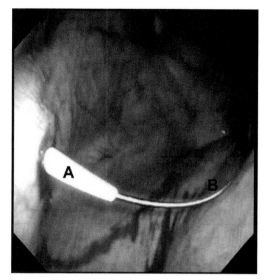

Fig. 11. Forceps can be used to "peel" the parietal pleural biopsies. It is thought that this method is safer than "punching" and allows for more immediate recognition of any bleeding that may occur.

Fig. 12. If an indwelling catheter is being placed along with medical thoracoscopy, it can be performed under direct visual guidance. A dilator (A) is being used over a guidewire (B) in this image.

Usually, multiple biopsies are obtained from the abnormal site. Anywhere from 2 to 6 samples are usually obtained and sent for pathology and culture as indicated.

○ After biopsies have been acquired, the pleural space must be visualized to confirm there is no bleeding. Hemostasis must be assured before proceeding.

○ If indicated, talc pleurodesis can be performed at this time.

○ After the procedure is completed, a chest tube is inserted into the pleural space to drain residual fluid or air. An indwelling pleural catheter is often selected in scenarios that feature pleural malignancy. With the thoracoscope in the pleural cavity, the indwelling pleural catheter can be inserted under direct visualization (**Fig. 12**). Usually, entry and exit sites of the indwelling pleural catheter are distinct from the trocar insertion site of the thoracoscopy.

○ All the access sites should be closed with sutures and dressed appropriately.

○ Usually, postprocedural fluoroscopy or chest radiography is performed to assess for immediate complications and chest tube positioning.

RECOVERY AND REHABILITATION

Generally, MT is an outpatient procedure. If pleurodesis is performed, the patient may have to be admitted for the management of associated discomfort. If a chest tube is placed, it is removed based on local practice patterns and indications for placement. Patients who have had an indwelling pleural catheter (IPC) placed can be discharged with the device in place. A follow-up appointment should be arranged in the appropriate time frame, typically for suture removal.

TRAINING

Training in MT varies across the globe. It is more commonly performed in centers across Europe than in the United States. It is thought that a minimum number of 20 procedures is required to establish procedural familiarity.[61] Similarly, 10 to 20 procedures per year help maintain competency. The American College of Chest Physicians recommends that at least 20 thoracoscopies with or without biopsies as a threshold number for initial competency.[71] In the United Kingdom, British Thoracic Society guidelines assign competency levels based on the complexity of the procedure = level 1 (basic diagnostic and therapeutic, including talc administration) through level III (surgical thoracoscopy, including lung resection).[72] The Executive Summary of the Multisociety Interventional Pulmonology Fellowship Accreditation Committee states a requisite annual institution case volume of 20 MT per year for accreditation of an IP fellowship program.[73] In the United States, IP training or board certification is usually required to perform MT independently.

BILLING AND REIMBURSEMENT

Within the United States, Current Procedural Terminology code 32601 can be used for a diagnostic MT used to evaluate the pleural space, lungs, mediastinum, or the pericardial sac.[74] Additional relevant Current Procedural Terminology codes and related Work Relative Value Units can be found in **Table 2**. Diagnostic thoracoscopy has a 0-day global period; subsequent procedures as well as evaluation and management can be billed separately. Compared to other procedures commonly performed by pulmonologists and IP in the United States, MT reimburses well (**Table 2**).[75]

OUTCOMES

MT is a very safe procedure. Overall, the morbidity and mortality profiles are more favorable than bronchoscopy with traditional transbronchial biopsies.

In a study of 168 thoracoscopies, only one death was noted.[76] Significant complications occurred in 6% of patients. The 2010 British Thoracic Society guidelines state that LA MT is a safe procedure. An analysis of over 4700 cases of LA MT showed a mortality rate of 0.34%. In a subset of patients who underwent only diagnostic thoracoscopy, mortality was 0% (0/2421).

Table 2
Comparison of coding and billing information for medical thoracoscopy and common bronchoscopic procedures (within the United States)

Description of Code	Current Procedural Terminology Code	Work Relative Value Units
32601	Thoracoscopy, diagnostic (separate procedure); lungs, pericardial sac, mediastinal or pleural space, without biopsy	5.50
32609	Thoracoscopy; with biopsies of pleura	4.58
32650	Thoracoscopy, surgical; with pleurodesis (ie, mechanical or chemical)	10.83
32651	Thoracoscopy, surgical; with partial pulmonary decortication	18.78
32653	Thoracoscopy, surgical; with removal of intrapleural foreign body or fibrin deposit	18.17
31652	Bronchoscopy, rigid or flexible, including fluoroscopic guidance, when performed; with endobronchial ultrasound-guided transtracheal and/or transbronchial sampling (ie, aspirations/biopsies), 3 or more mediastinal and/or hilar lymph node stations or structures	4.46
31653	Bronchoscopy, rigid or flexible, including fluoroscopic guidance, when performed; with endobronchial ultrasound-guided transtracheal and/or transbronchial sampling (ie, aspirations/biopsies), 3 or more mediastinal and/or hilar lymph node stations or structures	4.96
31628	Bronchoscopy, rigid or flexible, including fluoroscopic guidance, when performed; with transbronchial lung biopsies, single lobe	3.55
31631	Bronchoscopy, rigid or flexible, including fluoroscopic guidance, when performed; with placement of tracheal stents (includes tracheal/bronchial dilation as required)	4.36
31630	Bronchoscopy, rigid or flexible, including fluoroscopic guidance, when performed; with tracheal/bronchial dilation or closed reduction of fracture of the tracheobronchial tree	1.53

Nineteen of the studies involved the use of talc poudrage, which had a combined mortality of 0.69% (16/2315). It should be kept in mind that 9 of the 16 deaths were from a large, randomized study of talc poudrage using ungraded talc.[72]

The most worrisome complication in MT is bleeding. In an analysis of 4736 cases of LA MT, major complications such as empyema, hemorrhage, port site tumor growth, pneumonia, bronchopleural fistula, or postprocedural pneumothorax or air leak occurred 86 times (1.8%).[72] Although proven to be a safe procedure, the risk of intrathoracic bleeding is yet another reason that a subset of patients with pleural disease are managed within a collaborative atmosphere between IP and thoracic surgery.

SUMMARY

MT is a safe and effective procedure that has a variety of indications among various pleural diseases. When performed by an adequately trained operator, complication rates are low, and diagnostic yield is high. It is a procedure that can be performed with LA (usually with some form of moderate sedation) and spontaneous ventilation.

It should be recognized that there are some overlapping indications between MT and VATS. Owing to visualization capability, surgical control, and ability to acquire larger biopsy pieces, an open thoracotomy provides the most exposure and maneuverability within the pleural space. VATS is the usual surgical approach for pleural disease management, it has largely replaced open thoracotomy.[4,77] Through VATS, the exposure to the pleural space is excellent. However, this often requires the use of general anesthesia and lung isolation. There have been descriptions of VATS being performed without intubation and using a regional or epidural anesthesia.[78–80] However, MT remains the least invasive method to visualize the pleural cavity safely. Further study of these approaches may continue to blur the procedural lines between VATS and MT.

CLINICS CARE POINTS

- Medical thoracoscopy is a safe procedure that has both diagnostic and therapeutic indications in a variety of pleural diseases
- Unlike traditional video-assisted thoracoscopic surgery, general anesthesia is not required to perform medical thoracoscopy

- Inability to access the affected pleural space is an important absolute contraindication for medical thoracoscopy
- There are no robust data that suggest superiority between semirigid and rigid thoracoscopy
  - A majority of the published medical thoracoscopy literature that speaks to the treatment of complicated pleural space infection documents the use of a rigid thoracoscope and VATS

DISCLOSURE

The authors have nothing to disclose.

REFERENCES

1. Barré L. Complément du Dictionnaire de l'Académie Française. Paris: Firmin Didot frères; 1842.
2. Hoksch B, Birken-Bertsch H, Müller JM. Thoracoscopy before jacobaeus. Ann Thorac Surg 2002; 74(4):1288–90.
3. Jacobaeus HV. Uber die Moglichkeit, die Zystoskopie bei Untersuchung seroser Hohlungen anzuwenden. Munch Med Wschr 1910;40:2090–2.
4. Bhatnagar R, Maskell NA. Medical pleuroscopy. Clin Chest Med 2013;34(3):487–500.
5. Hawes JB 2nd, Stone MJ. Closed pneumolysis, or Jacobeus Unverricht operation as an aid in artificial pneumothorax. N Engl J Med 1930;203(8):366–7.
6. Marchetti GP, Pinelli V, Tassi GF. 100 years of thoracoscopy: historical notes. Respiration 2011;82(2): 187–92.
7. Fischer GW, Cohen E. An update on anesthesia for thoracoscopic surgery. Curr Opin Anaesthesiol 2010;23(1):7–11.
8. Duneesha D, Bhatnagar R, Nick AM. Local anaesthetic (medical) thoracoscopy services in the UK. Respiration 2018;96(6):560–3.
9. Madan K, Tiwari P, Thankgakunam B, et al. A survey of medical thoracoscopy practices in India. Lung India 2021;38(1):23–30.
10. Shaikh F, Lentz RJ, Feller-Kopman D, et al. Medical thoracoscopy in the diagnosis of pleural disease: a guide for the clinician. Expert Rev Respir Med 2020;14(10):987–1000.
11. Skalski JH, Astoul PJ, Maldonado F. Medical thoracoscopy. Semin Respir Crit Care Med 2014;35(6): 732–43.
12. Hooper C, Lee YG, Maskell N. Investigation of a unilateral pleural effusion in adults: British thoracic society pleural disease guideline 2010. Thorax 2010; 65(Suppl 2):ii4–17.

13. Saguil A, Wyrick K, Hallgren J. Diagnostic approach to pleural effusion. Am Fam Physician 2014;90(2):99–104.

14. Garcia LW, Ducatman BS, Wang HH. The value of multiple fluid specimens in the cytological diagnosis of malignancy. Mod Pathol 1994;7(6):665–8.

15. Grosu HB, Kazzaz F, Vakil E, et al. Sensitivity of initial thoracentesis for malignant pleural effusion stratified by tumor Type in patients with strong evidence of metastatic disease. Respiration 2018;96(4):363–9.

16. Wang Z, Xu LL, Wu YB, et al. Diagnostic value and safety of medical thoracoscopy in tuberculous pleural effusion. Respir Med 2015;109(9):1188–92.

17. Zhang X, Wang F, Tong Z. Application of Narrow-Band Imaging thoracoscopy in diagnosis of pleural diseases. Postgrad Med 2020;132(5):406–11.

18. Ishida A, Ishikawa F, Nakamura M, et al. Narrow band imaging applied to pleuroscopy for the assessment of vascular patterns of the pleura. Respiration 2009;78(4):432–9.

19. Wang F, Wang Z, Tong Z, et al. A pilot study of auto-fluorescence in the diagnosis of pleural disease. Chest 2015;147(5):1395–400.

20. Puchalski J. Advances and controversies in thoracentesis and medical thoracoscopy. Semin Respir Crit Care Med 2019;40(3):410–6.

21. Hallifax RJ, Corcoran JP, Psallidas I, et al. Medical thoracoscopy: survey of current practice-How successful are medical thoracoscopists at predicting malignancy? Respirology 2016;21(5):958–60.

22. Grosu HB. Rapid on site evaluation of pleural touch preparations in diagnosing malignant pleural effusion in patients undergoing pleuroscopy. National Library of Medicine; 2021. Available at: https://clinicaltrials.gov/ct2/show/NCT03868579. Accessed 06/09/2021.

23. Dhooria S, Bal A, Sehgal IS, et al. Pleural cryobiopsy versus flexible forceps biopsy in subjects with undiagnosed exudative pleural effusions undergoing semirigid thoracoscopy: a crossover randomized trial (COFFEE trial). Respiration 2019;98(2):133–41.

24. Shafiq M, Sethi J, Ali MS, et al. Pleural cryobiopsy: a systematic Review and meta-analysis. Chest 2020; 157(1):223–30.

25. Sasada S, Kawahara K, Kusunoki Y, et al. A new electrocautery pleural biopsy technique using an insulated-tip diathermic knife during semirigid pleuroscopy. Surg Endosc 2009;23(8):1901–7.

26. Wang XB, Yin Y, Miao Y, et al. Flex-rigid pleuroscopic biopsy with the SB knife Jr is a novel technique for diagnosis of malignant or benign fibrothorax. J Thorac Dis 2016;8(11):E1555–9.

27. Yin Y, Eberhardt R, Wang XB, et al. Semi-rigid thoracoscopic punch biopsy using a hybrid knife with a high-pressure water jet for the diagnosis of pleural effusions. Respiration 2016;92(3):192–6.

28. Khan MAI, Ambalavanan S, Thomson D, et al. A comparison of the diagnostic yield of rigid and semirigid thoracoscopes. J Bronchology Interv Pulmonol 2012;19(2):98–101.

29. Rozman A, Camlek L, Marc-Malovrh M, et al. Rigid versus semi-rigid thoracoscopy for the diagnosis of pleural disease: a randomized pilot study. Respirology 2013;18(4):704–10.

30. Dhooria S, Singh N, Aggarwal AN, et al. A randomized trial comparing the diagnostic yield of rigid and semirigid thoracoscopy in undiagnosed pleural effusions. Respir Care 2014;59(5):756–64.

31. Bansal S, Mittal S, Tiwari P, et al. Rigid mini-thoracoscopy versus semirigid thoracoscopy in undiagnosed exudative pleural effusion: the MINT randomized controlled trial. J Bronchology Interv Pulmonol 2020;27(3):163–71.

32. McDonald CM, Pierre C, de Perrot M, et al. Efficacy and cost of awake thoracoscopy and video-assisted thoracoscopic surgery in the undiagnosed pleural effusion. Ann Thorac Surg 2018;106(2):361–7.

33. Wang XJ, Yang Y, Wang Z, et al. Efficacy and safety of diagnostic thoracoscopy in undiagnosed pleural effusions. Respiration 2015;90(3):251–5.

34. Casalini AG, Mori PA, Majori M, et al. Pleural tuberculosis: medical thoracoscopy greatly increases the diagnostic accuracy. ERJ Open Res 2018;4(1). https://doi.org/10.1183/23120541.00046-2017.

35. Bhatnagar R, Piotrowska HEG, Laskawiec-Szkonter M, et al. Effect of thoracoscopic talc poudrage vs talc slurry via chest tube on pleurodesis failure rate among patients with malignant pleural effusions: a randomized clinical trial. JAMA 2020; 323(1):60–9.

36. Tschopp JM, Bintcliffe O, Astoul P, et al. ERS task force statement: diagnosis and treatment of primary spontaneous pneumothorax. Eur Respir J 2015; 46(2):321–35.

37. Baumann MH, Strange C, Heffner JE, et al. Management of spontaneous pneumothorax: an American College of chest Physicians Delphi consensus statement. Chest 2001;119(2):590–602.

38. MacDuff A, Arnold A, Harvey J, et al. Management of spontaneous pneumothorax: British thoracic society pleural disease guideline 2010. Thorax 2010; 65(Suppl 2):ii18–31.

39. Tschopp JM, Boutin C, Astoul P, et al. Talcage by medical thoracoscopy for primary spontaneous pneumothorax is more cost-effective than drainage: a randomised study. Eur Respir J 2002;20(4):1003–9.

40. Clive AO, Jones HE, Bhatnagar R, et al. Interventions for the management of malignant pleural effusions: a network meta-analysis. Cochrane Database Syst Rev 2016;2016(5):Cd010529.

41. Inc BMP. STERITALC®. 2021. Available at: https://www.bosmed.com/en/interventional-pulmonology/steritalcr/. Accessed May 19, 2021.

42. Janssen JP, Collier G, Astoul P, et al. Safety of pleurodesis with talc poudrage in malignant pleural

effusion: a prospective cohort study. Lancet 2007; 369(9572):1535–9.

43. Nayak R, Brogly SB, Lajkosz K, et al. Outcomes of operative and Nonoperative treatment of thoracic empyema: a population-based study. Ann Thorac Surg 2019;108(5):1456–63.

44. Shen KR, Bribriesco A, Crabtree T, et al. The American Association for Thoracic Surgery consensus guidelines for the management of empyema. J Thorac Cardiovasc Surg 2017;153(6):e129–46.

45. Bilgin M, Akcali Y, Oguzkaya F. Benefits of early aggressive management of empyema thoracis. ANZ J Surg 2006;76(3):120–2.

46. Wait MA, Sharma S, Hohn J, et al. A randomized trial of empyema therapy. Chest 1997;111(6):1548–51.

47. Brutsche MH, Tassi G-F, Györik S, et al. Treatment of sonographically stratified multiloculated thoracic empyema by medical thoracoscopy. Chest 2005; 128(5):3303–9.

48. Ravaglia C, Gurioli C, Tomassetti S, et al. Is medical thoracoscopy efficient in the management of multiloculated and organized thoracic empyema? Respiration 2012;84(3):219–24.

49. Kheir F, Thakore S, Mehta H, et al. Intrapleural Fibrinolytic therapy versus early medical thoracoscopy for treatment of pleural infection. Randomized controlled clinical trial. Ann Am Thorac Soc 2020; 17(8):958–64.

50. Pahuja S, Madan K, Mohan A, et al. Medical thoracoscopy for pleural infection: are we there yet? Ann Am Thorac Soc 2020;17(9):1173–4.

51. Sumalani KK, Rizvi NA, Asghar A. Role of medical thoracoscopy in the management of multiloculated empyema. BMC Pulm Med 2018;18(1):179.

52. Mummadi SR, Stoller JK, Lopez R, et al. Epidemiology of adult pleural disease in the United States. Chest 2021. https://doi.org/10.1016/j.chest.2021. 05.026.

53. Segal A, Sterrett GF, Frost FA, et al. A diagnosis of malignant pleural mesothelioma can be made by effusion cytology: results of a 20 year audit. Pathology 2013;45(1):44–8.

54. Renshaw AA, Dean BR, Antman KH, et al. The role of cytologic evaluation of pleural fluid in the diagnosis of malignant mesothelioma. Chest 1997;111(1): 106–9.

55. Rakha EA, Patil S, Abdulla K, et al. The sensitivity of cytologic evaluation of pleural fluid in the diagnosis of malignant mesothelioma. Diagn Cytopathol 2010;38(12):874–9.

56. Committee BTSSoC. BTS statement on malignant mesothelioma in the UK, 2007. Thorax 2007; 62(Suppl 2):ii1.

57. Bibby AC, Tsim S, Kanellakis N, et al. Malignant pleural mesothelioma: an update on investigation, diagnosis and treatment. Eur Respir Rev 2016; 25(142):472–86.

58. Agarwal PP, Seely JM, Matzinger FR, et al. Pleural mesothelioma: sensitivity and incidence of needle track seeding after image-guided biopsy versus surgical biopsy. Radiology 2006;241(2):589–94.

59. Boutin C, Rey F, Gouvernet J, et al. Thoracoscopy in pleural malignant mesothelioma: a prospective study of 188 consecutive patients. Part 2: prognosis and staging. Cancer 1993;72(2):394–404.

60. Galbis JM, Mata M, Guijarro R, et al. Clinical-therapeutic management of thoracoscopy in pleural effusion: a groundbreaking technique in the twenty-first century. Clin Transl Oncol 2011;13(1): 57–60.

61. Ernst A, Herth FJ. Principles and practice of interventional pulmonology. Springer Science & Business Media; 2012.

62. Kindler HL, Ismaila N, Armato SG 3rd, et al. Treatment of malignant pleural mesothelioma: American society of clinical Oncology clinical practice guideline. J Clin Oncol 2018;36(13):1343–73.

63. Lee P, Colt HG. State of the art: pleuroscopy. J Thorac Oncol 2007;2(7):663–70.

64. Du Rand IA, Blaikley J, Booton R, et al. British Thoracic Society guideline for diagnostic flexible bronchoscopy in adults: accredited by NICE. Thorax 2013;68(Suppl 1):i1–44.

65. Mehta AC, Avasarala SK, Jain P, et al. A Blueprint for success: design and implementation of an ideal bronchoscopy suite. Chest 2020;157(3):712–23.

66. Chang SH, Krupnick AS. Perioperative antibiotics in thoracic surgery. Thorac Surg Clin 2012;22(1): 35–45, vi.

67. Koulelidis A, Anevlavis S, Nikitidis N, et al. Local anesthesia thoracoscopy with versus without midazolam: a randomized controlled trial. Respiration 2020;99(9):789–99.

68. Grendelmeier P, Tamm M, Jahn K, et al. Propofol versus midazolam in medical thoracoscopy: a randomized, noninferiority trial. Respiration 2014; 88(2):126–36.

69. Loddenkemper R, Lee P, Noppen M, et al. Medical thoracoscopy/pleuroscopy: step by step. Breathe 2011;8(2):156–67.

70. Hu W, Zhang J, Wang J, et al. [Advantages and disadvantages of preoperative artificial pneumothorax for medical thoracoscopy]. Zhonghua Jie He He Hu Xi Za Zhi 2018;41(10):793–8.

71. Lamb CR, Feller-Kopman D, Ernst A, et al. An approach to interventional pulmonary fellowship training. Chest 2010;137(1):195–9.

72. Rahman NM, Ali NJ, Brown G, et al. Local anaesthetic thoracoscopy: British Thoracic Society pleural disease guideline 2010. Thorax 2010;65(Suppl 2): ii54–60.

73. Mullon JJ, Burkart KM, Silvestri G, et al. Interventional Pulmonology Fellowship Accreditation Standards: Executive Summary of the Multisociety

Interventional Pulmonology Fellowship Accreditation Committee. Chest 2017;151(5):1114–21.

74. Desai NR, French KD, Kovitz KL. Basic and advanced pleural procedures. Chest 2020;158(6): 2517–23.

75. Mahajan AK, Bautista J, Hodson E, et al. Financial justification for interventional pulmonology programs. Chest 2020;158(3):1115–21.

76. Blanc F-X, Atassi K, Bignon J, et al. Diagnostic value of medical thoracoscopy in pleural disease: a 6-year retrospective study. Chest 2002;121(5):1677–83.

77. Guerra M, Neves PC, Martins D, et al. Surgery for thoracic empyema: personal experience and current highlights. Rev Port Cir Cardiotorac Vasc 2012;19(1):21–6.

78. Kao MC, Lan CH, Huang CJ. Anesthesia for awake video-assisted thoracic surgery. Acta Anaesthesiol Taiwan 2012;50(3):126–30.

79. Sunaga H, Blasberg JD, Heerdt PM. Anesthesia for nonintubated video-assisted thoracic surgery. Curr Opin Anaesthesiol 2017;30(1):1–6.

80. Zheng H, Hu XF, Jiang GN, et al. Nonintubated-awake anesthesia for uniportal video-assisted thoracic surgery procedures. Thorac Surg Clin 2017;27(4):399–406.

Section 6: The Future of Pleural Disease

Joining Forces
How to Coordinate Large, Multicenter Randomized Trials

Lance Roller, MS[a], Lonny B. Yarmus, DO, MBA[b], Robert J. Lentz, MD[a,c,d,]*

KEYWORDS

• Clinical trials • Randomized • Multicenter trial • Pleural disease • Research designs

KEY POINTS

- Multicenter trials are increasingly relied on to produce practice-changing advances in medical care.
- A multicenter trial requires data to be acquired from two or more facilities that are organizationally and administratively independent from each other, which are conducting a standardized intervention with uniform central data collection and analysis.
- Major advantages of multicenter trials include being highly generalizable, less prone to confounding or bias related to idiosyncratic local practices, and capable of recruiting participants quickly and potentially to large sample sizes.
- Major challenges in multisite research include greater logistical, administrative, and regulatory burdens, which generally require sufficient funding and time to overcome.
- Further development of research networks capable of fostering multicenter research is required to accelerate the pace at which practice-changing advances in the diagnosis and treatment of pleural disease are realized.

INTRODUCTION

Medical research has long sought to ascertain optimal diagnostic and therapeutic modalities for the management of human disease. The wholesale study of entire populations is rarely practicable, necessitating the study of a sample of individuals belonging to an overall population. Conclusions are then extrapolated back to the population at large. Study results are deemed "high quality" if they are likely to closely approximate the true effect size had the entire population been studied.[1] Various schemas have been developed to assess this concept, all of which consider the design of a study as foundational to estimating the likelihood that its result is applicable to the larger population. One widely used system, the GRADE guidelines, considers randomized controlled trials as "high quality" by default, although downgrading occurs if aspects of the trial introduce biases that make

Summary COI statement: No authors report any financial or nonfinancial conflicts of interest pertinent to this work.

Funding information: Nonfunded work.

Notification of prior publication/presentation: No aspect of this work has been previously published nor is under consideration by any other journals.

[a] Division of Allergy, Pulmonary, and Critical Care Medicine, Vanderbilt University Medical Center, 1161 21st Avenue South, T-1218 MCN, Nashville, TN 37232-2650, USA; [b] Division of Pulmonary and Critical Care Medicine, Johns Hopkins University School of Medicine, 1830 East Monument Street, Baltimore, MD 21287, USA; [c] Department of Thoracic Surgery, Vanderbilt University Medical Center, 1161 21st Avenue South, T-1218 MCN, Nashville, TN 37232-2650, USA; [d] Department of Veterans Affairs Medical Center, Nashville, TN, USA

* Corresponding author. Division of Allergy, Pulmonary, and Critical Care Medicine, Vanderbilt University Medical Center, 1161 21st Avenue South, T-1218 MCN, Nashville, TN 37232-2650.

E-mail address: robert.j.lentz@vumc.org

Twitter: @RobJLentz (R.J.L.)

Clin Chest Med 42 (2021) 767–776
https://doi.org/10.1016/j.ccm.2021.08.011

its result less likely to represent the true population effect.[1,2]

Randomized trials emerged from nonrandom alternate-allocation trial designs in the mid-twentieth century and rapidly gained prominence.[3] However, randomization by itself may not adequately mitigate threats to study validity. Although it should reduce the odds of an important baseline imbalance between groups, it cannot reduce selection bias imparted by regional cultural, ethnic, genetic, or exposure differences when a study is conducted at a single locale.[4] Multicenter randomized trials remedy this problem by recruiting participants across a broader range of the aforementioned categories, therefore bolstering the validity and generalizability of the trial results. Multicenter trials also importantly allow for faster recruitment and shared financial and sometimes regulatory burden.

Several networks dedicated to the multicenter study of important pleural conditions have developed, yielding practice-changing studies in pleural disease. In this review, we describe the importance of multicenter trials, major elements required for the conduct of such trials, and lessons learned from the ongoing development of the Interventional Pulmonary Outcomes Group (IPOG), a consortium of interventional pulmonologists dedicated to advancing diagnostic and management strategies in pleural, pulmonary parenchymal, and airway disease by generating high-quality multicenter evidence.[5]

DISCUSSION
The Case for High-Quality Research in Pleural Disease

Pleural conditions are common and exert a significant financial and resource burden on the health care system in addition to the morbidity and mortality imparted at the level of individual patients. Older data suggest more than 1.5 million new effusions are diagnosed annually in the United States alone, a number derived from the late 1990s and is almost certainly now higher.[6–8] Likewise, the often cited estimated annual incidence of malignant pleural effusions (MPE) of 150,000 to 175,000 in the United States and 100,000 in the United Kingdom date to the late 1980s and are almost certainly underestimates at present.[9,10] MPEs have more recently been estimated to account for 125,000 admissions annually in the United States with charges topping $5 billion per year.[10]

MPE, associated with cancer mortality and symptomatic burden during the final months of life, has been subjected to the most intense study in recent decades, including many multicenter randomized trials.[11–18] Despite this, recent American Thoracic Society, Society of Thoracic Surgeons, and Society of Thoracic Radiology guidelines rank the evidence in favor of seven issued statements as weak per GRADE guidelines, highlighting the need for ongoing high-quality research in pleural disease.[19]

Additionally, technological advances continue to promote the evolution of diagnostic and therapeutic procedures in the wider field of interventional pulmonology. This has recently been most notable in diagnostic bronchoscopy, where a range of new guidance technologies have come to market in the United States in the last decade, including robotic-assisted bronchoscopy platforms and systems capable of correcting for computed tomography body divergence using digital tomosynthesis.[20–22] Biopsy tools are also evolving. With rare exception, these and related recent technologies have been cleared by the Food and Drug Administration under the 510(k) pathway, in which a novel medical device classified as having low or moderate risk of harm is only required to demonstrate substantial equivalence to a commercialized predicate device. Applications require some evidence supporting a claim of substantial equivalence in safety and effectiveness, but clinical data characterizing the performance of the new device are not typically required. Proponents argue this pathway is vital for the timely introduction of practice-changing technological advances. However, there are notable examples of 510(k) devices proving neither safe or nor efficacious and data suggesting 510(k)-cleared devices are recalled more frequently than devices undergoing formal premarket approval, which requires trial data demonstrating safety and effectiveness. It is therefore incumbent on the academic interventional pulmonology community to study new 510(k)-cleared devices as they come to market, including those intended for use in the pleural space.

Definition of a Multicenter Trial

Clinical trials involve the prospective allocation of patients into multiple groups (one group is often a control or current standard-of-care arm), with the intent of assessing the efficacy (or risks) of a specific treatment, therapy, medical device, or other medical intervention intended to treat or diagnose human disease.[4,23] Randomized allocation into treatment and control groups is preferred for generating data from which causal inferences will be made.[4] Proper randomization results in recognized and unrecognized confounding factors to be balanced between study groups, greatly reducing the risk of spurious or confounded conclusions to result from the investigation. In some cases, random assignment of research subjects is not practicable or is unethical, necessitating alternative study design.

A multicenter trial requires three elements: (1) data acquired from two or more facilities that are organizationally and administratively independent from each other, (2) a standardized intervention and uniform data collection, and (3) central data collection and analysis.[4]

Advantages of Multicenter Trials

Multicenter trials offer many potential advantages over single-center investigations (summarized in **Table 1**). First, simultaneous recruitment at multiple sites allows for recruitment of a larger number of patients. This translates directly into greater statistical power and therefore a higher likelihood of correctly identifying a difference between experimental and control groups on a given outcome measure, assuming a difference actually exists. Statistical significance does imply clinical significance; trials should not be intentionally overpowered to detect a difference between groups that is not clinically pertinent. That said, a small benefit or detection of a difference in the incidence of a rare outcome may still be meaningful to individual patients, the health care system, or society. For example, a particular intervention found to reduce hospital length of stay by 1 day could be insignificant in some settings (following an operation with an average length of stay of 10 days) but significant in others (following a procedure with average length of stay of just 2 days, in patients with limited life expectancy, such as pleurodesis for MPE).

Second, multicenter trials have the capacity to recruit subjects more rapidly than would be possible at a single site. This has financial benefits, because ongoing studies require ongoing funding to maintain the research apparatus. Furthermore, more rapid completion of high-quality trials means new findings are reported and implemented into practice more expeditiously.

Third, multicenter trials tend to recruit subjects who better represent the at-risk population as a whole in terms of cultural, ethnic, socioeconomic, genetic, and environmental exposure variation, any of which could influence the results of a study performed in a sample that is more homogeneous than the at-risk population. This greatly enhances the generalizability of conclusions derived from multicenter data. Relatedly, multicenter trials are less subject to idiosyncratic practice variations at a single institution, which are also a threat to generalizability, particularly when the intervention is a procedure.

Fourth, related to larger sample sizes possible and more heterogeneous samples, large multicenter trials offer the opportunity for more robust subgroup analyses to investigate heterogeneity of treatment effect and generate hypotheses for future trials.

Finally, diffusion across multiple centers allows for studies to be designed in a more collaborative

Table 1
Advantages and barriers to multicenter RCTs

Advantages	Barriers

Large
  More statistical power
  More meaningful subgroup analyses
	Regulatory requirements
	  Multiple IRBs
	  Multiple contracts and data-sharing agreements
	  Variable requirements between institutions,
	    countries

Once enrolling, can accrue participants
  quickly
	Cost/funding
	  Relatively high cost
	  Little support in developing nations

More generalizable results
  More diverse sample
  More diverse intervention delivery
    settings
  Less prone to idiosyncratic local
    confounding
	Overmonitoring
	  Default monitoring level set to that required of novel
	    therapeutics seeking FDA premarket approval
	  AE monitoring can be overzealous
	  Monitoring has become an industry

Pooling of research resources	Overly complex protocol
	  Demands of multiple IRBs
	  Compromise through complexity
	  Nested substudies

Abbreviations: AE, adverse event; FDA, Food and Drug Administration; IRB, institutional review boards.

manner and for sharing of research resources. The former promotes protocols that are more inclusive of different clinical settings, populations, and small variations in local practices, all of which further enhances subsequent generalizability of the results. The latter helps reduce barriers to the actual conduct of a trial, which are often financial or resource-based.

Challenges of Multicenter Research

Although the benefits of well-conducted multicenter trials are clear, there are numerous costs, literal and figurative, to conducting multisite research, also summarized in **Table 1**. These include greater administrative demands, regulatory burdens, need for monitoring subject and data quality to protect against threats to study validity, potential for overcomplicated protocols, and logistic challenges related to applying a single intervention in different settings, among others. These challenges threaten to slow down trial progress and ultimately translate into increased trial cost.

Research regulatory requirements have become increasingly complex. Most multicenter trials require the interface of a single protocol with multiple local institutional review boards (IRBs), which may require or prohibit different elements. This generally results in numerous protocol amendments that must then be submitted across all sites to maintain core protocol uniformity. International research is further complicated by country-specific regulatory requirements. Contracts and data sharing agreements between institutions or industry sponsors further complicate the regulatory realm.

Multicenter trial protocols also have a propensity to be overly complex. This arises as a consequence of variable regulatory demands from different locales necessitating protocol amendments, the collaborative nature of protocol development in which compromise is sometimes accomplished through complexity in the form of added elements, and inclusion of nested substudies intended to maximize knowledge gained and academic output but which requires additional logistic and data support. Complexity increases cost, promotes protocol deviations, and may dissuade additional prospective sites from joining a study.

Diffusion of study responsibilities across multiple sites and a greater number of study personnel can imperil study validity by inadvertent enrollment of ineligible subjects by teams less familiar with the protocol or submission of erroneous or incomplete data. Typical safeguards include requiring redundant eligibility confirmation before randomization,

study monitoring to verify database entries match clinical source documentation, and audits. The entity performing these checks should be independent from the core research team, which therefore requires the engagement of a research coordinating service.

The costs of mitigating the previously mentioned challenges comes in the form of money and time. Dedicated personnel facile with the various regulatory processes and independent coordinating center staff require funding to engage, not to mention the cost of supporting the central research team and all local sites and their staffs. Additional time spent addressing these elements during the study planning phase threatens to offset a major benefit of multicenter trials: the more rapid accrual of participants during the active study period.

Research support infrastructure and study monitoring has become an industry. Current trial monitoring frequently defaults to the high level required for regulatory approval of novel medications, which represents overregulation for a study involving already-approved medications or comparing two standard-of-care procedures.[24] Evidence that current study monitoring strategies impact the validity or outcomes of multicenter clinical trials is also lacking.[24,25]

Elements of a Successful Multicenter Randomized Controlled Trial

We have divided the steps involved in conducting a multicenter trial into three sections: (1) the pre-enrollment planning phase, (2) the active enrollment phase, and (3) the postenrollment phase. Each involves multiple distinct processes presented in vaguely chronologic order, although most overlap rather than proceeding sequentially. The terminology used to describe various groups, such as "central coordinating center" (CCC) for the core group of researchers directing the study, may vary between institutions or research networks.

Pre-enrollment planning
Defining the research question A would-be primary investigator (PI) should have a firm grasp on the nature of a clinical problem and intimate knowledge of related existing literature. From this a research question can be developed, which if answered would inform medical practice above and beyond currently extant data. The Patient/Problem/Population, Intervention, Comparison, Outcome (PICO) format is commonly used to construct a precise research question around which a trial protocol may be developed.[26] The question is further refined using a framework, such as the FINER criteria, in which a good

research question is feasible, interesting, novel, ethical, and relevant.[27] An additional consideration specific to multicenter trials includes whether sufficient foundational research has been performed to inform the development of a large-scale trial, including whether reasonable estimates of primary outcome measures can be made based on prior research or pilot studies.

Developing the central coordinating center CCC is our terminology for the core group of researchers responsible for planning, conducting, and interpretating a multicenter trial. This group invariably includes the PI, coinvestigators (Co-Is), and study coordinators. Study statisticians tend to be included in this group. The CCC is often contained within one academic institution leading a multicenter trial or may be comprised of individuals at different institutions participating in a research network.

The PI is ultimately responsible for all aspects of the trial. This investigator tends to be the originator of the research question and the primary architect of the protocol. Multicenter research favors a PI with significant clinical trial experience who is well-connected and well-respected within a clinical or academic community, which facilitates a strong study protocol, identification and recruitment of additional centers, and acquisition of study funding. These traits also place the PI in a position to arbitrate disagreements and build consensus among a disparate group of investigators (eg, on matters related to the study protocol or data interpretation). The PI also provides the final word when problems invariably arise and takes ultimate responsibility for the safety and privacy of all study participants.

Central Co-Is tend to be other investigators with clinical backgrounds (including physicians, advanced practice providers, pharmacists, trainees) at the same institution as the PI, or who are senior members of an established research network or subcommittee. They often assist with protocol development, recruitment, and study procedures (if applicable) during active enrollment. In some of our multicenter studies, one Co-I along with the study coordinator have together been responsible for managing the day-to-day conduct of a trial, with input elicited from the PI when necessary. This is a particularly important role for junior investigators seeking experience in clinic trial design and management.

The study coordinator (variably described as research coordinator, trial manager, or similar) is a vital position whose importance cannot be understated. Although most CCC staff have clinical and other responsibilities competing for time and attention, the study coordinator provides full-time support to the research enterprise and is often the point person for day-to-day trial affairs. Responsibilities vary, but generally include input into trial development (especially logistics), monitoring or actively assisting in ensuring regulatory approvals and contracts are established, creating or monitoring budgets and billing plans, recruiting study subjects, data entry and fidelity monitoring, handling of biospecimens, follow-up visit tracking, and ensuring pertinent regulatory tasks are performed (eg, adverse event reporting). Our study coordinators also participate in data analysis and manuscript preparation as integral members of our research teams.

There has been considerable commentary in the literature about the often overlooked or underrecognized specialty role of the study coordinator, and the pressing need to recruit, train, and retain adept coordinators as clinical trials continue to grow in number. Several potential barriers to this have been identified, including gender-related inequalities, limited formal educational or training pathways, academic underrecognition, and typical salaries.[28] Regarding the former, prior work identified women as overrepresented in the coordinator role. A 1990 paper describing the components of a successful multicenter trial comments, "She, for it is seldom he, stands at the center of the trial."[29] More recently, it was estimated 80% of trial managers within major UK clinical trial units are women.[30] In contrast, women remain underrepresented in the role of PI, as funding awardees, at more senior levels of academic medicine, and in other areas of senior trial leadership.[31–33] This creates the potential for gender inequality to influence coordinator careers and research group productivity. Coordinators are also less likely to be recognized academically as coauthors for their crucial contributions to all aspects of the conduct of a published trial. Finally, coordinators are often absent from decision-making boards at research funding institutions. Prior work suggests one-third of trials remain unpublished or unreported 30 months after proposed completion.[34,35] As experts in trial conduct, coordinators in prominent positions within funding organizations might better identify studies likely to succeed and make results public.

Engaging statistical support is also vital early in the development of any trial. Power calculation and statistical analysis plans inform the feasibility of a trial and the development of the study protocol. Some groups use a separate data coordinating center, particularly for large trials, in which statistical, data management, and data fidelity expertise resides.

Finally, many institutions have personnel specializing in different aspects of governmental or institutional regulatory, budgeting, or contracting requirements, which are often engaged during the planning phase of a multicenter trial.

Funding Multicenter trials are often expensive, because of the large variety of personnel required to plan a study, secure regulatory approval, manage the database and the quality of the data therein, recruit patients, deliver whatever intervention the study is investigating, then follow for outcomes over time until data are analyzed to an interpretable result. Discussion of the range of funding opportunities for multicenter research is beyond the scope of this review and varies by locale, but generally includes governmental, academic societal, academic institutional, private philanthropic, and corporate funding mechanisms.

Prior work has estimated the cost of multicenter trials. A 2003 study of a mock phase III multicenter trial of a cancer drug estimated more than $6000 would be required to fund the proposed study per enrolled subject, with one-third of research time and money dedicated to regulatory affairs.[36] In 2021 dollars, the cost per subject would be almost $9500. Another study evaluated 28 phase III trials funded by the US National Institute of Neurologic Disorders and Stroke before 2000, totaling $335 million in funding. Despite the high price tag, the improvements to health resulting from these trials provided a net benefit to society after 10 years estimated at $15.2 billion, representing a substantial return on government investment.[37]

Multicenter trials do not automatically require a lot of dedicated funding. As examples, we recently executed and published two multicenter trials regarding therapeutic thoracentesis techniques (manometry-guided aspiration vs symptom-guided; manual syringe aspiration vs gravity drainage).[14,15] The first was supported by a modest amount of funding, whereas the second, conducted at 10 sites, was unfunded. These trials compared different standard-of-care techniques and therefore required no specific funding related to the interventions. Both used postdoctoral pulmonary fellows to assist at sites without dedicated study personnel, who were in turn recognized as authors and gained experience conducting participating in a multicenter trial. Although this low-cost model is not applicable to many interventions, it could be considered when evaluating variations on existing standard-of-care interventions. Any trainee involvement should be encouraged and acknowledged appropriately.

Recruiting local sites High-performing local sites recruit patients efficiently, input accurate data in a timely manner, and maintain regulatory compliance. Selection of local sites capable of these tasks is therefore crucial to the successful completion of a multicenter trial. The study team at a local site usually consists of a local PI, responsible for overseeing research conduct at the site, local Co-Is who assist with patient recruitment, and local study coordinators to assist with data entry and regulatory compliance.

Identification of prospective local sites might hinge on many potential factors. Involvement with specialty societies or participation in national or international meetings and the networking that often accompanies such events can play a significant role. Evidence of ability to recruit for prior trials, active pursuit of local research, and prompt responses to queries are favorable signs. Most centers, with modern electronic health record assistance, can precisely estimate the volume of pertinent patients seen or procedures performed on an annual basis. Red flags include local personnel who are difficult to reach, slow to respond, or unresponsive to specific requests.

It is not necessary to have all sites approved and ready to enroll simultaneously at the outset of a multicenter trial. Many studies open initially at the central or sponsoring institution with other sites coming online as regulatory approvals are obtained. This also allows for overt issues to be identified by central study personnel who know the protocol most intimately so they are rectified before broad multisite implementation. Agreements to participate between the central PI and prospective local PIs are advantageous to establish early in the planning stage, however, and building in excess capacity is favorable to lagging recruitment because of underperforming sites during the active phase of the trial.

Establishing a research network is another mechanism to ensure the interest and cooperation of multiple sites with a favorable track record of executing clinical trials. This is the driving motivation behind the recent development of the IPOG. The IPOG has facilitated a range of studies to date, including investigator-initiated, industry-sponsored, and National Institutes of Health–funded trials. Making connections with an established research network, such as IPOG, is also an avenue in which a center inexperienced in conducting clinical trials can begin to participate in the multicenter research process.

Protocol development The protocol details study rationale, procedures, outcomes, safety/regulatory issues, and analysis plan. It determines how study interventions are conducted, what data are collected, and preemptively details how that data will be used based on the hypothesis on which the study is predicated. It therefore requires consideration from multiple perspectives, including knowledge of existing medical literature and a specific clinical question or problem, study logistics, and statistical considerations.

The central PI is usually the primary architect of the protocol, with input from central Co-Is and often local PIs who are identified early in the planning phase. The latter also help identify issues arising because of difference in practice patterns at different institutions. Some groups use a formal Delphi process to bring about consensus during protocol development.[38] In-person meetings of key stakeholders in a developing multicenter trial are also helpful in coalescing around a specific protocol, albeit more challenging in the current pandemic.

Pilot studies may be instrumental to the success of a subsequent larger multicenter trial. Such studies are primarily intended to generate more informed estimates of the magnitude of outcome effect sizes, which then feeds into the power calculation of the subsequent multicenter trial. They can also clarify whether recruiting patients into a given intervention is feasible, especially if there are concerns about the logistics of a particular intervention. However, if effect size can be reasonably estimated from existing data and logistical barriers are perceived to be low, a pilot study may not contribute substantially but will cost time and money.

Finally, once the protocol is established, a protocol paper should be considered. This benefits the study group by ensuring all aspects of the trial have been well-deliberated. Additionally, if significant protocol changes are believed necessary during the conduct of a trial, the discrepancy between final reported methods and methods described in the protocol paper enforces the need for the transparency of a full explanation. The methods paper is easy to adapt from a mature trial protocol and represents the first of many publications from a well-designed multicenter trial.

Regulatory affairs Regulatory compliance is a source of significant costs (in money and time) in the pre-enrollment phase of a trial, magnified in a multicenter trial in which local regulatory approvals are also necessary at each participating institution. This includes matters related to central and local IRBs or ethics committees, data sharing agreements, contracts between institutions or institutions and industry sponsors, clinical trial registration (eg, clinicaltrials.gov), and at times federal agencies (eg, the Food and Drug Administration). More general data privacy and protection

laws, including the European Union's General Data Protection Regulation, must also be complied with.

In recent years, some research networks have developed central IRB review, in which a single institution's IRB is designated as the IRB of record by way of reliance agreements between local participating sites and the central site.[39] To date, many large academic medical institutions do not allow participation to ensure local oversight.

Training and standardization of trial procedures One major potential pitfall of multicenter trials is the diffusion of study responsibilities to personnel outside the immediate locus of observation and control of the central core of researchers most responsible for developing the trial. Standardizing study procedures such that they are performed as similarly as possible at all participating sites is of paramount importance. A detailed and unambiguous description of study procedures in the trial protocol, specific training for all study personnel delivered during a site initiation visit as each local site begins to enroll subjects, and monitoring incoming local data to identify sites in need of restandardization are strongly encouraged. In the COVID-19 pandemic, most site initiation visits have been performed virtually via teleconferencing.

Enrollment phase

In the enrollment phase of a trial, in which subjects are actively being recruited and study interventions performed, attention is directed to several core processes: enrolling new patients and ensuring study-related follow-up, maintaining regulatory compliance (eg, adverse event reporting), and monitoring data quality. Interim analyses may also be performed during this phase.

Subject recruitment The rate at which patients are recruited into a trial usually directly determines the duration of the enrollment phase and is therefore the main focus during this part of the trial. Quick recruitment across all sites also allows for time to be "made up" to offset the slower, more arduous regulatory processes entailed in multicenter research.

Recruitment efforts tend to fall on patient-facing research staff, including the PI, Co-Is, and study coordinator. Recruitment may be passive, in which prospective subjects are screened for inclusion after referral to a particular clinic or service, or active, which might include mailers, calls, emails, and/or social network outreach directly to patients or to other practitioners.[40] Active recruitment methods often require local regulatory approval, and cost. Lists of patients with specific diagnosis or procedure codes can often also be generated by querying electronic health records, which coordinators can use to screen charts for additional eligibility criteria.

Establishing monthly local recruitment targets, usually based loosely on annual volume related to the patient population in question, can help encourage ongoing recruitment. We tend to use a monthly trial newsletter, distributed to central and local PIs, Co-Is, and study coordinators, as a friendly reminder of ongoing efforts and targets (**Fig. 1**).

Data entry and monitoring data quality Large trials, particularly related to drugs or devices moving through the premarket approval Food and Drug Administration pathway, almost always engage the services of independent study monitors. These staff are responsible for verifying data in the study database are complete and are corroborated by the primary data in the medical record. This typically entails multiple visits to each local site and interfacing with local study personnel and electronic health records. Audits including detailed assessment of enrollment criteria and adverse event reporting are often conducted. Such intensive monitoring has been estimated by some to comprise 25% to 35% of the cost of a trial.[24] In the absence of this kind of intensive local monitoring, data being entered into the central database should be intermittently reviewed by central trial staff for missing data, nonsensical values, or other suggestions of impaired data quality, which should lead to prompt queries to local study staff for clarification.

Postenrollment phase

After active enrollment finishes, there is often a tail period in which subjects are still undergoing follow-up study examinations or procedures. During this time period, central and local coordinators no longer have the burden of pushing for subject accrual, freeing up time to further inspect the data for quality and completeness.

Much of the primary manuscript can be drafted while awaiting final data points to be entered. We suggest establishing a writing committee and setting expectations for authorship well earlier, however, ideally during the pre-enrollment phase. Once all data have been entered, statistical analysis commences according to the prespecified analysis plan, allowing for the results and

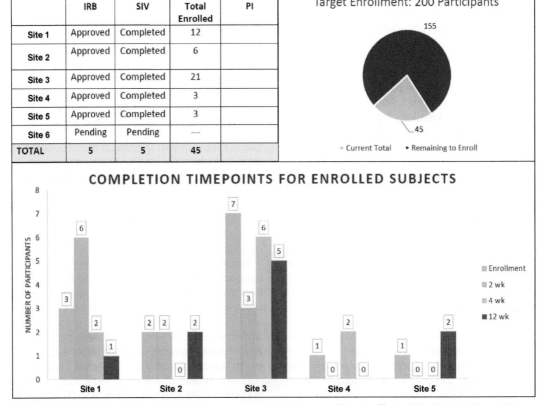

Fig. 1. Example of a monthly newsletter to encourage ongoing enrollment efforts. SIV, site initiation visit.

discussion sections of the primary manuscript to be completed. By drafting as much as possible in advance, the delay between close of accrual and manuscript preparation can be kept to a minimum.

A large, multicenter trial almost always collects more data than can be reported in the primary manuscript. Additional manuscripts, often drafted by local PIs, Co-Is, trainees or students, and other study staff, may not require tail data and can sometimes be published before the primary manuscript (although the decision to publish anything derived from the study should be reviewed by the central PI first). We encourage these side efforts, which can provide substantial additional value to multicenter trial participation and are another opportunity for junior investigators to show interest and productivity.

SUMMARY

Multicenter trials are capable of producing high-quality clinical research with the greatest degree of generalizability. They are increasingly considered the standard for generating practice-changing medical data. Conducting a successful multicenter trial requires significant time, money, and planning by a large group of disparate individuals, with numerous pitfalls as discussed. Despite their complexity, the benefits of conducting such trials seem to substantially outweigh the costs. As medical innovation progresses at an increasingly rapid rate, it will be vital to create more and enduring multicenter trial networks with expertise in studying new interventions at this high level.

CLINICS CARE POINTS

- Multicenter RCTs can accrue quickly, achieve large enrollment targets, and be highly generalizable; these benefits can be offset by cost, complexity, and high regulatory burden.
- Conducting a multicenter RCT involves distinct phases (pre-enrollment planning, active enrollment, post-enrollment) with unique demands.
- Developing or engaging a preexisting central coordinating center, including central PI and Co-Is, coordinator(s), and statistician(s) is crucial to a successful trial.
- The importance of research coordinator training, retention, and recognition appears to be under-emphasized.

FINANCIAL/NONFINANCIAL DISCLOSURES

No authors report any financial or nonfinancial conflicts of interest pertinent to this work outside the declared funding source for this trial (see below re: role of funding source).

FUNDING/ROLE OF SPONSORS

This study was not supported by funding.

ACKNOWLEDGMENTS

Guarantor statement: All authors take responsibility for the content of this work.

AUTHOR CONTRIBUTIONS

Study concept and design: all authors. Acquisition of data: n/a. Analysis and interpretation of data: n/a. Drafting of the manuscript: all authors. All authors participated in critical revision of the manuscript for important intellectual content and provided final approval to submit this version of the manuscript and have agreed to be accountable for all aspects of the work.

REFERENCES

1. Guyatt G, Oxman AD, Akl EA, et al. GRADE guidelines: 1. Introduction—GRADE evidence profiles and summary of findings tables. J Clin Epidemiol 2011;64(4):383–94.
2. Guyatt GH, Oxman AD, Vist GE, et al. GRADE: an emerging consensus on rating quality of evidence and strength of recommendations. BMJ 2008; 336(7650):924–6.
3. Bothwell LE, Podolsky SH. The emergence of the randomized, controlled trial. N Engl J Med 2016; 375(6):501–4.
4. Meinert CL, Tonascia S. Clinical trials : design, conduct, and analysis. New York : Oxford University Press; 1986.
5. Maldonado F, Yarmus L. Pragmatic studies in interventional pulmonology: two steps forward, one step back, but an imminent leap forward. Introducing IPOG, the Interventional Pulmonary Outcome Group. J Bronchology Interv Pulmonol 2019;26(3):150–2.
6. Light RW. Pleural diseases. 6th edition. Philadelphia: Lippincott Williams & Wilkins; 2013.
7. Owings MF, Kozak LJ. Ambulatory and inpatient procedures in the United States, 1996. Vital Health Stat 1998;13(139):1–119.
8. Feller-Kopman D. Therapeutic thoracentesis: the role of ultrasound and pleural manometry. Curr Opin Pulm Med 2007;13(4):312–8.
9. Marel M, Zrůstová M, Stasný B, et al. The incidence of pleural effusion in a well-defined region. Epidemiologic study in central Bohemia. Chest 1993;104(5): 1486–9.

10. Taghizadeh N, Fortin M, Tremblay A. US hospitalizations for malignant pleural effusions: data from the 2012 national inpatient sample. Chest 2017;151(4):845–54.

11. Rahman NM, Pepperell J, Rehal S, et al. Effect of opioids vs NSAIDs and larger vs smaller chest tube size on pain control and pleurodesis efficacy among patients with malignant pleural effusion: the TIME1 randomized clinical trial. JAMA 2015; 314(24):2641–53.

12. Bhatnagar R, Keenan EK, Morley AJ, et al. Outpatient talc administration by indwelling pleural catheter for malignant effusion. N Engl J Med 2018; 378(14):1313–22.

13. Davies HE, Mishra EK, Kahan BC, et al. Effect of an indwelling pleural catheter vs chest tube and talc pleurodesis for relieving dyspnea in patients with malignant pleural effusion: the TIME2 randomized controlled trial. JAMA 2012;307(22):2383.

14. Lentz RJ, Lerner AD, Pannu JK, et al. Routine monitoring with pleural manometry during therapeutic large-volume thoracentesis to prevent pleural-pressure-related complications: a multicentre, single-blind randomised controlled trial. Lancet Respir Med 2019;7(5):447–55.

15. Lentz RJ, Shojaee S, Grosu HB, et al. The impact of gravity vs suction-driven therapeutic thoracentesis on pressure-related complications: the GRAVITAS multicenter randomized controlled trial. Chest 2020;157(3):702–11.

16. Wahidi MM, Reddy C, Yarmus L, et al. Randomized trial of pleural fluid drainage frequency in patients with malignant pleural effusions. The ASAP trial. Am J Respir Crit Care Med 2017;195(8):1050–7.

17. Muruganandan S, Azzopardi M, Fitzgerald DB, et al. Aggressive versus symptom-guided drainage of malignant pleural effusion via indwelling pleural catheters (AMPLE-2): an open-label randomised trial. Lancet Respir Med 2018;6(9):671–80.

18. Mishra EK, Clive AO, Wills GH, et al. Randomized controlled trial of urokinase versus placebo for non-draining malignant pleural effusion. Am J Respir Crit Care Med 2018;197(4):502–8.

19. Feller-Kopman DJ, Reddy CB, DeCamp MM, et al. Management of malignant pleural effusions. An official ATS/STS/STR clinical practice guideline. Am J Respir Crit Care Med 2018;198(7):839–49.

20. Agrawal A, Hogarth DK, Murgu S. Robotic bronchoscopy for pulmonary lesions: a review of existing technologies and clinical data. J Thorac Dis 2020; 12(6):3279–86.

21. Aboudara M, Roller L, Rickman O, et al. Improved diagnostic yield for lung nodules with digital tomosynthesis-corrected navigational bronchoscopy: initial experience with a novel adjunct. Respirology 2020;25(2):206–13.

22. Katsis J, Roller L, Lester M, et al. High accuracy of digital tomosynthesis-guided bronchoscopic biopsy confirmed by intraprocedural computed tomography. Respiration 2021;1–8. https://doi.org/10.1159/000512802.

23. Fuhrer MJ. Conducting multiple-site clinical trials in medical rehabilitation research. Am J Phys Med Rehabil 2005;84(11):823–31.

24. Duley L, Antman K, Arena J, et al. Specific barriers to the conduct of randomized trials. Clin Trials 2008;5(1):40–8.

25. Prescott RJ, Counsell CE, Gillespie WJ, et al. Factors that limit the quality, number and progress of randomised controlled trials. Health Technol Assess 1999;3(20):1–143.

26. Davies KS. Formulating the evidence based practice question: a review of the frameworks. EBLIP 2011;6(2):75.

27. Hulley SB. Designing clinical research. Philadelphia: Lippincott Williams & Wilkins; 2007.

28. Buchanan DA, Goldstein J, Pfalzer AC, et al. Empowering the clinical research coordinator in academic medical centers. Mayo Clin Proc Innov Qual Outcomes 2020;5(2):265–73.

29. Warlow C. How to do it. Organise a multicentre trial. BMJ 1990;300(6718):180–3.

30. Beaumont D, Arribas M, Frimley L, et al. Trial management: we need a cadre of high-class triallists to deliver the answers that patients need. Trials 2019;20:354.

31. Penny M, Jeffries R, Grant J, et al. Women and academic medicine: a review of the evidence on female representation. J R Soc Med 2014;107(7):259–63.

32. Fitzpatrick S. A survey of staffing levels of medical clinical academics in UK medical schools as at 31 July 201. 36. Medical Schools Council, London, UK, 2012.

33. Zhou CD, Head MG, Marshall DC, et al. A systematic analysis of UK cancer research funding by gender of primary investigator. BMJ Open 2018;8(4):e018625.

34. Jones CW, Handler L, Crowell KE, et al. Non-publication of large randomized clinical trials: cross sectional analysis. BMJ 2013;347:f6104.

35. Gordon D, Taddei-Peters W, Mascette A, et al. Publication of trials funded by the National Heart, Lung, and Blood Institute. N Engl J Med 2013;369(20):1926–34.

36. Emanuel EJ, Schnipper LE, Kamin DY, et al. The costs of conducting clinical research. J Clin Oncol 2003;21(22):4145–50.

37. Johnston SC, Rootenberg JD, Katrak S, et al. Effect of a US National Institutes of Health programme of clinical trials on public health and costs. Lancet 2006;367(9519):1319–27.

38. Chung KC, Song JW. A guide on organizing a multicenter clinical trial: the WRIST study group. Plast Reconstr Surg 2010;126(2):515–23.

39. Burr JS, Johnson AR, Vasenina V, et al. Implementing a central IRB model in a multicenter research network. Ethics Hum Res 2019;41(3):23–8.

40. Carter Barry L, Gail A. Avoiding pitfalls with implementation of randomized controlled multicenter trials: strategies to achieve milestones. J Am Heart Assoc 2016;5(12):e004432.

UNITED STATES POSTAL SERVICE ®

Statement of Ownership, Management, and Circulation
(All Periodicals Publications Except Requester Publications)

1. Publication Title	2. Publication Number	3. Filing Date
CLINICS IN CHEST MEDICINE	000 – 706	9/18/2021

4. Issue Frequency	5. Number of Issues Published Annually	6. Annual Subscription Price
MAR, JUN, SEP, DEC	4	$396.00

7. Complete Mailing Address of Known Office of Publication (Not printer) (Street, city, county, state, and ZIP+4®)

ELSEVIER INC.
230 Park Avenue, Suite 800
New York, NY 10169

Contact Person
Malathi Samayan

Telephone (Include area code)
91-44-4299-4507

8. Complete Mailing Address of Headquarters or General Business Office of Publisher (Not printer)

ELSEVIER INC.
230 Park Avenue, Suite 800
New York, NY 10169

9. Full Names and Complete Mailing Addresses of Publisher, Editor, and Managing Editor (Do not leave blank)

Publisher (Name and complete mailing address)

Editor (Name and complete mailing address)

COLLEEN DETZLER, ELSEVIER INC.
1600 JOHN F KENNEDY BLVD. SUITE 1800
PHILADELPHIA, PA 19103-2899

Managing Editor (Name and complete mailing address)

PATRICK MANLEY, ELSEVIER INC.
1600 JOHN F KENNEDY BLVD. SUITE 1800
PHILADELPHIA, PA 19103-2899

10. Owner (Do not leave blank. If the publication is owned by a corporation, give the name and address of the corporation immediately followed by the names and addresses of all stockholders owning or holding 1 percent or more of the total amount of stock. If not owned by a corporation, give the names and addresses of the individual owners. If owned by a partnership or other unincorporated firm, give its name and address as well as those of each individual owner. If the publication is published by a nonprofit organization, give its name and address.)

Full Name	Complete Mailing Address
WHOLLY OWNED SUBSIDIARY OF REED/ELSEVIER, US HOLDINGS	1600 JOHN F KENNEDY BLVD. SUITE 1800 PHILADELPHIA, PA 19103-2899

11. Known Bondholders, Mortgagees, and Other Security Holders Owning or Holding 1 Percent or More of Total Amount of Bonds, Mortgages, or Other Securities. If none, check box ▶ ☐ None

Full Name	Complete Mailing Address
N/A	

12. Tax Status (For completion by nonprofit organizations authorized to mail at nonprofit rates) (Check one)
The purpose, function, and nonprofit status of this organization and the exempt status for federal income tax purposes:
☒ Has Not Changed During Preceding 12 Months
☐ Has Changed During Preceding 12 Months (Publisher must submit explanation of change with this statement)

PS Form **3526**, July 2014 [Page 1 of 4 (see instructions page 4)]   PSN: 7530-01-000-9931   PRIVACY NOTICE: See our privacy policy on *www.usps.com*.

13. Publication Title	14. Issue Date for Circulation Data Below
CLINICS IN CHEST MEDICINE	JUNE 2021

15. Extent and Nature of Circulation		Average No. Copies Each Issue During Preceding 12 Months	No. Copies of Single Issue Published Nearest to Filing Date
a. Total Number of Copies (Net press run)		391	338
b. Paid Circulation (By Mail and Outside the Mail)	(1) Mailed Outside-County Paid Subscriptions Stated on PS Form 3541 (Include paid distribution above nominal rate, advertiser's proof copies, and exchange copies)	228	208
	(2) Mailed In-County Paid Subscriptions Stated on PS Form 3541 (Include paid distribution above nominal rate, advertiser's proof copies, and exchange copies)	0	0
	(3) Paid Distribution Outside the Mails Including Sales Through Dealers and Carriers, Street Vendors, Counter Sales, and Other Paid Distribution Outside USPS®	117	92
	(4) Paid Distribution by Other Classes of Mail Through the USPS (e.g. First-Class Mail®)	0	0
c. Total Paid Distribution (Sum of 15b (1), (2), (3), and (4))		345	300
d. Free or Nominal Rate Distribution (By Mail and Outside the Mail)	(1) Free or Nominal Rate Outside-County Copies included on PS Form 3541	26	20
	(2) Free or Nominal Rate In-County Copies Included on PS Form 3541	0	0
	(3) Free or Nominal Rate Copies Mailed at Other Classes Through the USPS (e.g. First-Class Mail)	0	0
	(4) Free or Nominal Rate Distribution Outside the Mail (Carriers or other means)	0	0
e. Total Free or Nominal Rate Distribution (Sum of 15d (1), (2), (3) and (4))		26	20
f. Total Distribution (Sum of 15c and 15e)		371	320
g. Copies not Distributed (See instructions to Publishers #4 (page #3))		20	18
h. Total (Sum of 15f and g)		391	338
i. Percent Paid (15c divided by 15f times 100)		92.99%	93.75%

* If you are claiming electronic copies, go to line 16 on page 3. If you are not claiming electronic copies, skip to line 17 on page 3.

PS Form **3526**, July 2014 (Page 2 of 4)

16. Electronic Copy Circulation	Average No. Copies Each Issue During Preceding 12 Months	No. Copies of Single Issue Published Nearest to Filing Date
a. Paid Electronic Copies ▶		
b. Total Paid Print Copies (Line 15c) + Paid Electronic Copies (Line 16a) ▶		
c. Total Print Distribution (Line 15f) + Paid Electronic Copies (Line 16a) ▶		
d. Percent Paid (Both Print & Electronic Copies) (16b divided by 16c × 100) ▶		

☒ I certify that 50% of all my distributed copies (electronic and print) are paid above a nominal price.

17. Publication of Statement of Ownership
☒ If the publication is a general publication, publication of this statement is required. Will be printed
in the DECEMBER 2021 issue of this publication.   ☐ Publication not required.

18. Signature and Title of Editor, Publisher, Business Manager, or Owner

Malathi Samayan - Distribution Controller

Malathi Samayan   Date 9/18/2021

I certify that all information furnished on this form is true and complete. I understand that anyone who furnishes false or misleading information on this form or who omits material or information requested on the form may be subject to criminal sanctions (including fines and imprisonment) and/or civil sanctions (including civil penalties).

PS Form **3526**, July 2014 (Page 3 of 4)   PRIVACY NOTICE: See our privacy policy on *www.usps.com*

Moving?

Make sure your subscription moves with you!

To notify us of your new address, find your **Clinics Account Number** (located on your mailing label above your name), and contact customer service at:

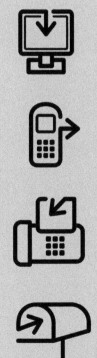

Email: journalscustomerservice-usa@elsevier.com

800-654-2452 (subscribers in the U.S. & Canada)
314-447-8871 (subscribers outside of the U.S. & Canada)

Fax number: 314-447-8029

Elsevier Health Sciences Division
Subscription Customer Service
3251 Riverport Lane
Maryland Heights, MO 63043

*To ensure uninterrupted delivery of your subscription, please notify us at least 4 weeks in advance of move.

Printed and bound by CPI Group (UK) Ltd, Croydon, CR0 4YY

08/05/2025

01864700-0010